TOTAL BODY TRANSFORMATION

TOTAL BODY
TRANSFORMATION

A 3-MONTH PERSONAL FITNESS
PRESCRIPTION FOR A STRONG, LEAN
BODY AND A CALMER MIND

STEVE ILG

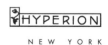

HYPERION
NEW YORK

Pregnant women are advised that special precautions may pertain to any exercise program they undertake. If you are pregnant, talk to your doctor before undertaking any exercises suggested in this book. The recommendations in this book are not intended to replace or conflict with the advice given to you by your physician or other health professional. All matters regarding your health require medical supervision. Consult your physician before adopting the suggestions in this book. The author and publisher disclaim any liability directly or indirectly from the use of this book by any person.

PHOTO CREDITS
Pages 20, 26, 72, 220, 222, 242, 260, 262 (WF student Dorman Balatazar in Virabhadrasana III), 265, 297: Ilg archives; page 21: Twilight Photography, Durango, Colorado; pages 23, 24, 149, 205, 218, 258: Marc Romanelli; page 39: image of Green Tara courtesy of Kapil at www.exoticindia.com; pages 71, 83: Kathy Ilg; page 237: Chris Kostman. All other photos: Wayne Williams, www.waynewilliams studio.com.

ISBN: 0-7868-6851-1

Hyperion books are available for special promotions and premiums. For details contact Michael Rentas, Manager, Inventory and Premium Sales, Hyperion, 77 West 66th Street, 11th floor, New York, New York 10023, or call 212-456-0133.

Book design by Richard Oriolo

FIRST EDITION

10 9 8 7 6 5 4 3 2 1

to Kathy . . .

thank you for your unconditional cheerfulness,

nonstop love and perspective,

and the stability of your faith in me.

You are such an adorable Light for so many.

You are my precious golden lotus.

You are my Namasté Way.

i bow to you.

ACKNOWLEDGMENTS

To my Students and readers who have contributed to this book through their heart and sweat and devotion. Thank you for recognizing and re-membering our humble but powerful tribe of crazy wisdom fitness warriors!

To my highly gifted agent, Susan Golomb. You sensed this book years ago and cultivated it. May many beings enjoy and benefit from our flower.

To my editors at Hyperion, Will Schwalbe and Mark Chait, for their sensitivity and artistic awareness within the emerging field of transpersonal fitness training.

To WF student Joe Glickman for embracing my wholeness principle and letting it radiate through you so well.

To my amazing photographers: Wayne Williams and Marc Romanelli.

i bow as deeply as my full lotus will allow me to the Masters of the inner path. Their spiritual efforts and Divine Blessings have allowed my own sacred journey to blossom from within.

To my family.

And, in fond remembrance of Stephan.

CONTENTS

Prologue

Don't just work out, work within.

—COACH ILG

WELCOME TO THE WORLD OF Wholistic Fitness®—a lifestyle fitness program that I have developed and honed over the past twenty years. If you're anything like the thousands of people whom I've taught during that time, this book may well be the best thing to ever happen to your long-term health and fitness. It outlines the routines used by my students and is designed to work in the same manner as if you had hired me as your personal trainer.

This program is unlike any you've encountered before, and this book will forever change the way you consider and perform fitness workouts. This unique workout course grew out of my personal experience as a world-class extreme multisport athlete who in mid-career healed myself from a catastrophic injury using yoga and meditation. Surprisingly, I found that these Eastern disciplines made me stronger than I had ever been and I went on to compete at levels even higher than I had achieved before. I have since incorporated them into a personal training program that has benefited thousands of people, including MVP hockey champion Michael Richter, Mount Everest mountaineer Gerry Roach, World Downhill Mountain Bike Champion Penny Davidson, and many, many more.

While my approach to fitness training may seem new and challenging to you, be assured that I don't do anything unless it's fun and tremendously effective. Wholistic Fitness (WF) is a lifestyle-based approach. It always has been. It can accommodate any time frame, ability level, or degree of intent you bring to it. My average Wholistic Fitness student has enjoyed formal WF practice for over eight years. Many of those students continue to integrate the WF philosophy and style into the rest of their lives. These statistics stand alone in a nation where most people, it has been shown, quit fitness programs within three months. I want to make myself perfectly clear right at the start: I'm not promising you another "Nine Minutes to Better Abs" workout. What I am promising you is a system that will transform your workouts into a path of personal growth and joy.

People around the world tell me that in addition to making them physically strong, WF keeps them "centered," "emotionally sound," and "moving enthusiastically forward in life." Others report a "very real sense of spiritual quality" affecting their lives from following this program. Certainly, the body/mind training effects enjoyed from my programs will vary with an individual's temperament, ability, purpose, and character. But I guarantee three things if you complete my program: a superior-looking and -functioning body, a more disciplined mind, and a heightened sense of well-being.

There are nine key characteristics unique to WF. They are my Five Fitness Disciplines (Strength Training, Cardio, Yoga, Meditation, Nutrition) and my Four Lifestyle Principles (Breath and Posture, Mindfulness, Appropriate Action, and Practice). These nine threads are woven into a fitness practice that ultimately allows you to consistently achieve a stronger, more supple, and leaner body supervised by a calmer, more controllable, and peaceful mind.

A key theme running through my work is *balance*. As a licensed multisport athlete, I've stood on top of podiums for strength and agility sports such as bodybuilding and competitive climbing and also gained podiums in endurance sports such as ultra-running and cycling. I have few peers in this regard. I have found it crucial in fitness training to balance muscle building with muscle lengthening, intense training periods with recovery periods, aerobic exercise with anaerobic, and to follow a whole-food diet that both cleanses and empowers the cells of the body.

But it is outside of athletic competition and training that I value balance perhaps even more. Buddha said, "The art of life is balance."

Balancing the demands of daily fitness with a satisfying career, with the steady perseverance of a responsible, caring husband or father or mother, for example, is truly high art, so important yet so underacknowledged in today's world. It is one of my visions for this book to encourage, acknowledge, and forward the nobility of balance in people's lives.

In my life, my best coaches taught me more than sport performance techniques. They taught me to see and use my fitness workouts as a tool in becoming a better human being. One of my early Nordic (cross-country) ski coaches, Scotty, refused to let me train with the team until I had completed my math lessons to his satisfaction. I had no choice. In Durango, Colorado, you see, our school system was so small that my math teacher also happened to be Coach Scotty. His tough love became clear to me, as under his care, I connected the dots that linked the discipline of ski training to the discipline needed to pass algebra and calculus.

> *What do you want to be, a "worrier" or a "warrior"?*
> —COACH ILG

Indeed, the entire foundation of WF is built upon balance: Balance between the Five Disciplines and the Four Principles, which leads to a whole personal training system. Cardiovascular fitness benefits tremendously from Strength Training. Nutrition patterns cannot be separated from the timing of training and recovery cycles. Flexibility work like Yoga keeps the body expressive and injury-free, while Meditation practice imparts depth, clarity, and calm control to physical fitness. Integrated into every aspect of life, this nine-limbed approach to fitness produces a comprehensive, balanced training effect. Inner strength—clarity, breath, balance, peace—results in the motivation and ability to achieve greater outer strength. And outer strength in turn fuels inner strength with improved power, esteem, and physical health. Eventually you'll discover, as I did, that the two—inner and outer strength—are one and the same.

> **Which dots are you not connecting in regard to your fitness training and your life? Do you consider your personal fitness efforts as a form of spiritual or personal growth endeavor? Why not?**
> _____

I've kept it a principal point in this book to draw the effects of good fitness training into the fabric of everyday life. As my Zen friends say, "How you do anything is how you do everything." How you enter a yoga pose, how you do a set of bench presses, how you eat your dinner, how you play with your children or make love to your partner—one informs the other and it all matters. Why? Because it all leads to an elevated state of awareness, which gives birth to balance, calm, strength, and, ultimately, peace of mind in life.

The trick you'll learn from this book is not to "do" your fitness, but to "be" your fitness.

> *Your workout is everywhere.*
> —COACH ILG

The inspiration for what became WF did not come fast or easy for me. I began a highly dubious career in outdoor and extreme sports back in 1978, long before the terms for those sports were coined and certainly long before the X-Games brought a huge amount of money into them. In the deep reaches of Colorado's rocky peaks, my training bros and I did exactly what the young extreme athletes are doing today. There were differences, however. We didn't have handheld cameras to video everything. Why would we? I recall feeling more humble than obnoxious, more appreciative of wildness than intrusive upon it. Without judging the present generation of extreme athletes, I think we may have practiced a bit more reverence for the wilderness back then. Probably because the equipment we used for our extreme sports was often clunky and prototypical, if not self-fashioned. Instead of helicopters swishing us up mountains, we climbed, often in a spirit of pilgrimage.

I began my journey as a sponsored athlete by nabbing a spot on the United States Junior National Nordic Combined Team at age sixteen. After that, I was consumed by an inner fire and made it my profession to gain and maintain sponsorship in as many different outdoor sports as possible. My favorite sports, of course, were those that came easiest. For me, those were the kinesthetic or skill sports, such as extreme skiing, ice climbing, rock climbing, alpine (downhill) ski racing, martial arts, and ski jumping. My devotion to athletic balance, however, required me to endure like a sled dog to succeed in my weak areas, namely, endurance sports: ultra-running, mountain bike and road cycling, Nordic ski racing, and sport snowshoeing.

When climbing dangerous mountain peaks, soloing rock or ice climbs, or when suffering through ultra-races, my stubborn, resolute attitude came to the fore. The worse I was getting beat or the more gnarly an external situation grew, the calmer, more focused, and more determined I became.

> *Racing is not about winning. It's about knowing yourself.*
> —COACH ILG

Intensity has always brought out the best in me. During long hours spent training for mountain or road-bike racing, I rarely took risks and often placed myself on "autopilot" for many of the required twenty to twenty-five hours spent training each week on a bicycle. But come race day and the firing of that start gun, I would take extreme risks on descents and passes. I loved attacking off the front of the pack, putting my head down, and forcing the suffering from guys chasing me down. Performing such acts of audacity mattered more to me than winning the race. One of my role models for competitive performance was Steve Prefontaine. This quotation of his remained tacked to the wall above my bed for many years: "I don't race to win, I race to see who has the most guts because if the race comes down to who has the most guts, I will win."

For a long and blessed while, everything was going great. I was actually holding sponsorship doing outdoor sports, crisscrossing North America in my sport pickup, climbing rocks and ice, racing bikes, ski racing, running mountain peaks—all of this during an age when getting paid to do that was very rare.

Then, in the mid-1980s, I fractured my lower back and smashed my pelvis during a horribly long climbing fall off the Diamond on Longs Peak in Rocky Mountain National Park, where I was attempting a winter ascent of a difficult route. I didn't really fall, but the Volkswagen-sized chunk of cliff I was climbing on sure did. The ensuing forty-foot, sixty-mile-an-hour crash into the Diamond's granite face paralyzed me and forced an epic self-rescue through a whiteout blizzard on the 14,000-foot peak. My recovery was accompanied by chronic and searing lower back and sacroiliac pain. Having already studied a little bit of yogic breathing and Tibetan meditation techniques to improve my outdoor athletics, I staunchly refused all pain pills and savvy sales pitches for back surgery. I was young and a bit naive about the serious nature of my spine injury. I wanted to prove the doctors wrong about my need for back surgery and I desperately wanted to compete again in outdoor sports: There was never a question in my mind that I would. I grew unshakably determined to overcome the pain, and the more I concentrated my mind on self-healing, the more interesting things became.

While sleeping and during some of my meditation sessions, I received images of arcane yoga postures, mantras, and other austerities. Entire training paradigms arose like blueprints of pain erasure and higher sport performance. Though most of these ethereal training prescriptions were far beyond my comprehension, some of them made sense to me. The WF programs that appear in this book are based in part upon these self-healing visions. So, what could have been the end of a career became a boon to it. Eventually, I rose above that injury to the highest levels of sport by developing a program that coupled yoga techniques with the steadfast application of Western fitness training. For instance, I found that yogic posture and breathing helped me reroute the neural drives to my lower back muscles, and the strength gained through my gym workouts helped my yoga postures. This complementary, integrated approach not only healed me but also allowed me to thrive. By the time I retired myself and my blown adrenal glands from sponsored outdoor sport at age thirty-four, I had competed in five World Championships in four different sports (a record still unmatched) and competed in national, regional, and state championships in three other outdoor sports.

I started teaching my style of fitness training to others in Boulder, Colorado. My method caught on like wildfire among the many world-class athletes who lived and trained there because it worked. In 1985, at the age of twenty-three, I authored my first book detailing my training approach to outdoor sports, *The Outdoor Athlete*. That book quickly became the bible of outdoor performance training. Because yoga was seen as so fringe at the time, my editor made me disguise those elements as "flexibility routines." By 1999, I was able to finally bring my yoga discipline out of the closet and included it in my next book, *The Winter Athlete*, which was geared to those seeking peak performance in my beloved winter sports.

These days, my lofty athletic ambitions have turned as mild as a Southern California winter, but I live a far better balance of physical and spiritual fitness. I remain a certified personal fitness trainer, licensed Expert Coach with the United States Cycling Federation, a registered yoga teacher, body-worker, energy-worker, and owner of Wholistic Fitness Personal Training, which is run through www.wholisticfitness.com. I prefer wearing a well-feathered cap: Not just one sport, all of them. Not just one fitness discipline, all of them.

While it took me thirtysome-odd years and a helluva lot of trials, tribulations, and joys to develop this program, it will require you only three months to complete the basic programs presented in this book.

Please read my Introduction very closely. I describe exactly what you will need to know about the Wholistic Fitness method, particularly the Five Fitness Disciplines and Four Lifestyle Principles. The Introduction gives you everything you need to get started: what to mentally prepare for, what equipment, what facilities, and what time allotment my program requires. The Wholistic Fitness Quiz at the end of the Introduction is a stylized version of my actual training application. The results from this quiz will identify your current "wholistic fitness" levels, from which you can gauge your workouts for the remainder of this book.

Part One presents my core program, the Green Tara. Think of Green Tara as our basic recipe upon which we will build. This core program deeply conditions joints and muscles while setting the pace for your WF journey. You have only four weeks to learn many new techniques and notions, so Green Tara will undoubtedly be your most difficult challenge. No need to be scared, though. Hundreds before you have pulled off Green Tara and I know you can too. After four weeks of Green Tara practice, I need you to take a recovery week—a well-earned seven-day vacation from structured training so joints, tissue cells, and mental vigor can be rejuvenated.

The reward for good workouts is more good workouts, so after your recovery week from Green Tara, you'll be ready for the next programs. Each is designed in the same format as Green Tara, but with far different training effects.

Part Two, the intermediate program, is the Cosmic Yang; this program develops fast-twitch power and inner balance.

Then it is time for Part Three, my advanced program, the Frugal Realm—a body/mind test piece for more than thirteen years. One student who emerged from its chambers described it as "Four weeks of Ilgonian torture that leads to enlightenment." Complete those three programs and you will truly know what genuine body/mind personal fitness is all about. You'll look and feel amazing!

To maintain your profound new level of fitness, Part Four, the Jeweled Lotus, has been culled from my archives to provide your maintenance program. The Lotus can be picked up at any time after completing the basic training programs and will keep all aspects of your fitness buzzing for up to two months.

What happens after you complete the programs in Parts One through Four? Well, for one thing, you'll probably be hooked on Wholistic Fitness! You will find that your exercise has now been transformed into a practice, after which there are many ways to deepen your practice. First, you can repeat the programs. There is much mastery to be attained in each training program. Often, it takes a good three weeks to really get each program dialed in. This is a good sign. I'd rather have students sad about leaving a program than completely bored with it. So my first suggestion is to go back and refine your performance on each of the programs. Just be sure to follow them in the same order as is presented and never remain on any of these programs longer than four weeks. *Always take a full week of recovery between programs.* Other options for continuing your WF Journey include exploring the many programs in my other books or pursue online WF training with a certified WF teacher at www.wholisticfitness.com.

Part Five, the Wholistic Fitness Sutras, features philosophical material that functions to open you to deeper layers of what the prior physical training is all about. Insights gained from periodically rereading this part change as your fitness matures from the physical toward the mental and even the spiritual. The thirty-five Wholistic Fitness Sutras presented here distill my method into kernels of body/mind wisdom.

Part Six, Questions and Answers, furthers the philosophical discourse I share with my students and contains dozens of actual questions, stories, and dialogues. It covers such terrain as injury counsel, funny anecdotes, spiritual ramifications from workouts, and transpersonal fitness insights.

Covering morning, midday, and evening mealtimes, Part Seven offers some of my most popular low-fat vegetarian dishes ideally suited for the Wholistic Fitness warrior.

Sources is a ground spring of valuable contacts I have found beneficial to those who not only seek personal growth through their fitness, but have found it.

Finally, please enjoy and use the vast and abundant Glossary and Bibliography sections. They reflect the depth and value of this book.

> Each of the programs found in Parts One, Two, and Three are formatted in the same manner. Each begins with a brief profile of the program and explains its goals. Then I describe all the Strength Training movements or techniques you will need for that program, and do the same for Cardio, Yoga, Meditation, and Nutrition. Thus, before you begin any program, you'll have all the tools and information you will need to crank those workouts! The actual fitness prescription for each part is found in the Daily Practice, a day-by-day description of your training schedule. Each part concludes with a Cycle Summation, reflective questions that can be used as a compass to guide you toward the next program.

> *This is getting ridiculous. I feel one quantum leap after another. The challenges are there, but everything is flowing. I feel very light and very strong right now.*
> —WF STUDENT SEAN MADINE, LOUISVILLE, COLORADO

Introduction

Through the discipline of training, life bears many dreams.
—COACH ILG

OUTWARDLY, THIS BOOK IS GOING to provide you with diamond-clear techniques and granite-hard programs that will transform each of your workouts into a path of overall excellence. Yet another and more inward purpose here is to offer a new way for you to maximize and enjoy all that is inside of you. I've designed this Path to break old patterns and to offer, through each new workout, an opportunity to change the things that restrict our bodies, our minds, and our spirits. I consider my workouts to be my sanctuary within—a place where I can breathe deeply, strengthen and nourish my body, and awaken my spirit. I teach, and have designed this book, from that same perspective.

For thousands of years, Eastern arts such as Tai Chi Chuan, Chi Gong, and from South India, yoga, were developed from "bodybuilding" disciplines that delivered peace of mind. They knew the key point: Spiritual endeavor, if it is to be genuine and effective, has to fortify the body before appreciable spiritual insight can be realized.

For the most part, here in the West we've gone a bit overboard on the physical, and often narcissistic, aspects of fitness training without honoring the link to its spiritual dimension. We go to church to do our "spiritual fitness" and then we go to the gym or lace up our running shoes to do our "physical fitness." We've not put a lot of effort into linking the two. We tend to only think of disciplines such as yoga and Tai Chi as spiritual and discount the spiritual qualities of bench presses and biceps curls.

This dichotomy comes from an old split in the American fitness scene. Typically, the yoga people scorned the grunting, iron-pumping gym people. Getting bigger muscles was, to the yoga people, the ultimate display of narcissism and mindless behavior. I suppose their India-tinted egos did not let them see that just because bench presses have not been around for 6,000 years does not make doing them any less sacred than doing the Upward Facing Dog yoga pose.

Then there are the puffy strong gym people who would not be caught dead inside a yoga studio. These self-named "gym rats" look strong, but the vast majority have very little functional strength. More than a few don't have the shoulder flexibility to comb their own hair. The tightness of their connective tissues suffocates their movement and physiology. In some cases, the restrictions present in their bodies have carried over into their attitude, making them appear to be a rather close-minded bunch. Besides not liking to stretch, they only do cardio work at gunpoint and associate meditation with being a wuss.

This separation between the yoga and gym worlds extends to other fitness disciplines. I have met numerous yoga teachers, for instance, who do not know much about the beauty of cardio training at all. In fact, many tell their yoga students not to run or cycle at all because doing so "tightens your muscles and ruins good yoga." I suppose they would rather all of us be like them: Overly flexible with all the verve of a potted plant? No thank you. Big deal if my *Marichysasana III* isn't as twisty curly as some white-bearded dude's from India. At least I can hammer my interval workouts and load up a heavy squat bar.

There is as much inner power to be gained from doing conventional fitness activities as there is in doing yoga poses. I think now that the initial rush of yoga has passed and "OM" T-shirts are passé, people are starting to realize that both schools are important, that yoga, with its emphasis on elongation, balance, and spirituality, goes hand in hand with the lean body-building look and power of doing gym workouts with cardio. People are now looking for the whole package; they want the best of the gym world and the best of the yoga world.

Recently some people have attempted to sprinkle dashes of yoga into Western fitness classes. These hybrid programs don't work. Like all hybrids, they are diluted versions of the real thing. A professional mountain biker doesn't race on a hybrid bike. Poking needles randomly into someone's skin is not acupuncture. Flippantly smashing one herb into another herb doesn't make an herbal formula healing. You've got to know the energetic properties of what workout you are doing and how they are best facilitated. For example, mindlessly mixing Taoist and Indian yoga into one class can be damaging, since each uses completely different energy systems in the body.

Wholistic Fitness is not a trendy hybrid of East and West. It is a trustworthy, intelligent, comprehensive program that keeps the purity of both energy systems separate while consciously blending fitness disciplines with lifestyle principles in a wisely structured, progressive, and cyclic manner, bringing you a new world of whole fitness, Wholistic Fitness.

SHIFT HAPPENS

Five short years ago, I started what turned out to become the most successful yoga program in the Los Angeles Valley. This program was not begun in a beautiful, incensed yoga studio surrounded by swaying palm trees and ocean breezes. My first students were not scantily clad, lithe young women. The program started right smack in the middle of a toxic, industrialized section of the Valley at Powerhouse Gym, Chatsworth, a famous bodybuilding hot spot where 80 percent of the members are huge, testosterone-loaded muscle heads. Yoga? Here? I never had a doubt. Yes, yoga. Yes, here. I knew if I could make yoga work here, it would work anywhere.

When I first approached the gruff owner of the acclaimed gym with my notion of teaching yoga there, he surveyed my 148-pound frame, scoffed and chuckled, "Yoga? Yoga will never work in a place like this!" Shaking his head and still chuckling, he motioned me away, but said, "Go ahead and try. Knock yourself out." So I did.

The first week four people showed up. Six weeks later, an average of twelve people were attending my High Performance (HP) Yoga classes. The buzz of how challenging the classes were caught on like baby oil in a pump-up room. Surfers and skaters showed up and loved the combination of strength, balance, and flexibility. Aging baby boomers were shocked by the difficulty of the practice but smiled with pleasure as their aching shoulders and lower backs were eased from chronic pain and stress. Like curious but shy lemmings, more and more of the steroid guys gathered outside my classes. A few even came in. But all of them saw the Light of Yoga. They saw me in the gym, cranking out weighted pull-ups and explosive jump squats. They sensed the difference between functional strength and barbell strength. Respect, if not total acceptance, was given to me from that point onward. Where once I felt like I was being judged by a grim high court, now a family took root. Where once yoga was nonexistent and ignorantly passed off, today Powerhouse Gym offers ten HP Yoga classes per week, averaging over fifteen students each. Steroid guys now study Patanjali's sutras. Oh, and the owner? He still has yet to come to my class, but he has built a whole new yoga studio inside the gym!

It's not a fluke that yoga has been around for thousands of years. It's been around for so long because it works. My students who are fully integrating both yoga and gym disciplines in their fitness regimen are having no problem pounding out 10 sets of 5 reps back squats, then transitioning into a slightly stiff but enjoyable *Paschimottanasana*. Students should never feel the need to take sides in their personal fitness or attachment to one fitness activity: It shouldn't be a mentality of gym versus yoga, but, rather, gym with yoga.

TO KNIT TOGETHER

The key to genuine fitness lies in the very word itself. "Fitness" comes from a Norse word meaning to knit together. Wholistic Fitness, therefore, knits together lifestyle principles and fitness disciplines for an unmatched level of body/mind fitness. The WF logo symbolizes the comprehensive balance of my method. It is the yin-yang symbol woven between a dumbbell. The yin-yang symbol expresses the harmony of paired opposites such as male-female, hot-cold, sun-moon. The horizontal and vertical lines are arranged in the manner of the zia of southwest Native America, which is a symbol that looks like the sun with lines radiating from it. The lines (or rays) of the zia represent rain, or abundance in all directions of life.

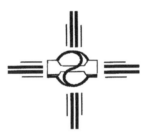

The benefits of cross training in yoga and gym workouts are clearly felt by anyone who does both. What must be understood is that one helps the other, and doing both brings balance of body and mind. Learning better breath and posture in yoga, for example, helps gym workouts. Gaining strength in the gym helps you hold yoga postures more easily. But it goes deeper than that.

HOW YOGA HELPS THE GYM RAT

For the gym enthusiast, yoga expands and makes pliable the fascial sheath that surrounds muscles. Lifting weights and doing cardio compresses the tissues of the body, causing this sheath to shrink as it contracts. Over time, this sheath virtually suffocates soft tissues of the body. The muscles do not grow in size, only in tightness.

Without doing yoga to expand and elongate our hard-earned musculature, the muscles actually atrophy due to poor nutrient transfer. Doing yoga also creates an alignment of optimal biomechanics; the pushing and pulling of our muscles becomes better synchronized. We stand, sit, and move with less pain, more efficiency.

A person with tight muscles should count this as a blessing as he or she begins a yoga practice. It is better to begin the yoga journey being strong but restricted rather than being weak and loosey-goosey. Muscle-bound or tight people will quickly grow more flexible and open. That is not a problem, it just takes time. But the core strength will be a great asset as your yoga practice matures. Stiffer, more restricted people can also more easily access the "edge" (the point of emotional "holding on" and slight physical pain) in a yoga pose, which is another blessing; not having to stretch very deeply to find an edge focuses the mind and engages mental concentration, which is the whole point of doing yoga. On the other hand, the hypermobile, "double jointed" students who have little deep-fiber strength make poorer yoga students initially. These people tend to collapse onto their joints because their core strength is virtually nonexistent. Since these natural Gumbys can just flop into many of the poses, their minds wander, because doing the postures does not grab their attention as it must in a stiffer student. To get to their emotional edge, they have to contort into extreme parameters of each pose, which invites overstretching of already lax connective tissue.

So basically, I am telling those of you who, like myself, come to your first experience of yoga with restricted and tight muscles to rejoice.

HOW THE GYM HELPS THE YOGI

The benefits of doing gym workouts for yogis (those who practice yoga) are equally obvious. Strong connective tissue is intrinsic to the integrity of a yoga pose. One must concentrate first on strengthening the ligaments and tendons that surround joint capsules. Aches, pains, and injuries can bother yogis who have not first developed the deeper fiber strength needed to protect the joints. In Santa Fe, a woman fractured a bone in her neck from doing too many headstands in the Iyengar style (which emphasizes precision alignment, not strength). This is a sad but common example of being injured because adequate deep-fiber, connective-tissue health has not been developed.

The traditional yoga forms of India do not take into account the North American physique, constitution, or culture, all of which necessitate categorically different "sun salutes" and asana transitions. It is not a lack of flexibility that hurts North Americans doing yoga, but a lack of strength. Arm balances, headstands, flow sequences, warrior poses, and standing balance poses all require more strength than flexibility. Many yoga teachers attempt to compensate for their students' lack of strength by having them rely on walls, blocks, bolsters, and straps. This is just addressing the symptom of muscular and psychological weakness; it teaches the yoga student to look externally for support instead of developing the strength component from within.

Gym workouts can develop the needed strength component for yogis quickly, safely, and effectively. The gym also sculpts and creates structural (and sexy) changes in body parts in a way that yoga cannot.

TIMING IS EVERYTHING

The Light of Yoga is a powerful one. But no less powerful is the Light of Western fitness training when we are taught a more spiritual attitude toward it. But something has to click for us to get that Light. That something is timing. Swami Mukunda said, "Time is God's way of preventing everything from happening at once." Currently, yoga is hitting mainstream consciousness in our country, but in my first book, *The Outdoor Athlete,* written over fifteen years ago, my editor would not allow me to even use the word "yoga." It would, he felt, "Scare readers away." Don Nielson, a three-time Olympic ski biathlete, told me a long time ago one of his training maxims, "Things take time." Things happen when they need to happen. Remember when you "hated working out"? Now you can't imagine your life without it. Soon you'll remember when you couldn't stand to stretch as an hour of yoga flies right by.

BEAUTIFUL BODY

The first goal of this book is to focus on the body. The rest will follow. Our focus will be on getting a beautiful and balanced body before anything else.

This beautiful body is, of course, a relative goal. By "beautiful" I mean a body that is under your control. It looks, behaves, and feels the way you want it to. It is a body you enjoy waking up in, looking at in the mirror, and moving in. By using this book, you will bring your body to its fullest potential. This can be accomplished at any age and with any prior fitness ability or lack thereof.

Along the way toward our more beautiful and balanced body, the mental and spiritual benefits will arrive. But for now we are not concerned with that. Even Patanjali, in his *Yoga Sutras,* which still remains the yogi's unquestioned blueprint to enlightenment after six centuries, refers to the body, ironically enough, as our first but necessary obstacle to enlightenment. If we cannot master the body, we stand not a chance for mastering the spiritual realms. There are no shortcuts around the body, no matter how "spiritual" we think we are or want to be.

We must work hard to gain a basic level of control over the physical body. This is an inescapable rule. But, things take time. So enjoy the process. As Pattabhi Jois said so exquisitely, "Just do your Practice, and all will be coming."

EIGHT THINGS YOU WILL NEED TO BEGIN

1. Prepare Yourself Psychologically

Everything that blocks us comes up rather quickly as we begin a fitness program: doubt, hesitation, impatience, disappointment, laziness, boredom, guilt. These are natural reactions. This is why nonwarriors quit fitness training. Their ego clamors on and on: This hurts, this is uncomfortable, and this is not fun. Instead of submitting to such ego games, warriors must accept and learn from these limiting thoughts so we may rise above them. Acceptance precedes transformation. Getting out the war paint works the best. Our ego is so strong; it requires a fierce program and a warrior student to subdue it. Fitness training is ideal ground for personal growth, better than psychological or psychiatric work. In this warrior path, we depend neither on pills nor pillow talk, we depend on workouts. Trust little counsel that does not arise from within your own breath and movement. Devote yourself to difficulty, because devoting ourselves to difficulty frees us from it. As Rumi hints time and again, we should welcome difficulty as a guest, for the difficulty may just be clearing us out "for some new delight . . . Be grateful for whoever comes, because each has been sent as a guide from beyond."

2. Practice with Humble Confidence

Don't expect to get this right from the start—be humble and patient. But be confident, because the techniques in this book have been heavily field tested. My meditation counsel to you, for example, does not take place merely on some fluffy zen pillow or come from reading New Age books. On the contrary, I tested my mental control by consistently free soloing (using no rope) difficult ice and rock climbs. My High Performance Yoga routines were not developed in pretty yoga studios with floaty music, but in training for extreme sports and healing from a devastating injury. This ferocity of spirit sets WF apart and spills into all my programs. You can't help but feel that confidence and be humbled by the intensity of these workouts. As the Sufis say, "Be noble for you are made of stars. Be humble, for you are made of dung." You are studying a noble path of self-transformation; be happy, feel the power, but remain humble and focused with intent to be all that you dare to be.

3. Embrace Your Weakness

You are about to train your whole person. Perhaps for the first time. There may have been fitness disciplines you have chosen to ignore or have resisted up to this point. Some of you are resisting yoga; others oppose the gym or cardio workouts. Many of you choose to ignore meditation, thinking that it is not "really a fitness discipline." But these very barriers block your development and are the keys to what you must work on. Strong in the gym? WF will challenge your flexibility. Strength without flexibility is restriction. Proud of your flexibility? WF will challenge your strength. Flexibility without strength is instability. Whatever is your weakest link in body/mind fitness, I will ask you to honestly bring it out of its protective ego, accept it, and watch your weakness transform into profound joy and inner power.

4. Pace Yourself

I want you to fall in love with the "Middle Way" of fitness. This means achieving at least nominal levels of balance in five different areas of fitness: endurance, mental focus, suppleness, agility, and strength. This takes work, but each step is rewarding and fun. I'll make sure of that! The programs will take three months to complete—so it's more of a marathon than a sprint. The going can get tough. To many of my students, "Ilg" is a four-letter word. However, by the end of this book, you will be a noble fitness warrior and better prepared for all of life's crazy circumstances and for any personal, athletic, or spiritual goal you wish to pursue.

5. Clear Your Schedule

Go to your schedule book right now. For the Beginning Program (Green Tara), you'll need to create an hour in the morning and an hour at night on the weekdays. Weekends you'll need around two hours on Saturday and two hours on Sunday.

For the Intermediate Program (Cosmic Yang), you'll need to create an hour in the morning, and one to two hours at night on the weekdays. Weekends you'll need two hours on one day, three on the other.

For the Advanced Program (Frugal Realm), you'll need to quit your job, renounce your family, and move to India. Just kidding. But you'll need an hour in the morning, and up to two hours at night on the weekdays. Weekends you'll need an average of three hours each day.

For the Jeweled Lotus Program, the range is the same as for Green Tara.

6. Tell Your Friends and Family

No matter how silly you might feel, tell your family and friends you are beginning a new fitness program and that some social and family events might need to be missed or rescheduled. Verbalizing your intent with this program is vital. Also, get creative with your workouts. You may be surprised at how willing your friends and family are to help you. If you have a Sunday gathering at your mother-in-law's house, then arrange to ride your bicycle over there and drive back with your family.

> Go! Do it now! Create the time in your schedule. You only live once, and Wholistic Fitness is calling you right now. If a three-month investment into something that will forever positively impact your long-term health, fitness, and spiritual growth isn't worth a few hours each week . . . what *is*?

7. Securing Your Training Facilities and Gear

Gym. Public or private. For most people, training with the collective energy of the gym *sangha* (community of like-minded people) is best. Make sure the facility is clean, has well-maintained quality equipment (mostly free weights), and is open a lot, if not twenty-four hours. Home gyms are great, but you need plenty of space and professional-quality equipment. The base minimum: power rack with Olympic bar and plates, flat bench, dumbbells from 5 to 40 pounds, dip bar, pull-up bar, lat pulldown machine, and an 8-pound medicine ball. (A good source for buying equipment is www.busybody.com.)

Yoga Gear/Studio. You won't need to join a yoga studio yet, but it's a wise option to have. If you are going to do yoga on a hardwood floor, you will need a yoga mat. Otherwise, all you will need is a carpeted, quiet practice space at least 8 feet square where it is least likely you will be interrupted while doing your practice.

Meditation Room or Space. When I lived with my college friends, I would often have to meditate in the bathroom in the early morning. I've also created meditation spaces right next to my bed, so I could just roll out of bed and sit. These days, I have a room in my home that I use for meditation, yoga, and bodywork. The key component to this space, regardless of size, is silence. Everybody that you live with should know that once you are in your Meditation Room or Space, you are off limits. No phone, no kids, no pets. You'll be working on developing sustained focus (*dhyana*) in this area, so make sure it's all yours and free of interruptions.

Sitting Cushion (Zafu). These meditation sitting cushions come in all sorts of fancy shapes and materials these days. If you are unable to comfortably sit in a cross-legged position (see page 115) due to surgery or a medical condition, then consider a "seiza" bench. Visit your local New Age center or www.huggermugger.com.

Bicycle. Nearly as vital as blood are bicycles to WF warriors. Get your road bike or mountain bike tuned up and ready to become a high priority in your life. All Wholistic Fitness warriors do their best to climb out of their cars and onto their bikes. Drop your bike off at your local bike shop for a tune-up and then go online and support the League of American Bicyclists, www.bikeleague.org.

Optional, Optimal, and Miscellaneous Sports Equipment. Quality running shoes (if you are a family warrior, then you might need a high-quality stroller to run with your kid), inline skates, hiking gear, Nordic (crosscountry) skis, rock climbing gear, swim gear, kayak gear, etc. Basically, if you've got it, we'll use it all in this path! If you don't got it, don't worry about it. The more fitness conscious you become, the more the universe will make these things appear in your life.

8. Herbs and Whole Foods

Dump the dairy, the meat, the junk food, and the fast food. Or at least start decreasing your intake of these culprits. Fish is okay a few times per week. Visit a whole foods market and get on a quality whole foods herbal program to replace any synthetic vitamin/mineral pills or engineered powders you might be taking. WF warriors will slowly shift (perhaps over decades—remember, take your time) to regenerative whole foods. And yes, tofu, rice, and lots of fruit and veggies will be a part of your staple diet. The whole foods and herbs that I use for myself and formal students of WF are purchased through Sunrider International. I've included some specific information about these herbs in Sources.

Here are the nuts and bolts of what you will need to know about my method of Wholistic Fitness Personal Training. There are nine key points in this approach: the Five Fitness Disciplines and the Four Lifestyle Principles. Let's check 'em out!

> The number of American youth ages twelve to nineteen who are overweight has nearly doubled in the last twenty years. Only 10 percent of our kids bike or walk to school these days, while nearly 61 percent of American adults are overweight or obese. The League of American Bicyclists is spearheading a program called Safe Routes to School and also lobbying to advance legislation for bicycle and fitness commuting in our country. Another superb contact is the website of Ron Jones, a Race Across America (RAAM) champion and my ultra-racing bro (see Sources). Ron works indefatigably to help turn our nation into a Tribe of Fitness Warriors: youth, elders, and all. Go to www.ronjones.org.

THE FIVE FITNESS DISCIPLINES OF WHOLISTIC FITNESS

Fitness Discipline 1: Strength Training

> *Resistance is the creator of all great things.*
> —HERACLITUS

First, let's nail down the appropriate term for this discipline. Gym workouts are called by a number of terms: weight training, weightlifting, resistance training, etc. I use the term "Strength Training" because it is a more powerful message to send to my students' subconscious than the other, more accepted terms. You may think this is trivial linguistics. It is not. In fact, it is key to long-term health to feed our psyches only those words, terms, and phrases that steer us toward a higher elegance. Our subconscious is always listening; it has no off switch. This is why many Hindi couples name their children with words that mean God. Every time they call their children, they are bringing the name of God into their cells. To the cellular body, the term "Strength Training" resonates with health and empowerment. Compare it to the other terms that slide right past the unaware fitness athlete: weight training, lifting weights, hit the

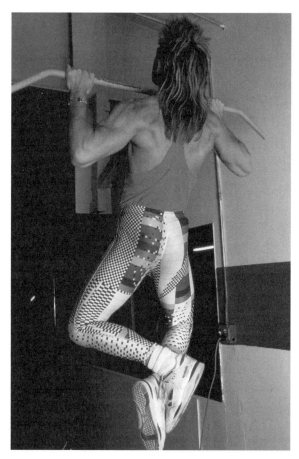

weights, etc. This attention to word choice is a hallmark of a WF warrior. Why? Because, as it is said, "God hides in the details."

True balance in personal fitness mandates getting into the gym and discovering the art of Strength Training. Getting our butts into the gym builds healthy lean tissue and deeply engraves into our posture a physical poise and presence that carries us into older age.

Many other benefits are also to be had within the Iron Temple, or the gym. There is no other fitness discipline that produces such a highly charged degree of self-reliance and confidence than Strength Training. People can do yoga for years without fundamentally creating a masterful posture or gritty determination or explosive power. The sinew one develops by knocking around the iron is invaluable, especially if done in the formative years of fitness training. With age it becomes even more important to delay and even reverse the entropic effects of gravity. Strength Training remains the most effective way to sculpt the body. No doubt about it. The way your body looks reflects the way you work on yourself. That sentence holds the clue to gym yoga: Barbells change more than the body. They change your mindset.

"It is only from the gym we reach and develop the deepest fibers of our inner power and spiritual valor." Coach Ilg, back in the day, getting frugal within the Frugal Realm training program.

Strength Training is so effective that after the initial muscle mass has been gained, doing it no longer needs to be a year-round endeavor. In fact, it shouldn't be. Cranking out high-intensity gym workouts for only a few consistent months or periodic bouts can maintain all the lean tissue and health benefits you need!

Fitness Discipline 2: Cardio

There is no truer test of lifestyle fitness than the integration of Cardio into our daily lives.
—COACH ILG

Cardio is any activity that elevates your heart rate and keeps it elevated consistently for at least twenty minutes. Not only is it a great and necessary activity to keep your heart, lungs, coronary, and respiratory health strong, but doing Cardio is also another way of meditating. In other words, I prescribe Cardio workouts to help pacify the mind, not agitate it.

When done mindfully, there is no finer meditation than the integration of Cardio into our daily lives. I gauge Cardio activities by what I call "an order of authenticity." By authenticity, I mean those Cardio activities that represent the most direct link between breath and movement. The most authentic Cardio activities have the least degree of "entertainment" for the ego. Running barefoot, for example, is the most direct, most authentic form of Cardio. There is nothing interfering with the directness of body, breath, and movement. To increase the personal or spiritual growth benefits of Cardio, engage in more authentic, natural forms of it. But remember, doing any Cardio activity is good, especially for weight management, fat loss, and coronary, pulmonary, and respiratory health. Here are Cardio activities listed in order of authenticity: running, walking, hiking, swimming, cross-country skiing, cycling, inline skating, indoor apparatus training, and indoor group exercise.

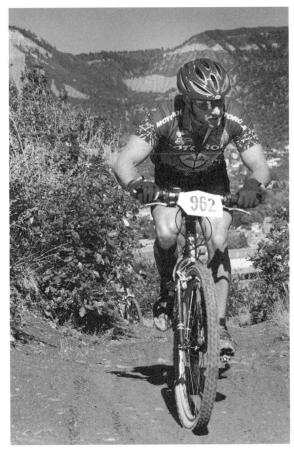

"The key component to WF Cardio is do the majority of Cardio workouts alone, without any music, partner, or other distractions." Coach Ilg racing in Durango, Colorado.

Limit the amount of mental distractions (ego attractions) while doing Cardio. Conventionally trained fitness people go to ridiculous lengths to distract themselves from Cardio training. You do the Stairmaster while watching soap operas, take aerobics to be entertained by the perkiness of the instructor, and endure indoor cycling workouts thanks only to the driving music.

All of this is okay, but the master of fitness knows that the primary direction in which to look during Cardio should be the same as in any meditation: within. Otherwise, Cardio loses its capacity as a vehicle for self-transformation.

I recall an early summer morning riding my mountain bike. My intent for the ride was to practice meditative Cardio. I had just topped out on a technically difficult, small chain-ring climb. Due to my elevated heart rate, my breath awareness became overwhelming. I kept riding through the rich sensation and merged my meditation into the turbulence of breath. Suddenly an elevated state of awareness dawned upon me. Me, my bike, the soft dirt were all mysteriously—no, *naturally* connected! It then seemed impossible to fall off my bike because the fabric of life felt so supportive. I struggle for words here because this was a spiritual, not logical, experience. Magic seemed all around.

When was the last time utter magic swept over you while Cardio training? I feel most fitness athletes do great disservice to their spiritual development by doing too many Cardio workouts with electronic gadgets plugged into their ears or monitors blinking at them. I don't even like to wear heart-rate monitors because I can feel their synthetic energy in subtle conflict with the seductive pulses of my own, natural electrical system.

The key component to WF Cardio is do the majority of your Cardio workouts alone, without music, input, partner, or other distractions. Not all of them, but most of them. I want you to really start going into your Cardio sessions, not around them. Let your breath be your music. And what is going to entertain you? Oh, you'll see. You'll have front-row tickets to the nonstop entertainment of your ego rebelling. That's okay. Soon, the noise of your rebellious ego will calm into a much more peaceful, healthy, and insightful silence. Then your true music will arrive. Remember, Noble Warrior, it is the silence between the notes that makes music.

Cardio is not as amenable to inconsistency as Strength Training; you must maintain an ongoing allegiance with it throughout the training year.

Fitness Discipline 3: Yoga

> *Stiffness is a disease of the unfit.*
> —WILLMANS AND SPERRYN, *SPORTS MEDICINE*

For Wholistic Fitness, I have created a style of High Performance Yoga that offers North Americans a fun, progressive, and challenging practice that prioritizes structural integrity of joints, organs, and mind. I created my style based upon Western exercise physiology principles while honoring the traditional science from India. To me, trying to make North Americans (especially tight, stressed-out ones) fit into a South Indian practice is a bit like trying to pound a round peg into a square hole (if you forgive the analogy). High Performance (HP) Yoga also elevates the often ignored aspect of engaged practice—finding and cultivating the yogic awareness in everyday life.

Most people associate Yoga with flexibility—the stretching into and holding of physical poses. They are not wrong; this physical yoga is called "Hatha Yoga." But Hatha Yoga represents only a few limbs from a much greater tree. The real Yoga is more about suppleness of mind than body.

Appropriately, Yoga is positioned midway through our Five Fitness Disciplines. It is the balancing act of all fitness endeavors. More than a physical component, Yoga is an endless practice of physical, mental, and spiritual expansion. In WF, it is a primary discipline that expresses our alignment, posture, and grace. I also use Yoga to prevent and/or heal injury by enhancing muscular and joint flexibility and proper energy transfer. It also improves mental fitness by heightening concentration, mental quietness, and emotional stability. Even contemporary medical doctors are finally coming around to the wonder of Yoga as preventative medicine. Dr. Bob Arnot, for example, directly experienced Yoga's ability to erase his chronic pain. Yoga changed his entire outlook on what "health care" truly really means. In his book, *Wear and Tear*, the good doc contributes nearly fifty pages of enthusiastic support to Yoga. It's been a long time coming, but I am very, very happy to finally see American medical doctors embracing Yoga. In fact, at least half of my private Yoga students are now medical referrals. (Appropriately enough, the American Medical Association's symbol—the staff of Aesculapius—is a Yoga energywork emblem.)

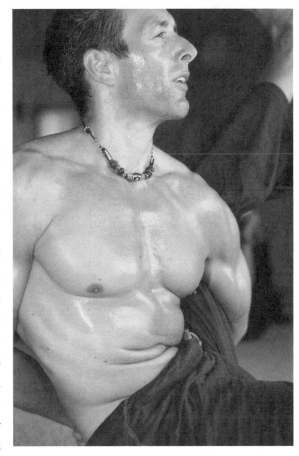

"But that's the beauty of yoga . . . it's not about what a pose looks like on the outside, but what is happening on the inside."—Coach Ilg

Before leaving this introduction to Yoga, I want to make the point that our most fundamental Yoga occurs not in a yoga studio or on a yoga mat. Wherever we go, there is Yoga. Yoga is in our breath and posture. It's the appreciation of the present moment. The practice of Yoga is the practice of allowing the moment to teach. It's letting the circumstances of our lives connect us more fully into the flow of life.

Yoga should be done throughout the year, in varying amounts.

Any activity that emphasizes balance, skill control, agility, and suppleness is really a kinesthetic (or yogic) discipline. Thus, all sorts of sports and activities can be considered yogic in essence: racquetball, basketball, climbing, wrestling, etc. Yes, even Strength Training could be classified as a form of Yoga. Wherever there is a conscious use of breath and movement, you've got yourself a yogic activity. What is funny is that whatever sports you do, Yoga will help. But hardly any sports help Yoga. All sports produce imbalance in the body. The higher the level at which you play a sport, the more pronounced the imbalance. Compare the arms of a pro tennis player or the upper and lower bodies of a pro road cyclist. Only Yoga irons out connective tissue restrictions and releases blocked energy within the compressed and imbalanced muscles of an athlete. Yoga is the only fitness activity completely balanced in neural, muscular, skeletal, and mental aspects. It's hard to say what is the most fun or rewarding part of Yoga—there are so many. But certainly the tremendous amount of energy that is released from tight bodies and overthinking minds has got to be a top pick. The more we learn how to let go through Yoga, the stronger, healthier, and more balanced we become. The highest quality moment in training is the one we invest in choosing softness over tightness. Don't try harder, try softer.

Fitness Discipline 4: Meditation

> *Warriorship is a continual journey. To be a warrior is to learn to be genuine in every moment of your life.*
> —RINPOCHE TRUNGPA

Meditation lies at the heart of Wholistic Fitness and is the glue that binds the Five Fitness Disciplines and the Four Lifestyle Principles into a complete body/mind training system. I prefer the Tibetan definition of Meditation, which is, simply, training the mind.

One of the many ways that Meditation helps our fitness is by developing emotional equanimity. A mind that has been stabilized through Meditation is not likely to get stressed out over missed workouts or lagging energy in the middle of the afternoon or a bossy coworker. Instead, we just stay present, accept it all as a teaching of inner elegance, and enjoy what is.

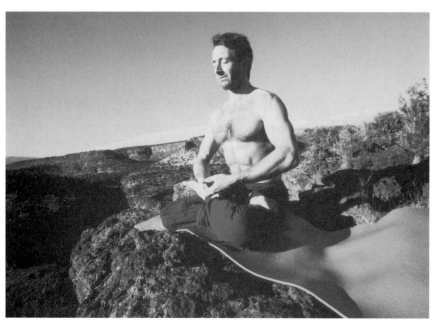

"Nothing but the accomplishment of the present gives form and function to the future."—Coach Ilg

I have spent many hours in formal Meditation. It has not made me a saint nor has it deleted any of my neurotic patterns. But it has made spending time with myself a lot easier and happier. If you were me, you'd realize how big a statement that is. I grew up in an angry household, lots of dysfunction. I was an angry kid confused by the contradictory messages and actions of my parents. Was I loved or not? Was I special or not? My family was not a touchy-feely, loving one. Attention, let alone affection, was rare. My adolescence was a storm season of anger turned within. "Why, I'll show them!" seemed to be my mantra. The "them" could have been anyone from my parents to my siblings to my schoolmates to any authority figure or institution. Anger often rushed my system, flooding my body with such force that anger-based hormones fueled me not just to one world championship in one sport, but five in four different ones.

That's a lot of need for attention. Fortunately, along the way, I found Meditation. In several ways, it saved my life. I know it can have a positive effect on yours.

Far from the popular conception of it as sentimental rumination, Meditation is the practice of performing one gritty mental workout after another. These dedicated sessions of sustained focus can transform normally stressful situations into opportunities for personal growth and even turn ordinary physical workouts into transcendental experiences. Before such transcendence, however, comes the initial ditch work of calming the fluctuating waves of thought long enough and often enough to rediscover our true nature (freedom and joy) instead of subservience to random thought (egoic desires and attachment).

Without a practice of Meditation in a personal fitness program, there can be no true long-term body/mind health. At Naropa University, in Boulder, Colorado, one of my Tibetan teachers defined Meditation as a "friend of wisdom." Although we live in a world administrated by distraction and mindlessness, each of us has an inner refuge, a sanctuary of stillness, and an entire world of wisdom that nourishes our spirit and heals every aspect of our lives. That sanctuary is Meditation. You will learn basic but very effective Meditation techniques in

Once, my expensive racing bicycle was stolen during a time when my Meditation sessions were at high volumes. I was practicing being aware of walking, eating, conversing, etc., as conscious forms of Meditation. I was all dressed to go for my daily mountain bike training ride and walked (consciously) down the flight of stairs to where my bike was locked in a garage. I recall looking up from watching my feet, and seeing only my broken bike lock instead of my beautiful bicycle. I calmly (and consciously) walked back up the stairs, reported the theft, and mindfully began preparing my back-up bike. During the ride, when my thoughts wanted to revisit the bike theft, I brought them at first back to my breath, then I practiced compassion for the thief and visualized my bike in the hands of some kid in a faraway land who was really enjoying it. The situation came, I acted appropriately, and let it go.

the programs that follow. Remember this for now: The training effect from Meditation is a quieter, more controllable mind.

Meditation must be done year-round.

Fitness Discipline 5: Nutrition

Our bodies are masters of regeneration, yet all our society dwells on is how quickly we age.
—COACH ILG

Most personal trainers discuss Nutrition with their clients in terms of grams, calories, and cholesterol levels as though our bodies were machines. Comparing a body to a machine shows little appreciation of the body's wisdom and dishonors our innate transformational capacities. Doing Yoga, for example, can completely alter endocrine and hormonal delivery function, restoring balance so that allergies, neurochemical disorders, etc., disappear. I've seen it happen to many of my students, as well as myself, but I've yet to see a machine change its nature from within. At a higher level of awareness and in accordance with yogic scripture, food represents Brahman—the Divine reality. When we eat "good" food, we are really eating "God" food. Since most dis-ease is traceable to not eating "good" food, we can see that poor nutritional choices are really sins—sins we commit against our higher Go(o)d!

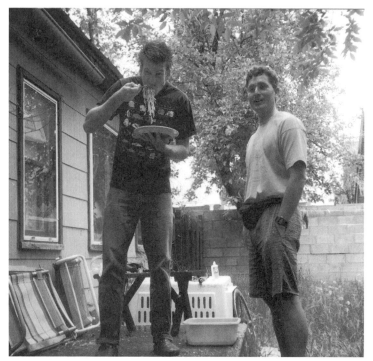

Hunger is the best spice, appreciation the finest of all wine. WF student Adam Moss carboloading while student Doug Milby supervises.

Conventional approaches to Nutrition are fickle, complex, economically driven, and as sterile as a textbook. WF Nutrition produces a path that is simple, joyful, and as durable as an eon. Proper "food combining," for example, is really nothing more than learning to eat foods that are the easiest for us to digest. However, this requires developing the art of inner listening, which means we must meditate.

Here is an example of WF Nutrition practice. At mealtimes, push yourself away from the dinner table while still slightly hungry. What! Yes, overeating is the single largest factor of poor health and disease. Eventually, I instruct my Master Students of WF that their stomachs should contain one-third food, one-third fluid, and be one-third empty. The resultant and delightful sense of lightness that you will feel from doing this is a well-documented and positive signpost in the yogic science of self-healing and is known as *Laghava*. Within a few months of undereating practice, as your stomach shrinks to a more natural size and digestive enzymes become more concentrated and thereby function better, the concept of undereating loses its emotional fear factor. This discipline is easier than you think, as you learn to feed the body accurately and with reverence.

Do not pay any attention to all those diet experts that propose crazy diets, zones, ratios, rations, and eating programs. Seldom are they successful over the course of one's life—let alone meaningful or sacred! I don't know which have come and gone more in my life, "revolutionary" diets or the promoters who peddle them. The simple fact remains, most diets and supplements only separate us from the Divine joy of appropriate Nutrition. That separation between our foods and our appreciation of them is what blocks most of us from beautiful and accurate and powerful Nutrition. WF removes that block to usher in a whole new dimension in the enhancement of health through the joy of Nutrition.

Nutrition is more than even a year-round discipline. It is an ongoing, moment-by-moment cultivation of what truly feeds us—physically, emotionally, and spiritually. Of all my Five Fitness Disciplines, this one remains the least coachable and most variable of all. I guess that is what makes Nutrition so much fun.

THE FOUR LIFESTYLE PRINCIPLES OF WHOLISTIC FITNESS

Throughout this book, various (and often peculiar) assignments are given to deepen your understanding of my Four Lifestyle Principles. The function of these principles is to connect your fitness training into your daily life. Please start becoming aware of them.

Lifestyle Principle 1: Breath and Posture

How we do anything is how we do everything.

Breath connects us with the spiritual plane while posture grounds our connection to the physical plane. Breath and Posture represent our immaterial and material realities. I think that Breath and Posture awareness is the most overlooked form of fitness, performance, and health care. Let me explain.

Breath

We began this life with an inhale. We will finish it with an exhale. All the stuff between we assume is life. If we are going to get to know anything in life, we should get to know (and love) our breath. It's what welcomed us here, and it's what will escort us "there." I bow to breath.

That paragraph took me forty years to write and a helluva lot of time spent breathing consciously. Like much of the material in this book, don't expect things that I teach you to make sense right off the bat. That would be far too easy. Spiritual warriors learn to cherish those things that must simmer within the conscious soup of *tapas*—or the burning desire to Rise Higher—before they can be truly known.

In many languages, the words for "breath" and "spirit" are the same. Breath ventilates, energizes, and calms both body and mind. Ramana Maharshi said, "One moment of conscious breathing is one moment of purity." How does this relate to physical fitness? If we can befriend an ally who can quell our fear, quiet our anxiety, and steady our resolve during sport performance, wouldn't we want to cultivate that friend?

Start by remembering Iyengar's famous quote, "Your mouth is for eating; your nose is for breathing." Don't breathe through your mouth. On an inhalation, inflate your belly as if making a mini beer belly. Upon exhalation, allow the belly to flatten. Do this a few times with your eyes closed. Notice a quality of lightness on the inhale? On the exhale, did you sense a heavier, calming feeling? Do it again. Rest your full attention just on the breath, nowhere else. Allow the breath its space.

Such a breath engages the respiratory diaphragm to work as a massaging mechanism for the spleen, stomach, intestines, and other organs. Diaphragmatic breathing also stimulates meridian, or energy, channels servicing the body. The curative and performance abilities of this area are so great that entire healing (*chi gong*) and athletic (*aikido*) systems are devoted to the breath. In India, breath is a science, studied for centuries, known as *pranayama*. "Pran" means life force and "yama" means extended, thus pranayama is the extension of lifeforce. Our American tendency is to disregard the simplicity of paying attention to our breath. Most of us simply suck air. This retards pranic flow and decreases vibrant living while increasing stress and tension throughout the body/mind.

Posture

Body-centered psychological therapists like Alexander Lowen, Moshe Feldenkrais, and Ron Kurtz were among the first Westerners to document how posture influences our well-being. Like breath awareness, postural integration profoundly affects our health and fitness. As we cultivate our posture, we cultivate our attitude. Whenever we submit to unconscious posture, a neural pathway is compromised. Muscular and chemical imbalance arrives. Through postural awareness, we can regain structural alignment, equanimity, receptivity to pran, and keep our busy minds anchored in the present moment. "Self-observation," said Dennis Lewis, "is the beginning of transformation."

1. *Stance.* Find where your upper thighs fall naturally straight down from their pelvic joint. Stand with your toes aligned under the knee, pointing straight ahead. This stance should be narrower than shoulder width for most people. This stance maintains the Q-angle, the most healthful angle formed by the femur and the pull of the patellar, or kneecap, ligaments.

2. *Foot Pressure.* Bring your awareness to the bottom of your feet. Feel the earth beneath. Lift the inner arches and toes. Feel all four "corners" of your feet distributed evenly upon the earth. Relax the arches and toes but keep the lifting sensation. You'll feel more inner thigh activity when you've got it.

3. *Knees.* Keep a slight bend at the knees. Never stand on hyperextended knees. "Track" the knees so they travel directly over the toes when they are flexed (bent).

4. *Pelvic Control.* Position the center of your hips over your heels. Be aware of anterior or posterior pelvic tilting; the former occurs when the butt sags down, the latter when the arch in the lower back is exaggerated. Keep the pelvis positioned between these two extremes, in a neutral position.

5. *Heart Center.* Make sure the heart is in front of your hips. Heart equals power and love. Hips equal fear. Lead from power and love, not fear. Drop an imaginary plumb line from your heart. Do your hips interfere with the line? If so, push them back and rotate the rear pelvis downward.

6. *Shoulders.* Gently pinch your shoulder blades together. This keeps the back of the heart (center of relationship energy) open and clear. Keep your shoulder girdle dropped, meaning don't hunch your shoulders or allow them to creep forward.

7. *Head.* Position the head as if it is being pulled from above. The head should be buoyant, the chin just a little heavy. Do not retract or protract the jaw. Eyes soft, spine straight.

It is not enough, however, to be aware of our posture for a moment, then forget it. From this point on, every workout, every washing of the dishes, every blow-drying of the hair, every shop-

I teach a "neutral alignment," which means adjusting the body so that the weight-bearing joints fall within the body's line of gravity. This do-it-yourself posture clinic teaches part-to-whole progression to attain proper postural alignment. The sitting and walking versions of this clinic maintain the same principles. I want you to practice this posture as often as possible, at the bank, in the grocery store, sitting at your desk, waiting in line at Disneyland. Your workout is everywhere.

Keep working with these guidelines until your new posture feels more comfortable. This may take several months. Don't be discouraged; you are reversing years of mindless posture. Suddenly you will realize how much effort is required to walk, sit, and stand with mindfulness and gracefulness.

ping errand should become an opportunity to cultivate elegant posture. In staying focused on posture, we attain physical and mental stability.

Wholistic Fitness uses Breath and Posture as the primary anchor for developing and maintaining structural and energetic integrity. When practiced consistently, this principle strengthens our connection between emotional and physical planes. It also sets the proper transformational training effect to reap the most benefit from Lifestyle Principle 2.

Lifestyle Principle 2: Mindfulness

> *Those who seek the easy way do not seek the true way.*
> —DOGEN

Mindfulness is the practice of being present. It is my second Lifestyle Principle and a natural offspring of Breath and Posture awareness. Mindfulness training reduces the streaming of random thought and assorted fictions of an uncontrolled mind. Where chaos describes the untrained mind, peacefulness describes both the nature and the effect of Mindfulness. As Ron Kurtz has said, "Mastery is the natural result of mindfulness."

On one level, the practice of Mindfulness carries with it pragmatic benefits for everyday life such as not misplacing keys, following through on things, driving safely, not breaking dishes, etc. On a more advanced level, Mindfulness changes the lenses of our worldview. We realize that increasing our focus while doing mundane activities tends to open whole new doors of spiritual perception.

I discovered only after retiring from hard-core training and sports performance that my years of "doing sports" were not so much about beating others, or standing on top of podiums, or collecting commemorative race T-shirts. It was the focused, Zen mind that I was chasing. Like all those who release stress through mindful activity—dancing, gardening, knitting, working crossword puzzles—athletes use the intensity of sport to calm their busy minds. Sixth-century Chinese philosopher Lao-tzu said, "Stillness in stillness is not real stillness. Stillness in activity—that is real stillness." Or consider Thoreau's great line regarding what seems to be an intrinsic desire for a pacific mind, "Many men spend their entire lives fishing, never realizing it is not fish that they are after."

Many fitness athletes have worked so hard on their bodies, yet still live their lives on autopilot. This is not an assumption, it is what my students admit during consultations. It is also how I lived much of my life—on autopilot, just going through the motions without really being them. No juicing of the moment. It is a shame to have no spiritual liaison with our workouts. I think that is why most people quit on fitness programs. No one is teaching them how to draw spiritual depth and emotional reward from their efforts.

Using my techniques, the student of WF cannot go on autopilot through their workout or through their day. After a shift occurs with Lifestyle Principle 1, you will find yourself enjoying paying deeper attention to what you are actually doing. That will be key. Until then, do this: Start witnessing yourself. Say to yourself, "I am brushing my teeth," "I am opening my car door," "I am listening to my child." Pay attention at any given moment. Keep paying attention until you forget. That is the way the spiritual game is played. We keep remembering and forgetting until we can make what was once unconscious, conscious. Sri Auribindo put it well: "Much of the spiritual journey is a process of continually falling down, getting back up, dusting ourselves off, looking up sheepishly at God, and taking the next step."

Just as Lifestyle Principle 1 transforms poor posture and shallow breathing into a trigger for unconsciousness, so too will our steadfast but often slow returning over and over again to Mindfulness become stronger until a lack of being present no longer feels go(o)d to us. When being present with that which is feels better than a busy mind, then we know we are making true spiritual progress. This cultivation of expanded awareness sets the stage for my third Lifestyle Principle.

Lifestyle Principle 3: Appropriate Action

Knowledge is the information you've got; wisdom is what you do with it.

Appropriate Action is the practice of performing action—mental or physical—from contemplative integrity. To be in accord with this lofty but attainable principle, all thinking, speaking, and doing must be the result of inner awareness, not of emotional or egoic reactivity. In WF mastery, we don't do something to achieve something, but we admit things to become animated through us as an expression of our highest self. It is very difficult to learn or apply this principle without sufficient training in the former two principles because Appropriate Action must come from inner spaciousness, not a crowded mind. Once we discover the joy that comes from performing each action as a step toward our highest self, little desire remains for superfluous antics of the ego such as overeating, drugging, unhealthy relationships, laziness, etc. Through Appropriate Action we create an inner environment conducive to personal growth. The fourteenth Dalai Lama, Tenzin Gyatso, articulated beautifully the epitome of Appropriate Action. He said, "Before performing any action or speaking any word, ask this question, 'Is it kind, true, and helpful?'" My Taoist yoga teacher, Sensei Kishiyama, taught me to always consider if opening my mouth was an improvement over silence. Usually, as I continue to discover, it is not.

Appropriate Action is difficult practice, but by the time we've arrived at her doorstep, we're already inside. In a sense, this principle is less a practice and more a fruit of the path. Fewer words and more direct experience describe this principle as well as our final one—Practice.

Lifestyle Principle 4: Practice

> *Practice and enlightenment are one.*
> —DOGEN

My fourth principle has two meanings.

The first is simply to practice the Fitness Disciplines and the Lifestyle Principles. Until the spirit of our personality animates these principles, they remain inert fabrications of the intellect. If we practice them with firm but gentle effort, however, self-transformation becomes a reality from which we learn each day. Qualities that once seemed far away—like inner peace, intuitive wisdom, equanimity, clarity, and profound appreciation—are now faithful allies along our journey. Practice in this first definition means to take each moment as it comes. To treat ourselves kindly with it, and not prejudge it as good or bad, happy or sad, beneficial or adversarial. Don't chop life up into judgments. Realize that your next lesson toward becoming a better human being lies in the acceptance of this instant.

The Practice principle also has a second meaning.

But that One is left up to you . . .

Wholistic Fitness Quiz

WHOLISTIC FITNESS HAS EARNED INTERNATIONAL recognition because it is more than just a method for physical fitness and health. It's a proven path to personal growth. Because of its wide-ranging impact upon a person's life, it is important for me to get a picture of a new student's fitness ability, attitude, and intent. Thus, before I begin working with a new student, I ask him or her to complete a training application. The way you complete this application gives me many clues about your "wholistic constitution" and helps me design an accurate program for you.

I have created a stylized version of my application in the form of a Wholistic Fitness quiz. Take a few moments right now, before we go any further, and complete it. There are no right or wrong answers. Answer each question honestly and without too much thinking.

Have fun. First thought, best thought.

Choose only one answer per question.

Wholistic Fitness Initial Quiz *Transformation Through Personal Training*

PART ONE: WHOLISTIC FITNESS DISCIPLINES

Section 1. Strength Training

1. Over the course of my year, I vary the amount, style, and intensity of my gym workouts
   every 4–6 weeks (1 point)   a few times per year (2 points)   hardly ever (3 points)

2. Over the course of my most recent gym workout, I focused my attention on my breath
   during and between each set (1 point)   only during each set (2 points)   hardly ever (3 points)

3. Over the course of my most recent gym workout, my priority for each set was
   to be elegantly strong and present (1 point)   to lift more weight (2 points)   to chat with babes (3 points)

Section 2. Cardio

1. Over the course of my year, I vary the amount, style, and intensity of my Cardio workouts
   every 4–6 weeks (1 point)   a few times per year (2 points)   hardly ever (3 points)

2. Over the course of my most recent Cardio workout, I focused my attention on my breath
   at least 75 percent of the workout (1 point)   maybe half the workout (2 points)   hardly ever (3 points)

3. Over the course of my most recent Cardio workout, my priority was
   to be elegantly strong and present (1 point)   to go faster/longer (2 points)   to get it over with (3 points)

Section 3. Yoga

1. Over the course of my year, I do Yoga an average of:
   3+ times/week (1 point)   1–2 times/week (2 points)   hardly ever (3 points)

2. Over the course of my most recent Yoga session, I focused my attention on my breath
   at least 75 percent of the session (1 point)   maybe half the session (2 points)   hardly ever (3 points)

3. I consider my tight and restricted body parts as an abode of
   sacredness and joy (1 point)   painful potential (2 points)   my neglected fitness (3 points)

Section 4. Meditation

1. Over the course of my year, I practice formal Meditation an average of
   3+ times/week (1 point)   1–2 times/week (2 points)   hardly ever (3 points)

2. I consider the value of Meditation in a personal fitness program to be

    most valuable (1 point)   considerably valuable (2 points)   hardly valuable at all (3 points)

3. My present attitude toward Meditation is most reflected by which statement:

    I crave it (1 point)   I usually force myself to do it (2 points)   I blow it off . . . it's too weird (3 points)

Section 5. Nutrition

1. Over the course of my year, I practice gratitude for my food

    before each mouthful (1 point)   before each meal (2 points)   hardly ever (3 points)

2. The last time I ate a meal or snack I ate it

    slowly, mindfully, and gratefully (1 point)   fast but mindfully (2 points)   gone in sixty seconds! (3 points)

3. My present attitude toward Nutrition is one of

    sacred joy (1 point)   necessity and occasional enjoyment (2 points)   gratification of hunger (3 points)

PART TWO: WHOLISTIC FITNESS PRINCIPLES

Section 6. Lifestyle

1. Over the course of this quiz, my posture has been

    strong, elegant, conscious (1 point)   in and out of my consciousness (2 points)   ooooops! (3 points)

2. When home, I usually

    am barefoot and sit cross-legged (1 point)   wear shoes and sit on furniture (4 points)

3. When home, I usually

    conserve water/electricity and recycle (1 point)   prioritize my comfort over conservation (4 points)

4. It has been _____ since the last time I rode my bicycle or other self-propelled, nonpolluting mode of transportation to work, school, or on an errand.

    less than 48 hours (0 points)   a week (4 points)   a month (8 points)   6 months (16 points) over 6 months (32 points)

5. It has been _____ since the last time I picked up a piece of litter.

    less than 48 hours (0 points)   a week (4 points)   a month (8 points)   6 months (16 points) over 6 months (32 points)

6. It has been _____ since the last time I considered that picking up litter, fitness commuting, or living lightly on the earth is an instrumental component of my personal growth, health, and fitness.

less than 48 hours (0 points)   a week (4 points)   a month (8 points)   6 months (16 points) over 6 months (32 points)

7. It has been _____ since the last time I gave a complete stranger a compliment or performed a random act of unconditional kindness.

less than 48 hours (0 points)   a week (4 points)   a month (8 points)   6 months (16 points) over 6 months (32 points)

8. It has been _____ since the last time I considered giving a complete stranger a compliment or performing a random act of unconditional kindness an instrumental component of my personal growth, health, and fitness.

less than 48 hours (0 points)   a week (4 points)   a month (8 points)   6 months (16 points) over 6 months (32 points)

9. It has been _____ since the last time I nurtured myself by one of the following: got a professional massage, took a vacation longer than three days, visited the wilderness at least one day without my cell phone

less than 3 months (0 points)   less than 6 months (16 points)   over 1 year (32 points)

SIX ESSAY QUESTIONS

(These questions are worth no points, but I still need you to answer them honestly.)

1. Identify the three most profound teachers in your life and their influence upon your life (these can be books, movies, people, animals, etc.).

   1st Teacher:

   Influence upon my life:

   2nd Teacher:

   Influence upon my life:

   3rd Teacher:

   Influence upon my life:

2. There are Five Fitness Disciplines in Wholistic Fitness: Strength Training, Cardio, Yoga, Meditation, and Nutrition. List them below from 1 to 5, with 1 being your most enjoyable and 5 being your least enjoyable.

   1.

   2.

   3.

   4.

   5.

3. Now give two reasons why you listed each of the five disciplines the way you did.

   1.

   2.

   3.

   4.

   5.

4. Wholistic Fitness does not cater to what we are good at but rather targets our weaker areas of fitness. How do you think you'll be able to handle this type of fitness philosophy?

5. There are many fitness and self-help books and many fitness trainers, why do you think you have been attracted to Coach Ilg's Wholistic Fitness method?

6. The only way to fall in love with your fitness training is to work out from love, not fear. Are you ready to accept your weaknesses and strengths, and use them to train for superior balance of body, mind, and spirit? Are you willing to be honest in your practice and learn to love the process of becoming who you really are?

Add up your total points for Parts One and Two here. Use the chart below to determine which Inka ("Certification") Level you are at:

Wholistic Fitness Inka Level

24 or less	=	Master Student
25–64	=	Warrior Student
65 or more	=	Novice Student

If you scored higher on Part One, you'll need to prioritize the softer disciplines of Meditation, Yoga, and Nutrition throughout the program.

If you scored higher on Part Two, you'll need to focus on stabilizing the consistency of your Strength and Cardio training throughout the program.

Training Hint: Watch for various options throughout this book relative to your Inka Level to maximize your Wholistic Fitness potential.

THE CORE PROGRAM:
THE GREEN TARA

Welcome to your first Wholistic Fitness program, the
Green Tara. As I told you earlier, this initial program
can be thought of as your basic recipe. I'm going to
give you all the ingredients that you will need, from
pivotal philosophies to exact exercise descriptions, to
do the actual workouts. After you have all the
ingredients, we'll pull it all together in Chapter 6, Daily
Practice.

I chose a popular deity of Tibetan Buddhism, Green
Tara, as the symbol for our opening work together. In
sacred literature, Green Tara represents the female
aspect of enlightenment. She encourages victory over
inner obstacles and fear. She reminds us that divine
grace demands self-sacrifice.

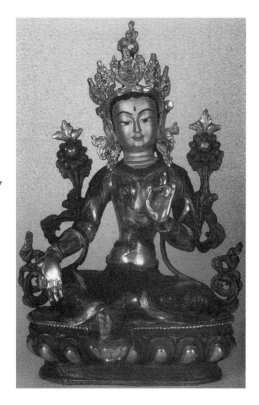

This powerful cycle will require Green Tara's blessing! For the next four weeks, I am targeting the physiologic and structural integrity of your body while developing a mental tenacity needed for success in the ensuing Cosmic Yang program. This routine is bombproof; profound personal growth lies within Tara's embrace—if you stay consistent with her challenges. I myself return time and again to this very program, for Tara never fails to teach me deeper lessons about who I really am.

> *The best way out is always through.*
> —ROBERT FROST

CHAPTER 1

Strength Training

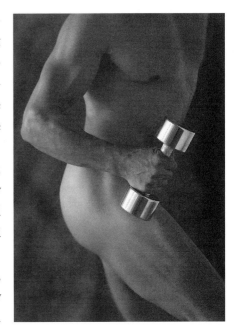

F ROM GREEN TARA'S STRENGTH TRAINING work-
outs you will gain mental and physical integrity. I'm going
to build your fitness from deep within your cellular and structural body. That means getting into the gym and strengthening ligaments, tendons, and associated connective tissue
before anything else. Basically, I need to make your posture
stronger than it is right now.

Besides developing structural and mental integrity,
these initial Strength Training workouts greatly reduce injury
potential. They prepare you for higher levels of fitness and
create a healthier bone mass so your "internal frame" will
forevermore be better equipped to handle the aging process.

I have copyrighted several intense gym techniques that,
unlike typical gym workouts, develop subtle but extremely
beneficial energy production components within your cells.

Learning techniques such as Ku Bottom Form or 3-Stage Technique will connect you to a hidden treasure of inner focus and physical strength. You will realize why WF students are so enamored with their training; they are motivated for what lies within, not ahead.

There are three meditations to prioritize in *all* of your gym workouts. These are the first things that determine—and define—a WF warrior in the gym:

1. Less Is More: Prioritize Elegance, Not Resistance

Each set in the gym should be done with an emphasis on elegance. Forget about the amount of weight you can lift. Shift focus to how you are lifting it.

The key to functional strength training is learning to make less feel like more. Such artful lifting reduces stress factors on the joints while maximizing electrical production within the muscles. One day at Powerhouse Gym, I was working out next to a group of young ballplayers. At first they were all into their typical heaving and grunting, each trying to be the one to lift the most.

By the time I had finished my "elegance-priority" style of working out, they tuned into the poetics with which I was lifting. A visible change could be seen in their approach to the weights, a much deeper awareness on lifting form, instead of lifting egos. Unfortunately, their beer-bellied coach was completely oblivious to the spiritual connection that was going on and gave me the evil eye while ushering the ballplayers away from me.

Always carry yourself elegantly, no matter what. You never know who is watching you and perhaps impacted by your radiant posture.

2. Establish Lifting Rhythm: Focus on the Yin and Yang

Every repetition in the gym should express three distinct qualities: yin (female), yang (male), and neutral (transition). Nearly every injury, as well as training staleness, in the gym is due to ignorance of this rule.

A yang, or male, phase is explosive and occurs on the concentric contraction—when the muscle fibers shorten as they contract. This happens as a barbell is lifted toward the chest during a barbell curl.

The yin, or female, phase is a slower, more controlled motion that occurs on the eccentric contraction—when the muscle fibers

GREEN TARA STRENGTH TRAINING

PHYSICAL BENEFITS
structural integrity maximized

weaknesses balanced

neuromuscular system enhanced

myofibrillization: contractile proteins; thicken, increase in number and enzymatic activity

TRANSPERSONAL BENEFITS
teaches patience and wholeness

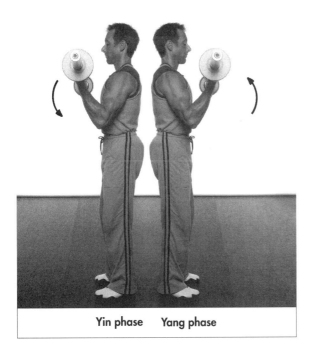

| Yin phase | Yang phase |

lengthen as they contract, like when the barbell is lowered from the chest during a barbell curl.

The neutral, or transition, phase links the yin and the yang together. It parallels *kumbaka* in yoga, or the moment between inhalation and exhalation.

3. Coordinate Breathing Rhythm: Merge into the Breath

Exhale on yang phases (explosive, concentric, shortening). Inhale on yin phases (slower, eccentric, lengthening). Since most yang phases occur as the weight is being lifting upward (as in the bench press, barbell curl, seated press, etc.), a good way to remember this principle is to blow the weight upward—exhale as you push. Inhale as you attempt to control the descent or the lowering of the weight.

Let's start exploring the strength training exercises of the Green Tara program. We'll begin with the lower body, move onto the midsection, and tie things up with upper body exercises.

Remember, you'll learn on which day and how many of these movements to do in Chapter 6. You can always refer back to this section later when working on the other programs. For now, study the following descriptions and visualize performing each of them with artistic, impeccable lifting form. I detail how to do each movement and also include "Wholistic Notes" for each movement, which offers more dimension to the specific exercise.

Remember, elegant and mindful lifting form is paramount in WF-style strength train-

PREPARATION FOR THE "IRON TEMPLE"

- Get a chronographic wristwatch if your gym does not have a lot of well-positioned wall clocks by which you can easily see the second hand. Several WF strength training techniques must be timed.

- Unless otherwise noted, all strength training movements must be carried to Failure of Elegance, the point where a collapse of elegant lifting form occurs.

- Unless otherwise noted, you are allowed only a 30-second recovery phase, the time spent between each set and each different exercise movement. Thus, the flow of your workout must be maintained from start to finish. No gossip, no water, no flirting. Just focus. World-class focus.

- Warm up before strength training. Master WF students often ride their bicycles to the gym. Lesser warrior options include 5 minutes or so on a treadmill or other cardio apparatus. You don't need to stretch before WF workouts because we prioritize elegance, not injurious herky-jerky form in the gym.

- Do a "focus set" before each movement. This means using the empty bar or very light resistance and closing your eyes and cranking off a fluid dozen or more reps before using your actual resistance. This increases the localized temperature of the respective joints of the body part being trained and prepares you mentally. Use focus sets to visualize how beautiful and strong you are going to be in the upcoming workout. Focus sets transfer into daily life and sport performance. You'll find yourself instinctively visualizing your actions before you do them. This is good *cinha* (positive sign of spiritual advancement).

- Be clean. Wear high-quality shoes that create stability to your lifting. Wear clothing that doesn't limit range of motion. And *always* conduct yourself as a WF representative in the gym; make it a point not just to put away your weights but someone else's as well. Not many are awake. You'll find numerous ways to practice elegance!

- Use no props. In WF, we meet the truth of the gym nakedly, with no gloves on. This means, literally, I don't want you to wear weight-training gloves. And don't use those silly foam bar sleeves during squats, or hand or knee wraps and straps. Don't dare put a board under your heels while squatting, if your heels come off the ground while squatting then by God get into yoga class so your hip flexibility increases. A weightlifting belt, if used at all, should *only* be used during heavy leg workouts and then, only during the actual set. External aids do not actually aid anything except ego—they furnish false support instead of internal structure and wise lifting form.

ing. Each set done in the gym should be done with as much concentration as a yoga pose. *There is no difference to the WF warrior between a yoga pose and a gym exercise.* "Yoga" means union, so unite the gym with the yoga studio. Do this, and you will quickly transcend the boredom and inconsistency that plague so many others.

LOWER BODY TRAINING

The strength of our lower body determines our connection to life.
—Coach Ilg

In Native Americana, humans are known as "the Two Leggeds." Our upright, bipedestrian locomotion distinguishes us from the world's other creatures. It should not come as a surprise to realize that our lower body is the site for a major confluence of subtle energetics. From a body/mind perspective, developing the power of our lower body can be intimidating. Fact is, many people shy away from leg training.

How long has it been since your bare feet have touched, let alone run, upon natural earth? Many of us have such weak, tender feet that we no longer consider wearing shoes as unnatural. How long has it been since you ate a meal sitting cross-legged on the floor? How long since you walked or biked to work, or squatted (without the support of a toilet seat) in the natural position to go to the bathroom?

Many us of have such tight, restricted hips from sitting in furniture, driving cars, and using contemporary toilets that we no longer consider such modern-day distortions as being unnatural. But they are. And because of such unquestioned acceptance, we've become a nation filled with lower back complaints, obesity, and a growing list of psychological "dis-orders." I say the only dis-order is ignoring the vital natural wisdom of moving more naturally upon Mother Earth.

In the gym, we can see this same lack of attention to the lower body. You know the type of gym member I am talking about: good chest, big biceps, but their skinny legs remain a secret hidden by baggy pants. Is it the intensity that frightens people away from hard lower body training? A fit lower body brings graceful symmetry to our physiques and helps to ground and balance us to move forward in our lives with an efficiency and flair that surpasses that of common man. Even kings and queens applaud the ballet dancer, commenting on the beautiful power of their legs.

A well-trained lower body conveys a particular poise. Developing a beautiful pair of well-muscled, lean legs beneath firm, shapely buttocks, however, demands high-intensity workouts and long-term determination. These days, people can buy themselves all sorts of body parts including new breasts and new faces. But a sexy butt and traffic-stopping legs? You still gotta work for those, baby! There is no intellectual defense for not cultivating a stronger, more supple and capable lower body. Following the programs in this book will give you that fit lower body, but before you head to the gym, I want you to know there is more to a good lower body than just a nice pair of stems.

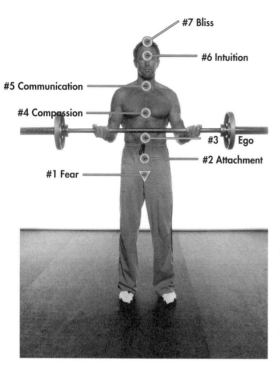

Chakra Energy Chart

#7 Bliss
#6 Intuition
#5 Communication
#4 Compassion
#3 Ego
#2 Attachment
#1 Fear

Spiritually, our lower body propels us forward into our lives and reflects how we feel about that movement and direction. Our legs are the external extension of our pelvis. This deep, bony bowl is situated between our hips and is home to the lower chakras. The chakras are vortices of energy located within the spine, not too different from the neural plexuses. Yogic science details seven such chakras, beginning at the root of the spine (muladhara chakra) and eventually moving to the crown of the skull (sahasrara chakra). The first two chakras are both located within the pelvis and are associated with fear, power, survival, manipulation, and ego protection. As if by anatomical irony, this body part is amply guarded by strong, thick, short ligaments that make tight, restricted hips so damned "sensational" as we try to increase their flexibility, such as in hip-opening yoga poses. The state of our lower body reflects movement from our inner levels to outer manifestation.

When the pelvis is out of alignment, so too is the spine and the energy running through it. Go to the chiropractor all you want, but as long as your pelvis is out of alignment, inevitably, so is the spine. Many of us feel so anxious and off-center all the time that we take drugs in an attempt to chemically recenter or elevate us. But really, it is structure that affects function. Get the structure of the pelvis aligned and balanced through wise gym and yoga training, and guess what? We become aligned and balanced. The hips and pelvis also house the sacred Kundalini energy of yogic anatomy that when stirred awake can ignite all the chakras, moving us toward higher levels of consciousness.

Injuries or issues in the lower body can be key points in body/mind education. The knees, for instance, represent *Maya*, or illusion. They are where we kneel to surrender or acknowledge a higher authority. Knees are known to buckle during overwhelming situations. If we are too arrogant or stubborn to refuse their psychological/emotional aspects, knees may reflect the lack of inner attention and become injured. If we are afraid of what higher work demands of us, we may also shut down this area and get injured here. Collapsed or flat arches, sensitive feet, or brittle toes long sheltered by shoes are proof that our entire body suffers from the lack of energy stimulation once naturally delivered by barefoot living. Becoming addicted to shoes can suffocate our internal organs, making them hard, lethargic, and predisposed to diseases. One of the greatest reasons to do yoga barefoot and to train the legs in the gym is a much-needed stimulation of energy to the lower body. In fact, doing yoga and lower body strength training is like giving yourself regular reflexology or acupressure sessions.

This was just a brief introduction to the body/mind value of our lower body. I hope I've given you reason to believe that there is a whole lot more going on "down there" than many of us may think. You have a wonderful amount of new birth awaiting you as my programs open and awaken latent potential within your lower body.

Stiff Leg Deadlifts

(see page 29)

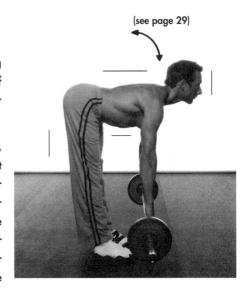

Stand upright in neutral alignment (see page 29) with a barbell resting at arm's length on the front of your thighs, palms facing your body. Puff out your chest a bit while slightly drawing shoulders back. Extend your neck, as if your head were being suspended from above.

Begin bending forward from the lower, not upper, back. This is a slow, mindful descent that does not allow your hips to move forward, but keeps them directly over the heels. Knees are kept extended while your spine strives to remain flat. Allow the barbell to drift away from your thighs during the descent. Genuine bottom position is reached as the flat back becomes parallel to the earth. Slowly begin to raise your upper torso from parallel, studying every centimeter of the ascent for possible postural flaws, until you're back to the starting position. The barbell will almost float toward the thighs on the way back up.

YANG PHASE: **None.**

YIN PHASE: **Both the lowering and the raising of the upper torso.**

WHAT YOU ARE PRIMARILY TRAINING: **Posture, lower back, hamstrings.**

WHOLISTIC NOTES: **You must be present to win on this one. Unique to this movement, both phases are yin, slow and controlled. The moment your back hunches over, self-correct to a flat back, and raise back to start again. Mental focus is key for this powerful posture conditioner. This movement was instrumental in my comeback from spinal injury. WF warriors do not pray for lighter burdens, we just create stronger backs.**

Finally, after all these years, I am beginning to see a lot of "gym rats" sucking it up and taking yoga classes. But I haven't seen many yoga teachers or devotees applying their treasured yoga to cranking out heavy back squats! I think it's time for that to change, don't you? Invite your yoga teacher to your next lower body workout in the gym.
—COACH ILG

Leg Extensions

Sit beautifully upright in a leg extension machine with ankles behind the lifting pads. Grip the bench by the sides of your body. Your knees should be bent, with legs forming a 90-degree angle or slightly more. Draw toes toward the shins. Select a resistance appropriate to your prescribed repetition range.

Powerfully extend your legs by lifting with the ankles. Top position is when your knees are just shy of full extension and your toes are pointing toward the sky. Initiate a slow descent by really controlling the first several inches. Upon reaching the starting position, make a smooth transition into another powerful extension. Repeat.

YANG PHASE: Extending the legs.

YIN PHASE: Lowering the legs.

WHAT YOU ARE PRIMARILY TRAINING: Quadriceps, sitting posture.

WHOLISTIC NOTES: Refrain from overgripping the seat handles. Use your hands only to sit more beautifully, not to lever the weight up. Anchor your focus on contraction of your quadriceps (frontal thigh), especially toward the end of a set when it's easy to get sloppy with your form. My master students can do entire sets with their hands resting on their thighs while listening to the stingingly sweet sonata arising from the quadriceps.

Leg Curls

Choose either a seated, prone, or standing leg curl apparatus. This description relates to the prone version. Situate yourself as elegantly as possible within the context of the machine. Nestle the backs of your ankles behind the lifting pads. Your knees should be free from any compression and have a slight flexion. Borrowing a Pilates technique, precontract your gluteal (buttock) muscles and the abdominals. Grip the apparatus to support only elegance, not leverage. Feet and toes should track directly under the knee.

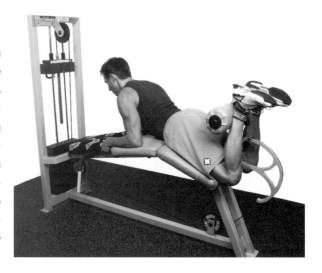

Without fidgeting the hips or losing the precontracted state, evenly curl both heels toward the glutes until your legs form a 90-degree angle. Lower slowly to the starting position.

YIN PHASE: Lowering the weight.

YANG PHASE: Curling ankles toward glutes.

WHAT YOU ARE PRIMARILY TRAINING: Hamstrings.

WHOLISTIC NOTES: Keep the upper body quiet and pinch your glutes continuously. Purity of movement comes when you heighten the integrity of the muscles and their attachments. Energetic sciences tell us the thighs represent movement in our lives. Issues that we may have about body image, sex, or financial security, are all examples of undigested emotional energy often held within hamstrings and illiotibial bands (the long strap of connective tissue that makes up the lateral thigh). Strengthening our thighs while increasing their flexibility is a tremendous journey, affecting many aspects of our lives. Leg curls help facilitate such inner work.

Back Squats

Using a power rack, situate a barbell across the back of the neck, low on the trapezius (upper back) muscles. Assume a stance wider than shoulders, toes pointing slightly out. Knees are never locked out, but remain just shy of extension. Grip the barbell with palms facing out at a comfortable, steady position several inches wider than shoulders. Look straight ahead.

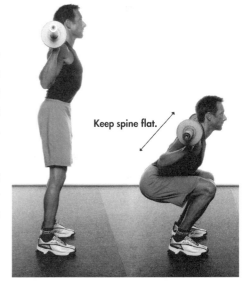

Keep spine flat.

Begin a controlled descent, tracking the knees over the toes. Do not allow the heart center to collapse forward. When the tops of your thighs are parallel to the ground, begin an explosive phase up to the starting position—without bouncing in the low transition phase.

YIN PHASE: Lowering the weight.

YANG PHASE: Rising from bottom position to top.

WHAT YOU ARE PRIMARILY TRAINING: The "power chain" musculature—hips, thighs, midsection, erector spinae muscles of the spine.

WHOLISTIC NOTES: Back squats single-handedly develop enormous reservoirs of inner power, spiritual tenacity, and mental focus. There are a million ways to cheat or take it easy during a set of back squats. Take responsibility for the nuances of this lift. Character, remember, can be lost by a single act. If your heels come off the floor during the descent, widen your stance, and beef up your yoga practice to increase hip flexibility. Never pause at the top or bottom positions—just commit to the flow.

Leg Press

Leg presses must be done on a leg press apparatus. Sit in the machine and place your feet on the foot plate in a shoulder-width stance. Heels in, toes slightly turned out. Make sure the seat is positioned so your legs are bent at a 90-degree angle or slightly less. Grip the handles at your sides. Relax your spine into the padded support.

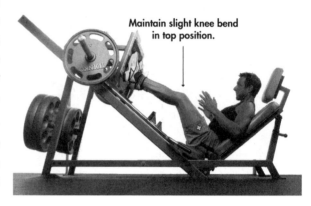

Maintain slight knee bend in top position.

Press forward against the foot plate, straightening your legs until they are just shy of complete extension. Without pausing in this top position, initiate a controlled, slow return to the starting position.

YIN PHASE: Lowering the foot plate.

YANG PHASE: Raising the foot plate.

WHAT YOU ARE PRIMARILY WORKING: Quadriceps, glutes, and lifting cadence.

WHOLISTIC NOTES: Track your toes in line with your knees during execution. Sit with as much presence as a god upon a throne, for this apparatus is truly a temple empowering all spiritual athletes to look deeply within. At extreme moments only breath remains, like a mountain stream, steady in tempo, leading to panoramic awareness.

Jump Squats

Take a standing position with your feet spread apart, just wider than your shoulders, with your toes pointed just slightly outward. Interlace your fingers behind your head, and keep your elbows wide. Do not push your head forward.

Drop into a half squat and explode upward as high as possible. As your feet leave the ground, focus on leading from the heart to keep your spine as upright as possible. The moment your feet contact the ground, explode upward again. Repeat for the required amount of reps.

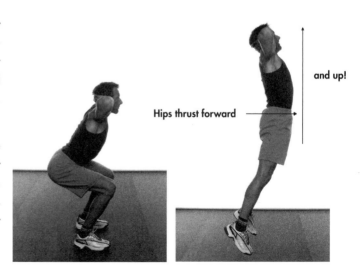

and up!

Hips thrust forward

YIN PHASE: Falling toward the earth.

YANG PHASE: Exploding away from the earth.

WHAT YOU ARE PRIMARILY WORKING: Fast-twitch fiber development, hips, thighs, core postural muscles, and increase of pain threshold (ego slaying).

WHOLISTIC NOTES: Do not overattenuate the landing; land nearly flat-footed then jump as fast and high as possible. Imagine doing this movement with bare feet on a ground of redhot coals! As the reps go on, your upper body will want to collapse—don't let it. This is key. Work those postural muscles. Allow pain to come. When everything is comfortable, we get complacent. There is no spiritual growth in complacency.

Standing (or Seated) Calf Raise

I'll describe the standing calf raise since it is more traditional; however, the same principles apply for the seated calf raise. The difference between the two movements is that the seated calf raises place more specific stress onto the calf complex, while the standing calf raise is more of a wholistic movement for the knee and ankle joints.

Stand in a standing calf raise "sled" apparatus and place your feet hip-width apart, pointing straight ahead, on the foot platform. Settle your hips and lower back into the respective area on the rear pad. Grip the handles at the sides of your body. Keeping your spine erect, bend your knees, exhale, and squat the weight upward. Stop at the top of the motion. Carefully readjust your stance so only the balls of your feet press into the foot platform and your heels are in the air, off the back of the foot platform.

Rise all the way up on your toes. You'll feel your calf muscles reach a peak of contraction. Then slowly lower your heels until they break parallel to the foot platform. In this bottom position, you'll now feel what should be a not unpleasant stretch to your Achilles tendon area. From there, rise again to the top position and repeat with poetic, not jerky, cadence.

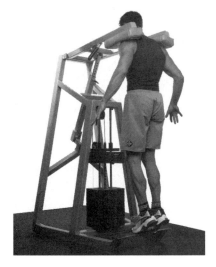
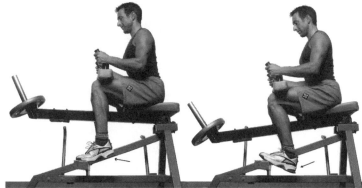

YIN PHASE: Lowering the heels.

YANG PHASE: Raising the heels.

WHAT YOU ARE PRIMARILY WORKING: Lower leg muscles, integrity of ankle and knee joints, and mental concentration and determination.

WHOLISTIC NOTES: Really pinch the top position—visualize squeezing "calf juice" from the calves in that top position. This movement is fantastic and, for athletes, critical to injury prevention. One reason I excelled for years in mountain races is because I could hammer the steep, tricky downhill sections faster than my non–strength-trained competitors. Why? Because calf raises gifted me with ankle joints that have connective tissues the strength of aircraft cable. It will do the same for you, too. But remember, poetic form is an absolute must.

MIDSECTION TRAINING

Move from the core of who you are, radiate your energy from your solar plexus.
—COACH ILG

We're about to visit an area of the body that keeps a lot of fitness athletes in a conundrum of correct training. I am referring to the midsection, or what is generally misnamed "stomach training." Stomachs are digestive organs. Our abdominals, however, are those frontal plane muscles responsible for maintaining posture and transferring power through the hips. Though it's completely natural for a stomach to distend while digesting, a well-trained set of abdominals should always be flat and strong. Having said that, I perpetually see people overtraining the abdominals without first conditioning the internal organs of the midsection. The intestines, for example, must be intelligently squeezed, compressed, and twisted so their attachments become better suited to handle progressive abdominal training. Because WF includes yoga in the overall training strategy, I do not prescribe a lot of direct abdominal work in beginning programs. The yoga will impart the graduated strength and suppleness to what I like to call our "internal lacing." Also, I think it is important to keep the abdominals strong but not risk overtraining them. I've seen too many lower back injuries occur due to people going crazy with abdominal training. I do not ignore direct lower back work—the other half of midsection training. I include lower back work during leg training, however, because it makes better biomechanical sense to do so.

If we consider midsection training from an energetic standpoint, we find a very important energy center lying behind the navel. This is the "jeweled city" of the third chakra, manipura. The energies associated with this solar plexus center revolve around ego identification, attachment, personal power, will, and esteem. Keeping a good set of abs often helps keep manipura tuned up. Thus, our self-confidence and willpower function better. Too much fat covering this area can be symbolic of too much ego attachment. When we cling to things, fat tends to gather here. It's easy, especially in this country, to become third chakra gluttons; attractions to those things that delight the senses but are not truly needed are all tests of third chakra fitness. To keep manipura in balance, material goods must be kept in check. When manipura is purring, we are free from worrying about our kids, jobs, cars, houses, all that stuff that accounts for so much anxiety in our lives. As manipura comes into condition, we find ourselves trusting our gut feelings more and more. We balance our intellect with our intuition.

For Green Tara, I've selected two fundamental training movements that strengthen the "internal lacing" to support more advanced abdominal training later. These two movements will also complement the yoga postures in the program that develop the spiritual aspects of manipura.

Medicine Ball Crunches

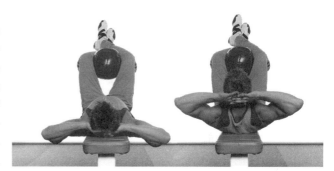

Lie supine on the floor or on top of a flat bench with your fingers interlaced around the back of your neck. Float your lower leg bones so that they are parallel to the ground. Place and then squeeze a 4 to 8 pound medicine ball between your knees. Note: If your lower back arches into the air, or if your lower back feels uncomfortable while squeezing the medicine ball, do this exercise without an actual ball. Options include a "physioball" and your imagination of a medicine ball!

Curl your upper torso toward the medicine ball while pressing the lumbar spine downward. Keep curling the upper torso upward until your abs reach their peak contraction and your shoulder blades attain the greatest height from the starting position. After attaining that top position, lower to the starting position. Without pausing, begin the next repetition and repeat for the prescribed amount of repetitions.

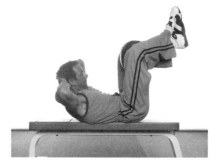

YIN PHASE: **Lowering the upper torso.**

YANG PHASE: **Raising the upper torso.**

WHAT YOU ARE PRIMARILY WORKING: The core musculature; the abdominals and their stabilizers and assistives (external obliques, internal obliques, transverse abdominus, multifidus, erector spinae, quadratus lumborum, etc.).

COACH ILG ON CORE TRAINING

Thanks in large part to ridiculously expensive and ever redundant fitness conventions, "Core Training" has stormed center stage within the fitness industry. Scores of young, perky personal trainers fresh from "Stability Ball Training 101" workshops are now gleefully consuming precious space in the gym with their giant "physioballs" and other unrecyclable gizmos. According to product literature, I need these gadgets to improve my "balance, agility, functional strength, and coordination." Hmmm. I thought that's what yoga did. Or practicing a handstand or mountain biking or climbing up a rock. Modern Core Training is nothing more than quirky spinal stabilization movements. They are physical therapy exercises gone wild. Some of the stuff is fun and helpful in a novel way, but I also find it questionable for long-term effectiveness. Core Training is no more effective than my strength training techniques such as Staccato, Swan Medicine, and 3-Stage, and it is infantile compared to the yogic sciences of asana, internal locks, and pranayama. Professionally, I think Core Training is great for injury rehabilitation, youth and senior fitness, and novelty. But doing it day after day can actually overuse and weaken the very muscles and neural fabric it intends to strengthen. I don't do much "core" stuff in the gym. Personally, I like to pump iron. I rely on yoga for my "Core Training." By the way, anyone know the half-life of a plastic "Stability Board"? Maybe the fitness convention people do.

WHOLISTIC NOTES: Squeezing the medicine ball adds more resistance to the muscles and also draws energy toward your core—what in yoga is known as Mula Bandha or a "root lock," referring to the root of the spine. If holding the medicine ball between your legs is too much, place a rolled-up towel in the same spot. Why this basic movement when modern gyms are heavily adorned with expensive abdominal machines? Because true character comes through on simple movements. Developing character is like glass—even a little crack shows. Draw your focus inward, don't become distracted.

Suspended Leg Raises

Prop yourself into a suspended leg raises apparatus by gripping the handles with palms facing each other, forearms resting on the padded bars. Press your lower and mid spine into the rear pad and let your legs become suspended beneath you. Lift your spine out of the hips and drop your shoulders away from your ears. Put a slight bend into your knees, and press both knees and ankles together. Flex your toes toward your face.

Swing both legs up to horizontal from the hips. Let them hover parallel to the ground for a moment before slowly lowering them back down to perpendicular.

YIN PHASE: Lowering the legs from horizontal.

YANG PHASE: Raising the legs to horizontal.

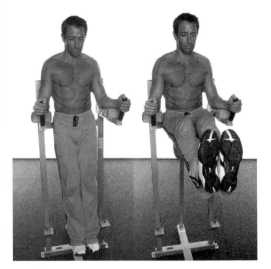

WHAT YOU ARE PRIMARILY WORKING: Rectus abdominus, pelvic stabilizers, core movement.

WHOLISTIC NOTES: Always lower your legs slowly with control coming from the abdominals to prevent inelegant swinging. This movement annoys most people when they cannot control the dynamic balance involved. This is precisely why they should keep practicing it. To decrease intensity, this movement can be done lying supine or, to increase the intensity, it can be done using an AbOriginal Strap hung from a pull-up bar with your elbows looped through the straps.

Oblique Twists

Lie supine on a bench press apparatus. Stabilize your upper body by grasping the upright support bars. Raise your legs to a perpendicular position. Bring your ankles and knees neatly together and slightly flex both knees. Press as many vertebrae of your spine as possible down into the bench.

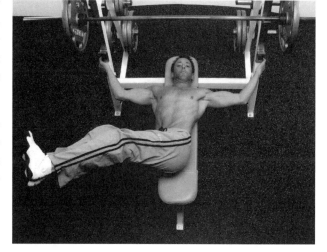

Slowly lower both legs to your right side. Your left hip will rise away from the bench. Counteract the downward action as your legs attain a parallel position to the floor by raising them back to start position. Lower to the other side and repeat.

YIN PHASE: Lowering the legs.

YANG PHASE: Raising the legs.

WHAT YOU ARE PRIMARILY TRAINING: Upper torso rotators, obliques, and serratus (a muscle that rotates, protracts, and abducts the scapulae). Also affords an internal massage to the intestine and colon, increasing digestive power.

WHOLISTIC NOTES: Visualize internal organs being squeezed and wrung like a wet towel. This movement not only enhances all power through the hips but additionally cleanses and strengthens visceral connective tissues.

Lift ain't no fun without big "guns."

Our upper body is our showcase. Lean, symmetrical muscles here are highly sought after because a good-looking upper body attracts eyes. Immature fitness athletes tend to overtrain their upper body and undertrain the lower body. This could be due to the fact that the upper body contains our doing and thinking centers and, as a society, we prioritize doing and thinking over movement, which is the responsibility of the lower body.

The chest, back, shoulders, and arms represent our "doing center"—the place where we turn our inner desire into outward expression. Good chest development is the foremost lure of the upper body. Lying opposite the chest is the upper back. Development here gives a beautiful V-shape to the upper body and makes the waistline appear smaller. Training the chest and back can awaken the potential energy within anahata chakra, the energy center of love, balance, healing, and relationships. Unfortunately, most people pay too much attention to the chest and not enough to the mid and upper back. This can create an imbalance within the heart center, reducing the love and balance in our life. I specifically design WF strength workouts to balance and liberate chakra energies.

Balancing the chest and back are the shoulders, a very attractive body part that tells the world how well we are able to carry our burdens and provide for a potential mate. Our arm development personalizes and refines the flow of inner energy outward. Injuries or issues with the wrists can be examples of trying to hold on too hard to things we really cannot control. The final three chakras—vishuddha (throat center), ajna (brow center), and sahasrara (crown center)—are only indirectly influenced by strength training, breath (stimulates vishuddha), focus (stimulates ajna), and surrender (stimulates sahasrara). This is appropriate because opening those chakras requires meditation, forcing the fitness athlete to sit quietly and learn how to still the mind.

Pull-ups

Grasp a pull-up bar using an overhand grip slightly wider than your shoulders. Lift both heels off the floor, crisscross your ankles in back of you, and curl your heels toward your butt.

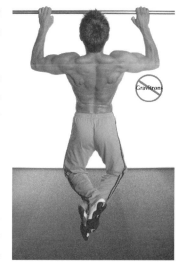

Using an explosive upward movement, pull your heart—not your chin—toward the bar and draw your elbows out to the sides. Reach your maximum height—be it two inches or your heart touching the bar—then lower yourself with control until your elbows are only slightly bent. Repeat for prescribed repetitions.

YIN PHASE: Lowering down from the bar.

YANG PHASE: Rising toward the bar.

WHAT YOU ARE PRIMARILY WORKING: Latissimus dorsi (major muscle of the back connecting the lower and upper extremities), rhomboids (muscles that stabilize the scapulae posteriorly and adduct it), teres complex (muscles that stabilize the head of the upper arm bone, humerus, in the shoulder joints), spiritual tenacity, and humility.

WHOLISTIC NOTES: Initiate your pull from the back of the heart. Don't overgrip. Have faith. You must have a clear purpose here and know precisely what you are targeting. How do you expect to master your life if you cannot master a pull-up? Pull-ups bring forcefulness to life. Each set, you will push yourself to the point of giving out. That is fine. Giving up, however, is *not* fine. As UCLA basketball coach John Wooden taught, "Never let what you cannot do interfere with what you can do." Do not let me catch you *near* that damned Gravitron machine. Face your inner dragons nakedly beneath the simplicity of a pull-up bar. If my wife trained herself to do eight pull-ups, so can you!

V-Handle Pulldowns

Attach a V-handle to a lat pulldown apparatus and sit in the machine holding the V-handle above you with your palms facing each other. Place both knees solidly beneath the knee pad, making sure you are firmly connected to the machine. Lean back (away) from the machine. Emphasize the natural curve in your lower spine and keep your head pulled up.

Pull the V-handle to your chest. Allow the heart center to come forward to meet the V-handle, and squeeze your shoulder blades toward

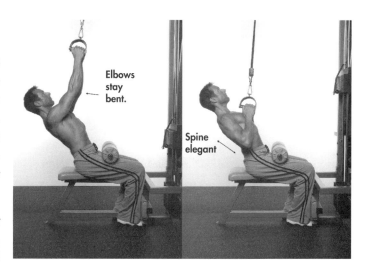

Elbows stay bent.

Spine elegant

your spine. After a slight pause in this bottom position, slowly control the ascent of the V-handle until your elbows are nearly locked out but not quite. Do not pause in the top position, but elegantly transition into another downward pull. Repeat this pattern for the prescribed amount of reps.

YIN PHASE: As the V-handle moves up and away from the heart center.

YANG PHASE: As the V-Handle moves toward the heart center.

WHAT YOU ARE PRIMARILY WORKING: Same muscles as pull-ups but at a different angle. This exercise also helps to break down resistances and adhesions in the scapular and shoulder area, freeing the heart chakra's energy.

WHOLISTIC NOTES: Where pull-ups contribute width to the back, this movement adds depth and stability to it. I like to raise my heels to drive my knees more solidly beneath the knee pads. Use mental focus to limit the amount of hip movement.

Hang Cleans

Assume a hip-width standing position with your knees slightly flexed, holding an Olympic barbell at arm's length against the top portion of your thighs. Grip the barbell with your palms facing your thighs, just wider than your shoulders.

Bend both knees to store some momentum before literally jumping up while simultaneously shrugging your shoulders toward your ears. Allow the hips to extend like you are lifting too heavy a box onto too high of a counter. No timidity here—both feet should

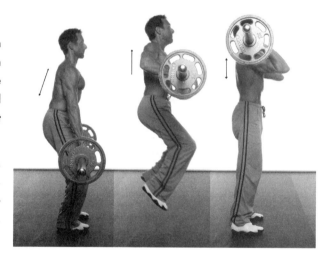

explode off the ground. This "jump phase" imparts velocity to the upward movement of the barbell. As the barbell rockets toward the ceiling, keep your elbows high and pointed toward the ceiling so your arms do not interfere with the upward line of the barbell. As the barbell travels up, it should remain close to the body. Next comes the "catch phase." As the barbell reaches maximum height (almost throat level), quickly squat under the barbell and catch it on the upper chest by flipping your elbows quickly underneath the barbell. Stand up, keeping the barbell sandwiched between your throat and upper shoulders. Finally comes the "drop phase" where you essentially drop the barbell back to the starting position by quickly drawing both elbows back past the midline of the body. The barbell will "fall" onto your lap, and you are ready for the next rep.

YIN PHASE: Not much yin to it, but it occurs during the "drop phase."

YANG PHASE: As you jump the bar up between your shoulders and throat. Doesn't get much more yang than this!

WHAT YOU ARE PRIMARILY WORKING: The "power chain" muscles—the hips, thighs, and upper torso. Also, fast-twitch fiber development and motor skills coordination.

WHOLISTIC NOTES: My antivenom to the modern gym machines . . . no apparatus on earth can duplicate the majesty and power of a Hang Clean. Be quick with the feet. A sublimely technical lift, second only to back squats for developing full-body power. When you "get it" the barbell skyrockets toward the ceiling effortlessly. This movement makes a "Warrior 3" yoga pose feel like recess and I've seen several Pilates teachers shuffle away from this lift baffled, dazed, and confused. So, take your time, and be patient with the initial bewilderment. I'm looking to develop your neural and spiritual tenacity more than anything here. It will come. Go ahead—scream, grunt, groan! Don't be afraid to go out on a limb on this one. That's where the fruit is.

Dips

Start by pressing yourself to arm's length above a dip bar apparatus. If you have a choice, a dip bar with handles that flare outward instead of parallel to each other is best. Drop your chin onto your chest and curl your heels toward your butt.

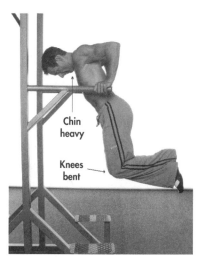

Chin heavy

Knees bent

With control, bend your elbows and gracefully lower your chest toward the handles. The moment your upper arm bones break parallel to the ground, aggressively extend your elbows by pushing down on the handles until a top position is attained where elbows are just shy of complete extension (locked out). Without pausing, begin lowering into your second rep.

YIN PHASE: Flexing the elbows, lowering the torso toward the ground.

YANG PHASE: Extending the elbows, raising the torso away from the ground.

WHAT YOU ARE PRIMARILY WORKING: Chest, shoulders, triceps, and conviction.

WHOLISTIC NOTES: Keep a steady, tigerlike gaze on the ground. Never waver the chin away from your chest. Use breath vigorously and you'll create a beautiful dance of functional strength. A dynamic remedy for those with little faith in their own power. Do not go *near* any assisted resistance dip machines like a Gravitron. Far better to develop your true, naked spirit by just bending your elbows two inches for two years on a real dip bar instead of submitting onto those expensive crutches.

Dumbbell Flyes

Lie supine on a flat bench holding a pair of dumbbells above your chest at arm's length, palms facing each other. Press as many vertebrae of your spine as possible into the pad beneath you, including those that make up the back of your neck. Raise both feet into the air and bend the knees so legs form a 90-degree angle (this is the "yin leg position"). Bend both elbows ever so slightly. Curl your chin toward your chest, looking toward your knees.

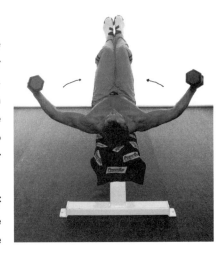

Lower both dumbbells with simultaneous control to the sides of your body. Do not flinch your elbows. Once the dumbbells are flush to your chest, retrace their descent path perfectly back to the top position in aggressive but disciplined manner. Repeat.

YIN PHASE: Lowering the dumbbells down from top position, toward the ground.

YANG PHASE: Raising the dumbbells up from bottom position, toward the sky.

WHAT YOU ARE PRIMARILY WORKING: Both upper (clavicular) and lower (sternal) chest, some shoulders, and lifting artistry.

WHOLISTIC NOTES: Dumbbell flyes are one of the most aesthetic strength training movements when executed mindfully. The arm motion here is like hugging a very large tree trunk. Some personal trainers describe the arm position like the spread wings of a bird. The key point is to keep both elbows slightly bent, yet fixed, through the range of motion. My "floating feet" technique is known as the "ultra yin foot position" in WF. It purifies lifting form to activate every fiber in your chest, as well as working core muscles (see sidebar, page 54).

Dumbbell Bench Presses

Lie supine on a flat bench holding a pair of dumbbells above your chest at arm's length, palms facing toward your legs. Press as many vertebrae of your spine as possible into the pad beneath you, including those that make up the back of your neck. Raise both feet into the air, use an ultra yin foot position, and bend the knees so legs form a 90-degree angle. Curl your chin slightly toward your chest, looking toward your knees.

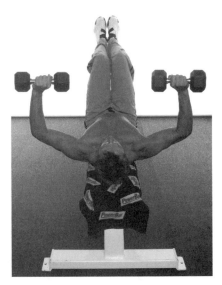

Slowly lower both dumbbells simultaneously to the sides of your upper chest by deeply bending the elbows. As the dumbbells draw flush with your chest and with the palms still facing toward the legs, press the dumbbells up by extending the elbows in a slight arcing motion. As they near the top position, the two dumbbells just "kiss" each other above your chest. Without pausing, repeat.

YIN PHASE: Lowering the dumbbells from top position, toward the ground.

YANG PHASE: Raising the dumbbells from bottom position, toward the sky.

WHAT YOU ARE PRIMARILY WORKING: Both upper (clavicular) and lower (sternal) chest, some shoulders, and lifting artistry.

WHOLISTIC NOTES: Forget about how much you can bench and focus on how beautifully you can utterly torch your pectoral muscles. Keep your legs and lower spine completely quiet. If your hips are moving about, you are decreasing the electricity needed to really "zap" the chest. This is precisely why we use the ultra yin foot position described in dumbbell flyes. This overpopular lift is often sloppily performed from ego reiterating attitudes that sever true inner power development. Be different: Lift purely and with sensitivity to breath and inner, not egoic, energetics.

Bench Press

Lie supine on a bench press apparatus holding a barbell at arm's extension above the chest, palms facing the legs. Take a grip slightly wider than shoulder width. Press as many vertebrae of your spine as possible, including those that make up the back of your neck, into the pad beneath you. Raise both feet into the air and bend the knees so legs form 90-degree angles.

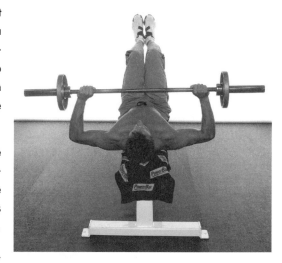

Flex both elbows cleanly out to the side, slowly lowering the weight until the barbell just touches the chest between the nipples and the clavicle (collarbone). Without pausing, press the barbell up by powerfully extending the elbows. As the elbows almost reach complete extension, lower the barbell and repeat.

YIN PHASE: Lowering the barbell from top position, toward the ground.

YANG PHASE: Raising the barbell from bottom position, toward the sky.

WHAT YOU ARE PRIMARILY WORKING: Both upper (clavicular) and lower (sternal) chest, some shoulders, and honesty (by way of strict form).

WHOLISTIC NOTES: Be brave and honest enough to just say no to any hip involvement. Don't change your wrist position during the lift. Look for your own natural neural groove to develop over time so that the barbell hits the same place on your chest each rep. A good hint to stay focused on strict form is to keep your eyes on the barbell as it moves up and down.

Seated Dumbbell Press

Sit on the edge of a flat bench with an upright spine, feet at shoulder width, knees bent so legs form a right angle. Toes point forward. Gripping a pair of dumbbells, raise your elbows laterally to your sides (90-degree shoulder abduction). Position your lower arm at a right angle to your upper arm (90-degree elbow flexion). Both upper arms are parallel to the ground, lower arms are perpendicular to the ground, and palms face forward.

Slowly extend your arms overhead as if pushing the dumbbells into the sky. Keep extending your arms until they are directly overhead, not pushed forward. Slowly lower the dumbbells by bending the elbows directly out to the side, not collapsed forward, until they have reached the starting position.

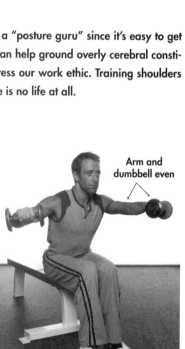

YIN PHASE: Lowering the dumbbells.

YANG PHASE: Raising the dumbbells.

WHAT YOU ARE PRIMARILY WORKING: Deltoids (shoulders), triceps, torso stabilizers, and postural awareness.

WHOLISTIC NOTES: Use a mirror and your reflection in it as a "posture guru" since it's easy to get sloppy with all the angles involved during this movement. This exercise can help ground overly cerebral constitutions by bringing them into the shoulders, where we develop and express our work ethic. Training shoulders in the gym can be a bit repetitive, reminding us that life without discipline is no life at all.

Seated Dumbbell Lateral Raises

Sit on the edge of a flat bench and press your knees together. Keeping your spine flat, draw your navel toward the front of your thighs. Grasp a pair of dumbbells under your hamstrings, palms facing each other, elbows flexed at about 60 degrees. Look forward and lengthen your spine as much as possible.

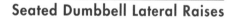

Raise both dumbbells laterally by lifting your upper arm out to your sides. Keep lifting until both elbows pass parallel to the ground and your palms completely face the ground. Slowly lower the dumbbells back to the bottom position.

YIN PHASE: As dumbbells are lowered toward the ground.

YANG PHASE: As dumbbells are raised away from the ground.

WHAT YOU ARE PRIMARILY WORKING: Deltoids (shoulders), spinal stabilization, and coordination.

WHOLISTIC NOTES: In the top position make sure your elbows are even with, or slightly higher than, your hands. Very little, if any, activity occurs at your elbows, but a lot at the shoulders. Shoulders remain dropped away from the ears. Stay fluid, and allow a personal rhythm to emerge. This movement is good for dissipating inner conflict and stress regarding the direction in your life.

Barbell Curls

Stand beautifully upright in a hip-width stance and with knees slightly flexed, feet pointed straight ahead. Puff out your heart center a bit and keep it in front of your hips. Draw both shoulders back. Pull your head upward, giving length to the neck. Hold a barbell at arm's length near the top of your thighs with your palms facing outward, shoulder width apart. Elbows pressure the sides of your body.

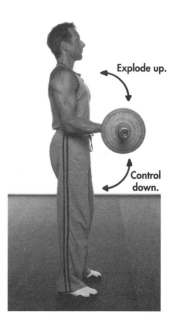

Explode up.

Control down.

With controlled verve, bend your elbows forcefully to raise the barbell toward your throat. Nearing the top, elbows naturally elevate, but limit this elbow sway to a couple of inches. As you feel the biceps on the front of your upper arm reach peak contraction, extend your elbows and pin them back to the sides of your body as the barbell floats down to the starting position, providing deep stretch to the biceps. Before reaching complete elbow extension, begin the next repetition by again flexing the elbows. Repeat.

YIN PHASE: As the barbell is lowered toward the ground.

YANG PHASE: As the barbell is raised away from the ground.

WHAT YOU ARE PRIMARILY WORKING: Biceps, forearms, and postural elegance.

WHOLISTIC NOTES: Tense the abdominals, tighten your buttocks, and curl the tip of your tailbone under you to protect your lower spine against compaction. Use a mirror and watch your posture like a hawk, keeping your shoulder girdle even and the dance of your repetitions smooth. Our arms express how we choose to reach out and grab life. As you perform this movement, realize that the poise with which you do this exercise can help you elegantly strengthen your actions in daily life. Be enthusiastic, but your form must drive the enthusiasm.

Two-Bench Triceps

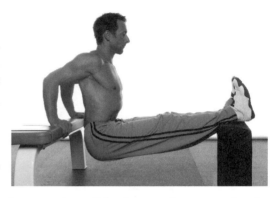

Suspend yourself between two flat benches at arm's extension. On the bench in front of you, rest your feet, ankles and knees together, with your heels near the middle of the bench. Position your palms on the inside edge of the second bench, fingers gripping the lip of the bench under you. Hands should be placed beside each hip. Lengthen your spine, drop the shoulders away from the ears, and pull your head up.

Begin your set by flexing your elbows. This will lower your hips toward the ground. Feel your front shoulders stretch due to the deep elbow flexion. As your upper arm bones reach parallel to the ground, start extending the elbows in an effort against gravity to raise the hips until the arms reach extension. Make sure you complete this arm extension in the top position; don't cheat the range of motion. Repeat by again bending the elbows.

> YIN PHASE: **Lowering the hips.**

> YANG PHASE: **Raising the hips.**

> WHAT YOU ARE PRIMARILY WORKING: **Triceps, muscular endurance, concentration.**

> WHOLISTIC NOTES: **This difficult movement is made easier by moving from your core, trusting the breath, and keeping your eyes soft. Use my time-honored "escape plans" to finish your sets during this movement, but never quit. Escape Plan A: Put one foot on the ground and use it. Escape Plan B: Put both feet on the ground and use them. Escape Plan C: Just hold the top position, pause, pray, and hammer out reps as best as you are able.**

WHOLISTIC FITNESS STRENGTH TRAINING TECHNIQUES

World Class strength training techniques created by a World Class athlete and coach, what more do you want?
—*SPORTS WEST* MAGAZINE

The following Strength Training techniques, which I introduced in 1982, were intended to transform the sterile and predictable gym workout into a colorful, challenging, and creative explosion of inner and outer strength. They did just that, and still do. These techniques are divided into two categories: Stimulative Phase Techniques, which are used during the actual lifting of weights, and Recovery Phase Techniques, which take place in between sets. These techniques are copyrighted, but please share them with your training partners. Have fun exploring these techniques and may they bring you rich insight and high performance!

Stimulative Phase Techniques

The art of life is to know how to enjoy a little and to endure much.
—WILLIAM HAZLITT

Envelope Technique

Increases muscular endurance and deep fiber recruitment. Teaches perseverance and mental stamina.

"Open the envelope" by performing the first set for 1 minute. Recover for 30–45 seconds. Then perform 2 heavy sets of 6–8 reps. Recover for 30–45 seconds. "Close the envelope" by doing a final set for another minute. Try to time each set to end with momentary failure. This takes inner art and practice.

Staccato Technique

Designed to enhance capillarization of muscle tissue, associated hypoxic mechanisms, and to teach elegance through difficulty. Improves mental concentration, as well as breath and postural awareness.

Set is performed for 1 minute, divided into 10-second "splits." Begin the set by "sticking" the first rep in the top position and holding it there for the 10-second split. Then, "move" during the next 10-second split by performing the exercise movement through its full range. Repeat this procedure until the 1 minute point is reached. Staccato techniques always begin with a "stick" and finish on a "go" phase.

3-Stage Technique

Created to improve mental focus, lifting form, rhythm, and postural awareness during work output.

Exercise is performed for 1 minute, divided into 20-second "splits." Perform first split, or "stage," by executing only the top half of the movement. Second split: Train only the bottom half of the movement in accelerated tempo. Third split: Perform the movement throughout its full range with total conviction.

Shivaya Technique

A pre-exhaustive technique to fatigue a specific muscle within its strongest contractile range.

Choreography of set: First 3 repetitions, full range; reps 4 through 9, train only the top half of the movement; reps 10 to failure, full range (the optimal rep range in this final set should be 5 to 6 reps).

Swan Medicine Technique

Grace and fluid movement are two aspects of Swan Medicine. This technique increases mental concentration while promoting muscular endurance and isometric strength.

For use with dumbbells (or machines with independent arm levers). Select a resistance so that failure will be reached within 6 reps. While one limb holds the resistance in the top or mid or bottom position (contraction intensity high), the other limb does the standard range of movement for the exercise. Upon failure of the working limb (around 6 reps), repeat sequence in opposite manner.

Recovery Phase Techniques

Without haste, but without rest.
—Life motto of Johann Wolfgang von Goethe

Ku Technique

Method. Upon the completion of a set, keep holding the weight as effortlessly as possible. Hold this position for 5 nasal breaths in one of the two positions:

Ku Top Form—The exercise movement is held at its top position. For example, when doing a front lat pulldown, take 5 nasal breaths while holding the bar at arm's extension.

Ku Bottom Form—The exercise movement is held at its bottom position. For example, when doing a front lat pulldown, take 5 nasal breaths while holding the bar at the chest.

Meditation. The word "Ku" is Sanskrit for the void. Feel the inner power now under attention. "He who has never failed somewhere, that man cannot be great," Herman Melville knew, "and it is better to fail in originality than to succeed in imitation." Find your truth in this originality, in this failure.

Entre Nous Technique

Method. After performing the final repetition of a set, set down the weight but maintain a contact of the weight. Just touch it. The point is to maintain touch with your apparatus on the physical level to access the spiritual level. Take 5 nasal breaths, and begin the next set.

Meditation. Be at one with the movement. By maintaining touch with the apparatus, you keep the mind from wandering. Just you, your apparatus, and your breath. That is all. Work to eliminate distracted mind.

CHAPTER 2

Cardio

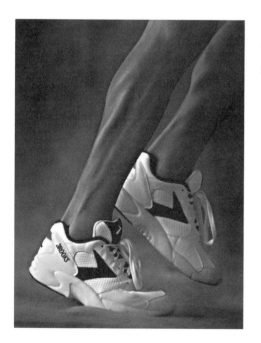

STARTING WITH THE GREEN TARA program, there are two things to get you on track in regard to your Cardio fitness:

1. Cross train as much as possible among a variety of Cardio activities. Run, bike, hike, do the "stairs," take group exercise classes, skate, swim. Make it a point over the next three months to learn or renew at least two new Cardio activities or sports. Life is short—change it up!

2. Be prepared to practice both aerobic and threshold (or interval style) Cardio workouts. The aerobic workouts will be your lower-intensity but steady-state sessions that function as fat-burner workouts. My threshold or high-intensity Cardio workouts will include dastardly effective "interval" sessions that will build inner character, more power production, and, well, a great looking butt.

The rest of this chapter reveals my philosophy behind these two points and details the specific Cardio workouts that are part of your Green Tara daily routine.

CROSS TRAIN

Let's say you enjoy running. That is fantastic, but don't be a compulsive runner. It'll only shorten your Achilles tendon, tear down your joints, and degenerate your overall (balanced) fitness. Only professional or sponsored runners should run every day. Everyone else should intersperse running with other Cardio activities. I don't mean to pick on runners. Same thing goes for swimmers, walkers, group exercisers, or cyclists. Don't be addicted to one fitness discipline. There is no balance in that. I'll show you a much more effective way to a higher, safer, and way more fun level of fitness.

> Aerobic (low to moderate intensity) workouts work best for fat burning when done for longer periods, not necessarily more intensely. Very little fat is actually being metabolized for the first 20 to 30 minutes of any Cardio workout, regardless of intensity. It's mostly a sugar-based metabolism up until that point. However, the more time you spend doing Cardio beyond 30 minutes, the more stored body fat you will be liberating to fuel your effort.

The Cardio Training in a fitness plan should encompass a wide spectrum of activity and intensity. In WF philosophy, cross training is mandatory. Too many people do the same Cardio workouts all the time then wonder why they get bored and injured. They wonder why their physiques and fitness levels never change. Why? Because you were born to dance, baby! You gotta dance the Cardio spectrum! Specificity is for insects, not Wholistic Fitness warriors.

Whatever Cardio activity you are good at or do most often, change it. If you are a good swimmer, ride a mountain bike. If you are a club racquetball player (a questionable Cardio activity in the first place), start indoor cycling classes. If you are great at "locomotive activities" like running, cycling, paddling, or hiking, but lack lateral movement skills, it's time for you to begin racquet sports, kickboxing, soccer, or basketball.

If you really want some beneficial karma and to earn points toward WF mastery, start getting in some of your Cardio workouts by becoming a fitness commuter—one who walks, runs, skates, or rides their bicycle to work or school or errands. That is real WF warriorism. The point is, as in any true spiritual work, you must push the edge of your comfort zones.

I emphasize the "wholeness" factor in Cardio training because of this fitness paradox: The better you are at a given Cardio activity, the fewer calories you burn and the smaller the training effect. Summer Sanders, an Olympic medalist in swimming, would burn a million calories less than me if she and I swam the English Channel. Why? Because Summer is so perfectly trained in swimming that she slices through the water like a trout whereas I flop about in the water like a wing-shot duck.

COACH ILG ON THE ULTIMATE ATHLETE

There is still no international competition that truly tests Cardio fitness. People say that Ironman races (2.3-mile swim, 112 miles bicycling, 26.2-mile run) are the ultimate cardio test. Not even close. Ironman competitions only test endurance (aerobic), not threshold (anaerobic), fitness. A Wholistic Fitness version of "Ironbeing" would start with a gnarly 1-mile steep uphill run, followed by a 10-kilometer inline ski race (to incorporate upper body strength endurance), before going all out in a four-hour time-trial bicycle race! That would be a truer test of overall Cardio fitness than the current Ironman races.

But to discover the "ultimate overall athlete in the world," we need the World Wholistic Fitness Games—a single-day, three-part event testing three physiologic categories: strength, flexibility, and endurance. It would work like this:

Event 1: Yin Energy Competition (Flexibility). The athletes perform judge-selected yoga poses that are timed and judged for style and strength points as the competitors move into and must hold backbends, forward folds, spinal twists, inversions, arm balance, and standing balance poses. This event also functions as a warmup for the following two events. Right off the bat, muscle-bound power lifters will get their ass kicked and I don't think endurance-specific athletes would fare much better.

Event 2: Yang Energy Competition (Strength). Athletes compete in pull-ups, dips, and jump squats to determine strength-to-weight fitness before performing one-repetition-maximum tests in bench press, back squat, and deadlifts to decide maximal strength. The so-called Ironmen that made it through the first event will now see their endurance-specific legs buckle in this event. But if they can hold on, their turn comes next. The muscle heads, on the other hand, will shine in this second event. But their confidence will be shortlived as the WWF Games move to the final event.

Event 3: Ultra Mountain Bike Race (Endurance). To close the day, the tired athletes compete in a 3.5-hour mountain bike race. Why mountain biking? I want these games to be fun and safe. If this final event was a footrace, the training would damage the joints when training for the other two events are considered. Cycling produces no concussion on the joints. Besides, mountain bike racing with lots of climbing really pushes the competitors and makes for excellent spectating.

Now *that* would be "Reality TV" worth watching. My games would determine functional, broad-spectrum athletic fitness. A shorter, more frequent version could be created: The Sunday Night WF Games. That would get people psyched for their weekly workouts. I have never understood why the world seems to reward specialization and not versatility, particularly when it comes to athletics.

But because I suck at it, swimming is a better fitness tool for me than it is for Summer. She's too good at it. A key to higher levels of fitness is to do things you suck at. By exchanging Cardio activities that you are good at for ones that are more challenging to you, you'll burn more calories, become more fit, and develop a fuller dimension to your body/mind energy. Your ego might take a licking, but that will turn out to be a good thing over the long term. I promise.

Injuries and imbalances occur by doing the same thing over and over again. You were not designed that way. Life was not designed that way. Everything always changes. Life is a dance. You were designed to be a dancer. So I say, let's dance.

CROSS TRAIN TO BRING LESS PAIN

Cross training in Cardio is also much more healthy for your body. One reason my wife, Kathy, and I have never had a serious training injury in a combined thirty-five years of professional fitness and outdoor sport instruction is that we shuffle around our Cardio training. Kathy teaches everything: HP Yoga, Krav Maga combat fighting, indoor cycling, step aerobics, and more. My Cardio includes mountain biking, road cycling, snowshoeing, Nordic skiing, trail running, etc. Kathy and I are constantly flipping between Cardio activities. Our cross training keeps us mentally refreshed and puts less physical stress on our joints.

INTERVALS: THE BUDDHA OF INTENSITY

To give anything less than your best is to sacrifice the Gift.
—STEVE PREFONTAINE

A magazine interviewer once asked me what the largest difference was between a serious athlete and a recreational one. Without hesitation, I answered, "Intervals." Any real athlete does interval training—repeated bouts of high-intensity Cardio exercise sandwiched between short recovery periods. Intervals, though very difficult to do, create a huge reservoir of cellular power, what I call "threshold fitness." Once you attain a degree of threshold fitness, your whole life seems charged. It is a tremendous feeling, and sadly, so many people lose out on ever feeling this magnificence within them.

Threshold fitness is the type of explosive vigor that enables Lance Armstrong to attack his cycling competitors halfway up a mountain pass, shatter the group, and do it again and

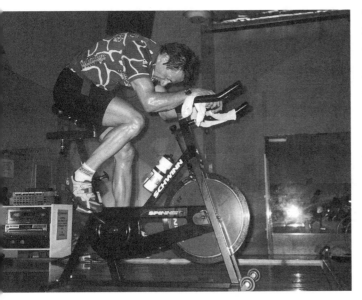

again until only he remains by the time the finish line is reached. You may have done threshold and interval training during elementary school P.E. classes when your coach made you do "wind sprints." Our modern technology has not updated the methods nor the pain factor you probably still associate with those wind sprints. I can't make doing intervals fun for you, but they'll surely transform your fitness and your life energy.

From the intensity of intervals drips the precious and rare spiritual medicine: honesty. If fitness is religion, then intervals are our prayers.

Why is doing intervals so important in my program? Because intervals make you a better person, period. They make you familiar with physical failure but immune to spiritual failure. You want to know failure? Ask a champion from any walk of life, they'll tell you. How many tennis balls did Pete Sampras hit into the net or outside the lines? How many bike races did Lance Armstrong lose, compared to the ones he has won? Ask any well-known author how many rejection slips he or she received before that first book contract. The only thing that fails the mediocre man is his will. Interval training toughens your will.

With each interval workout done, your inner character develops an ego-cutting acid. This affects the spiritual fiber of your being. Sugar Ray Robinson, the champion boxer, once said, "If you want to see a great fighter at his best, watch him when he is getting licked." Interval workouts "lick us" every time. Intervals force us to face all sorts of inner dragons and magnify our weak mental areas. Intervals are like meditation sessions on steroids; they really zap you into the moment like nothing else can. By the end of this book, if your practice is strong and sincere, something will change about your presence. There will be an unmistakable confidence in your step and in your eyes. In an age filled with gossip, false images, unconsciousness, and fickleness, you will be a WF warrior, beaming with light, love, and a deep-seated compassion born from the humility of interval training.

HOW INTERVALS SHOULD BE DONE

Do your interval workouts alone and in as controllable an environment as possible. Limit external factors that could interrupt your interval session. If you are going to do your interval

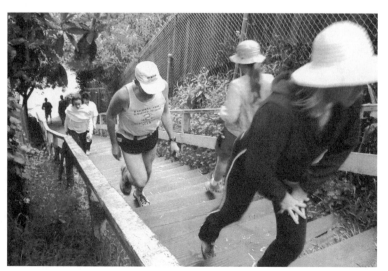

workouts on a treadmill or indoor stationary cycle, make sure you don't gossip, and that you push yourself to the limit without embarrassment. I know that sounds silly, but I don't see a lot of people in gyms really, truly digging down deep. Embarrassment comes from the ego, so if you are concerned about

WF Master Student Kit Johaneson running the Santa Monica stairs during a Private Training Intensive with Coach Ilg in Los Angeles.

your appearance in the gym, you're going to have to deal with that element of your ego. That's why I like to do my intervals out in the mountains where I feel free to grunt, groan, and howl along with the screaming sensations in my lungs . . . I can let my e(eeee)-go!

If you are going to do your interval sessions outdoors while running or cycling, make sure you limit the impact of traffic concerns, dogs, terrain changes, road debris, etc. If your joints can take it, running intervals at a local track is a great spiritual workshop. You'll be surrounded by other fitness warriors and the vibe to rise higher will be strong.

A good alternative to track running is powerwalking up and down a flight of outdoor or stadium stairs. In Boulder, I would lead a group of us to run the Colorado University stadium stairs every Tuesday. It was great looking across the field and watching your fellow fitness warriors running up and down the long stairs. In Santa Monica, California, hundreds of fitness warriors gather like Zen monks to climb a flight of old, rickety wooden stairs barely tethered to the California Incline as the Pacific Ocean glimmers a short distance away.

In this book, I have prescribed a variety of diverse interval workouts for you: Hill Repeats, Minutes Are Forever, Cruise Intervals, 15 × 15's, and Assigned Intervals. For now, let's take a look at your initiation into interval training, which appears in the Green Tara Daily Practice. For our first jump into this sacred arena of self-growth, I've selected Assigned Intervals. Here's how to do them:

ASSIGNED INTERVALS

In your Green Tara Daily Practice (see Chapter 6) you will see this on your Friday prescription:

Cardio of Choice

Assigned Intervals

> 20 minutes @ Zones 1 and 2
>
> 5 sets x 1-minute intervals @ Zone 4 w/1-minute RI
>
> 5 minutes RP
>
> 3 sets x 3-minute intervals @ high Zone 3 w/2-minute RI
>
> 20 minutes @ Zones 1 & 2

Now let's break it down.

Friday

This is the day of the week that you are scheduled to do your intervals.

Cardio of Choice

This means you can use any Cardio activity you desire, with adjustments as described above (no group exercise classes; must be done alone; must be in a controlled environment). If using any indoor apparatus or outdoor machine like a bicycle, make sure you can control your heart rate while using it and can keep it sustained without interruption. Be sure of your handling skills if using a bicycle, inline skates, etc. The best forms of Cardio activity for interval training are those that are highly manageable, such as indoor trainers, treadmills, or tracks. Stadium stairs are great for intervals. If you are doing intervals outdoors, be very careful of your terrain; limit all traffic, dogs, intersections, etc. You'll be very woozy during interval workouts so keep the logistics simple and safe. Use a chronographic wristwatch for interval workouts.

20 minutes @ Zones 1 and 2

This is basically your warmup. It means doing your Cardio activity for 20 minutes at an easy pace, between 60 to 72 percent of your maximum heart rate. Basically the effort level here means you can easily speak but can't really sustain a long whistle. (See Table 2.1.) For example, I like to ride my mountain bike to my favorite interval hill at an easy, Zone 1–2 pace as my warmup. It takes about thirty minutes, and when I arrive at the bottom of my interval hill, I'm ready to rock and roll.

5 sets x 1-minute intervals @ Zone 4 w/1-minute RI

This means that you need to time yourself while doing 1-minute high-intensity efforts between 86 to 90 percent of your maximum heart rate. Basically the effort level during Zone 4 intervals means you are mouth breathing and your effort is so difficult that it feels like you are sucking goose eggs. Immediately after each 1 minute of Zone 4 efforts, you bring your intensity level to almost nothing for 1 minute. Once the 1-minute recovery interval (RI) ends, you must blast off into your next interval. Repeat until you've done five 1-minute intervals linked by five 1-minute RIs.

5 minute RP

This is a gift. It means you are granted 5 luxurious minutes of a Recovery Phase or "RP." During RPs, it is best to keep moving slowly, don't stop completely (unless you are ready to pass out). Enjoy!

3 sets x 3-minute intervals @ high Zone 3 w/2-minute RI

This means that you now need to time yourself while doing 3-minute moderately high-intensity efforts between 80 to 85 percent of your maximum heart rate. Basically the effort level during the higher end of Zone 3 intervals means you are hurting hard and the effort level is forced but sustainable. It's the "time trial" mode; you are dancing the edge between sustainable effort and blowing up. Immediately after each 3 minutes of high Zone 3 efforts, bring your intensity level almost to nothing for 2 minutes. Once the 2-minute recovery interval ends, you must blast off into your next 3-minute Zone 3 interval. Repeat until you've done three 3-minute intervals linked by three 2-minute RIs.

20 minutes @ Zones 1 and 2

This is a repeat of how you began your workout. Before, it served as a warmup. Now it serves as a cooldown. It means doing your Cardio activity for 20 minutes at an easy pace, between 60 to 72 percent of your maximum heart rate. Basically the effort level here means you can easily speak but can't really sustain a long whistle. For an example, I like to ride my mountain bike back home from my favorite interval hill at an easy, Zone 1–2 pace as my cooldown. It takes about twenty minutes. By the time I arrive back home, the drama of the interval session has been replaced by a feeling of tranquility. Anything that was stressing me out before my intervals seems magically trivial afterward.

2.1 Cardio Zones

ZONE	% OF MAXIMUM HEART RATE	INTUITIVE GAUGE
Zone 1	> 65% (aerobic)	recovery/warmup/cooldown: can easily speak and whistle
Zone 2	65–72% (aerobic)	can speak but winded; can't sustain a whistle
Zone 3	73–85% (aerobic/threshold)	forced but sustainable effort
Zone 4	86–90% (threshold)	high intensity up to 3 minutes; breathing difficult
Zone 5	91–100% (threshold max)	maximum effort up to 30 seconds; hurts so bad you're ready to hurl

CARDIO COMMUTE

Also appearing in your Green Tara Daily Practice will be an option called Cardio Commute. On days when this assignment pops up on your Daily Practice Sheet, you are instructed to ride a bike, inline skate, run, or walk to work, school, the gym, the yoga studio, or on an errand.

If that is too tough for you, other honorable WF Warrior efforts include using mass transit or carpooling.

How simple, how noble can one fitness assignment be? Do you have what it takes? This is one assignment that makes or breaks genuine spiritual fitness warriors.

CHAPTER 3

High Performance Yoga

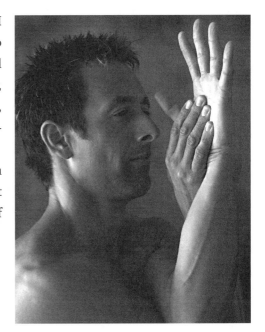

NOW IT IS TIME TO have some barefooted fun! I plan on complementing your Strength and Cardio benefits with Yoga. Among the training effects you will notice from this component will be enhanced flexibility, improved organ function and health, injury prevention, mental focus, less stress, and an increased sense of well-being.

Are you starting to get an idea of exactly why a Wholistic Fitness lifestyle is so powerful? There is just nothing like the comprehensive and delightful balance of this path. Let's go, Noble Warrior! Onward and upward!

Better buckle up. I'm going to shear seven centuries of a highly evolved, complex Eastern science of enlightenment into a few paragraphs. I'm navigating us through some immense intellectual terrain, keeping only the shining kernels so there will be knowledge, substance, and power in your Yoga practice.

> *Yoga is not learned by technique,*
> *It is a gift you are given by the guru*
> *and you spend the rest of your life*
> *trying to understand.*
> —MUKUNDA

Yoga is the world's original body/mind fitness training system. "Yoga" means union, or yoke. What are we supposed to unite? Well, in classical yoga, we deal with two levels of union. On one level, we are uniting body with mind. On another, we are uniting the individual self (what the yogis call *atman*) with the universal self (*brahman*). There are about a million different interpretations to what I just wrote in that sentence. What is most important to realize is that unlike Strength and Cardio, Yoga is a very old, vast, and precise science of mental control, self-healing, and spiritual endeavor. Because of its great depth and age, 99 percent of what Yoga is is far beyond the scope of this book. But that doesn't matter. We've got plenty of things to work on, believe me.

The earliest evidence of Yoga dates back to the second millennium B.C.E. Some teachings have been found preserved on petrified palm fronds. Yoga began not as physical training but as a highly evolved system of mental and sense control, all tinged with spiritual ramifications. Around the tenth century B.C.E., the physical practice of "Hatha Yoga," or "physical yoga," begins appearing as an established element of Yoga.

> I have a feeling that you and I were once ancient Yogis. I think you and I were initially attracted to working out because in former lifetimes, our souls discovered something that just felt right about staying fit. We have carried over that "karmic" attraction toward fitness into this lifetime so that on a soul level, we can continue our learning and injoyment. What was the deeper reason behind your purchase of this book? What is the true motivation behind you wanting a new way to improve your fitness?

Sometime about 200 B.C.E., a sage (or some say sages) known only as Patanjali systematized all the existing yogic knowledge into a treatise, the *Yoga Sutras*. Patanjali presented an eight-step scientific layout of how to become enlightened through Yoga. His work was so unflinchingly complete and clear that his system is now known as Classical Yoga and he is considered "the grandfather of Yoga." In the *Yoga Sutras*, Hatha Yoga is affirmed as the best way to make a yogi's physical body fit and worthy enough for advanced spiritual work.

To me, anyone who enjoys working out is a Hatha Yogi. We enjoy moving, breathing, and being in our bodies. It makes complete sense to us to stay in shape instead of out of shape. We find it easy to understand that the only true wealth is health. Keeping our bodies healthy makes us happy.

Similarly, we find it sad to see so many unhappy people who don't enjoy being in and caring for their bodies. How could anyone ever be truly happy over the course of a lifetime in a body that is unfit, restricted, and not fun to move around in?

Yogis consider that a happy, comfortable body makes for a happy, comfortable mind.

As I said earlier, Hatha Yoga is an integrated part of Patanjali's eight-limbed path of Classical Yoga. The first two limbs, *yama* and *niyama*, are five ethical and five personal disciplines to be practiced as best as possible throughout our lives. These timeless guidelines encourage us to get our act together and get in harmony with society before beginning spiritual work. The yamas and niyamas train us "to become a somebody before becoming a nobody," as Ram Dass liked to put it.

Today's commonly accepted images of fat-bellied spiritual teachers, of people going to church then smoking or eating junk food immediately afterward, would make no sense to a Hatha Yogi of old. They would probably study our society for a few days and ask how can one endeavor to control one's spiritual life before even being able to control a bag of Doritos or a pack of cigarettes? B.K.S. Iyengar, the most well-known Hatha Yoga Master of modern times, is attributed with saying, "One cannot hope to master the spiritual realms with the body of a weakling!"

The third and fourth limbs of Classical Yoga are what we are most familiar and concerned with in this book, for it is the combination of these two limbs that make up Hatha Yoga. The third limb, *asana*, is Sanskrit for seat, but the common interpretation of the word is "posture." Asanas are stretching-like poses that are performed either fluidly (as in Tai Chi) or statically. Asana brings strength to the body and focus to the mind.

The fourth limb, *pranayama*, means extended "breath" or "life force" and refers to mindful breathing techniques, which amplify the life force of an individual.

Asana prepares the body to handle more *pran* (life force), and *pranayama* amplifies the *pran*. Just doing *asana* without *pranayama* is not doing Yoga at all, but is instead just a form of gymnastics or calisthenics. The deep nasal breathing technique you will learn in this book is a form of *pranayama* that is used in conjunction with yoga postures, or *asana*.

After *pranayama*, the fifth limb of Classical Yoga is *pratyahara*, which requires the gradual lessening of external or materialistic desires and attachments. It means to "draw within" yourself and control the appetite of your various senses. The final three limbs are considered as one, the quest for enlightenment: *dharana* (concentration), *dhyana* (sustained concentration or meditation), and *samadhi* (enlightenment).

Patanjali, as well as all the Yoga Masters, has always urged strict adherence to becoming better and more consciously evolved, and in control of your passions and emotions through the yamas and the niyamas, before moving deeper in Yoga. The reasoning is that as your spiritual energy increases, you must use your growing radiance to help others along the way and not misuse powers gained in Yoga.

HATHA YOGA DETAILED

If someone says that they do Hatha Yoga, the next question would be, "What kind?" Any Yoga class that combines holding or flowing postures with breathing is a Hatha Yoga class. There are numerous styles of Hatha Yoga, and ever since America has gotten her monied hands on Hatha Yoga, it seems, the list grows weekly. America's penchant for inventing and reinventing things certainly did not stall when Yoga became the new fitness fad. The established methods—basically the styles in place before Madonna started doing yoga—include Iyengar, ashtanga (Madonna's reputed practice, by the way), vinniyoga, kripalu, ananda, kundalini, integral, anursara, and Bikram.

Some Hatha Yoga styles are very slow and methodical and others are dynamic and free-form. Some styles, such as kundalini, focus more on pranayama while others really emphasize asana, such as Iyengar and ashtanga. It's like the martial arts: There are plenty of different schools (Tae Kwon Do, Hap Kido, Tai Chi), but their objective is still *kara te* (way of the empty hand). Ideally, there should be no competition among the various styles of Yoga, especially given the spiritual philosophy from whence Hatha Yoga came and points toward. However, just as in any other sport or discipline I have studied, certain styles and teachers start power-tripping and proclaim, "My yoga is better than your yoga!" It's crazy; it's like monks having a meditation competition and having a fight break out, "I am the most serene!" "No, I am more serene than you!"

All I know is that different styles and teachers of Yoga appeal to different personalities and at different times during life. In this book, you will be introduced to my style of Power Yoga, known as High Performance Yoga. And my style is definitely better than anyone else's! (Just kidding!)

HOW HATHA YOGA WORKS

Think of Hatha Yoga as the Physical Education Department within the overall science of Yoga. In Hatha Yoga, each posture (*asana*), when combined with the breath (*pranayama*), is designed to eventually rid the body of all weakness and all disease, while stabilizing the mind and emotions.

Yoga postures work similarly to the way acupuncture does. But instead of using needles to unblock energy lines and dams, yogis use their bodies and breath to compress, cleanse, and strengthen the tissues and glands. Instead of having someone else stick needles into us, we stick our own elbows, heels, heads, feet, you name it. The Wholistic effect from a wise choreography of poses practiced at a reasonable level of intensity and frequency affects our long-term health in three main ways:

1. structurally, to align the physical body

2. organically, to cleanse, balance, and empower the organs and glands

3. energetically, to concentrate mental energy and to condition the subtle network of vessels (nadis) and energy centers (chakras) to accommodate an increase and eventual manipulation of life force (pran).

There, that's about all I wanted to cover before getting to your specific Yoga practice. Don't be intimidated by the upcoming Sanskrit words and terms. Yogic anatomy and physiology are just much more expansive, embracing, and inwardly evolved than is our Western analytical approach. But both perspectives work quite well with each other, as is being demonstrated each passing year in the fields of psychoneuroimmunology, fuzzy logic, nucleicbioquantum fields . . . whatever, dude! Be it pran or wavicles, the blending of the great Eastern traditions with the youthful exuberance of the Western mind is going to make the dance even more exquisite.

HIGH PERFORMANCE YOGA

I created a brand of Hatha Yoga called High Performance (HP) Yoga. It is based on my experience with many styles through the years, but it most largely honors the ashtanga tradition. It is a

POWER YOGA

"Power Yoga," of which there are many versions, including my own, is linked historically and thematically with the ashtanga tradition of Mysore, India. This vigorous, challenging style was developed through Sri Pattabhi Jois, a modern-day Hatha Yoga master. Coincidentally, it has been alleged that Jois was so impressed by Western gymnasts who happened to be performing at the Mysore Palace, he integrated their athleticism into his style of Yoga. The gymnastic flavor will surely not escape the attention of anyone who has taken a true Ashtanga Yoga class. It's nice to think that America is not so disconnected from Yoga after all!

Through Yoga, I became not only a better athlete, but a kinder, more compassionate, and wiser human being. I've seen it quickly accomplish these qualities in many others as well, from ages twelve to seventy-eight, and in many who never, ever thought they'd do Yoga. Whoever you are, however old, whatever you do, Yoga will help. It complements every sport, every activity, every occupation, and interferes with no religion or faith. Its eons-old science of self-healing has consistently destroyed disease, retarded aging, and transformed average people into enlightened beings.

> A lot of people remark about how "different" I teach and how effective HP Yoga is compared to many other styles. All I can say is that I created HP Yoga to help me stay alive in the high, extreme mountains. I had to rely on HP Yoga to train my mind and my body to free-solo difficult rock and ice climbing routes where one wrong move or hesitation or lack of strength and flexibility meant "lights out" for Ilg. I used HP Yoga to get me to the tops of podiums in several sports, safely and confidently. I think you'll feel this power and faith in the routines you will be practicing.

Power Yoga style, and its main difference lies in my sequences and choreography. It's the only system that is based on Western periodization, or cyclic training, principles.

I designed HP Yoga especially for stiff, restricted, and injured bodies like mine, and for those of us who won't stop going to the gym or doing Cardio just because of Yoga. My routines provide safe and progressive strengthening and limbering effects on the joint abilities of North American—not South Indian—physiques. HP Yoga is therefore particularly well-suited to fitness warriors.

And for competitive athletes? One magazine called HP Yoga "the secret weapon for enhanced sports performance." It is easy to see why fitness people are attracted to HP Yoga. All HP Yoga sessions begin easily and build into a vigorous, strength-oriented warmup that offers a Cardio-training effect. Then, after our bodies are warm and operating at their peak elasticity, specific postures from general categories, such as backbends, forward folds, spinal twists, hip openers, etc., are practiced. The session always finishes with a relaxing meditation phase.

If you had only one chance to work out in a day, an HP Yoga session is the clear choice. One session gives you a daily dosage of strength, cardio, flexibility, and meditation. Perfect!

CHECK YOUR EGO

Although these are entry-level HP Yoga routines that appear in this book, they will challenge and bring body/mind reward to anyone. Even hard-core ashtanga and other Power Yoga devotees will benefit from these routines.

Athletes, especially those unaccustomed to dedicated flexibility or bodyweight strength moves, will have to immediately tone down their driven nature when it comes to HP Yoga. My first encounter with even the basic poses humiliated me due to my lack of flexibility. Some of

> Remember, do *not* push the edge of where you feel sensation. Do not compete! Just practice!

the hip opener poses truly infuriated my ambitious drive. I was forced to temper my driven nature. Yoga does that to everyone. These days, my humility remains (I still seem light-years away from many of the advanced poses), but my ambition in Yoga has been supplanted by acceptance and respect. I encourage you to let your breath guide you into and out of the postures, not your ego. The likelihood of reaching some goal in Yoga should become meaningless. The goal and the path of your Yoga practice should merge into one.

TWO KEY POINTS OF PRACTICE

Here is what you'll need to practice during your Green Tara program Yoga sessions.

1. *Breathe Through Your Nose.* As you practice the following Yoga routines, refrain from mouth breathing. Nose breathing creates an internal heat that warms the tough connective and muscle tissues. This heated air makes the body more elastic and helps cut through various restrictions. After getting used to nasal breathing, you are ready to amplify the pran (life force) by doing ujjayi pranayama. To do *ujjayi* breathing (which means the "victorious breath"), continue nasal breathing but slightly constrict the back of your throat making a Darth Vader–type of sound. Ujjayi will sound like a pretty loud hiss for the first few years. With practice, ujjayi matures toward a more subtle, deeply hollow breath.

   Try incorporating nasal and ujjayi breathing into everyday life and into your other workouts (except interval sessions). You'll be pleasantly surprised at how effectively it brings calmness to the mind and energy to the body. Ujjayi is great to use during Strength Training to keep the joints warm and the muscles more powerful.

2. *Dance Your Edge.* Strike a balance between effort and ease during each Yoga posture. I call this spot "dancing your edge." It is an intuitive place just before pain and is the place of progress in Yoga. Get to your edge, then soften the sensation of the edge by ujjayi breathing. Enter into and away from your edge by using your breath. Yogis never move without the breath. Think of the last time you hurt yourself. Were you breathing consciously? Probably not. It's nearly impossible to hurt yourself when you let your breath guide your action.

Your ability to combine the above two practice points will dictate your progress in my Yoga routines. Good luck, have fun, and remember, don't push the river of your progress—just let it flow instead.

High Performance Yoga: Because elegance during difficulty is beautiful.

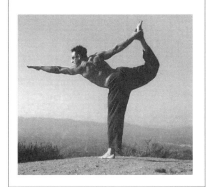

Not much. To do the following HP Yoga routine, you'll just need some empty, clean space in your home. If this space is carpeted, make sure it is deep cleaned. On carpet, the balance poses might be a little more challenging, but that's okay. You will sweat, so to prevent sweat from making your carpet smell like a gym, wipe off frequently with a towel.

If your practice space is a hardwood floor, a yoga sticky mat or a woven Ashtanga rug (a woven cotton rug that absorbs perspiration) is suggested. Your local yoga studio will usually sell them. Sweat management tends to be an ongoing issue in Power Yoga styles, especially for beginners. To avoid slipping, use a towel frequently.

Practice in a place where you are not likely to be interrupted by phones, kids, pets, etc. This is *your* time. Turn off the phone, turn off your "doing" mode, and slip into your "being" mode. This ability is a trainable component of your mental fitness and will become easier to do with practice.

Practice in comfortable clothing that does not interfere with movement or breathing.

Practice on an empty stomach. For most people, this means not eating for two and a half hours before your session.

No shoes, no socks. Reasons for doing this include stimulation of reflexology points on the bottoms and tops of the feet.

Drink filtered water adequately before and a lot after your Yoga practice, but never during. Drinking during a practice douses the beneficial internal heat and cools your internal system, negating many of the physiologic and energetic benefits.

Quickly shower, when possible, before your Yoga session to rinse off lotions, perfumes, etc. Do not apply anything to your skin or face. Do not wear any jewelry. After your session, it is fine to go dandify yourself if needed, but not before.

Some poses are followed by an additional option pose. I've also given variations to some of the poses. Don't think you have to do them. Do not compete. Asana practice can be a fountain of youth for the body or as damaging to it as professional bull riding if you force yourself into poses where you don't yet belong. Don't do an option pose unless (1) you can do the main pose with smooth, steady nasal breathing and (2) the option pose feels appropriate to your body with no sharp pains or unusual sensations. Grow into your repertoire of asana gradually. *Never force a pose.*

Rest when you need to rest. The moment you consistently notice any of the following signs during a Yoga session, take a few moments to rest in Child's Pose (see photo, page 100) before resuming your practice:

- mouth breathing, gasping, or grunting instead of steady nasal breathing

- "muscling" the postures and trying too hard

- difficulty concentrating

- nausea, dizziness, racing heart rate, or sudden pain

If resting in Child's Pose does not alleviate those signs, stop your practice for the day. You'll come back stronger next time. If the signs continue over the course of several sessions, consult a yoga-knowledgeable doctor.

GETTING TO KNOW THE POSES

Let's take a look at the specific HP Yoga routine that you will practice over the next four weeks. The whole routine will take between 45 and 90 minutes, depending on your level of ability, desire, and time availability.

It is a great routine that I still use and teach often. I'll use the rest of this chapter to break it down for you, posture by posture.

This first cycle, I'll remind you, is the most challenging one of the book because it is our basic recipe. Take your time to learn it.

HP YOGA: THE GREEN TARA PRACTICE

Sun Salutation Warmup

This warmup achieves similar effects as any warmup does before exercise: It increases the temperature of the body so that joints become lubricated, tissues become more supple, and the mind can start becoming focused on the workout. In HP Yoga, there are five different Sun Salutation series. It's pretty easy to memorize all of them, but I've illustrated each series so you can set this book in front of your practice area and follow them.

> 3 x Ardha Surya Namaskar (Half Sun Salutation)
>
> 2 x Series A Modified
>
> 1 x Series B (both legs = 1 set)
>
> 1 x Series C (both legs = 1 set)
>
> 5 x Series A

Begin your Yoga session by flowing through Ardha Surya Namaskar (Half Sun Salutation) three times, then do two rounds of Series A Modified, one round of Series B—remembering that you have to do both legs to complete one round—one round of Series C, which also requires you to do both legs, and finish with five rounds of Series A. Although this will only take about 20 minutes, you'll be sweating and ready to do the following poses, which, unlike the Sun Salutations, are held statically for 30 to 60 seconds each.

High Performance Yoga Sun Salutations
(Ardha Surya Namaskar Half Sun Salutation)

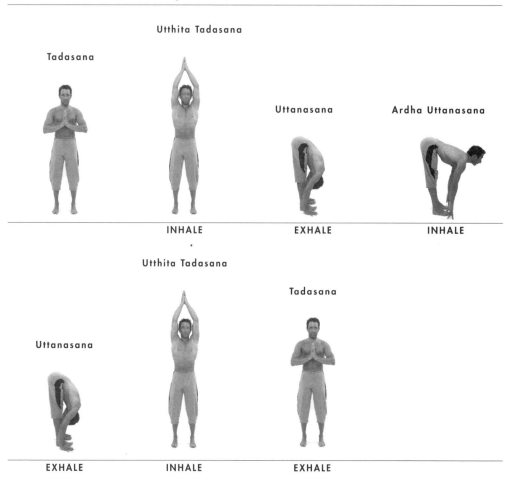

High Performance Yoga Sun Salutations, Series A-Modified (No Jumping Required) (Circled pose can be held for several breaths to develop stamina)

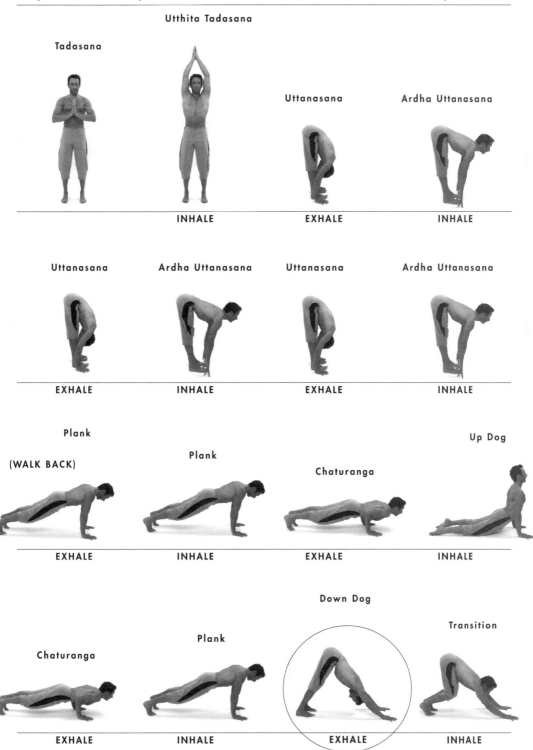

Tadasana

Utthita Tadasana

Uttanasana

Ardha Uttanasana

INHALE   EXHALE   INHALE

Uttanasana   Ardha Uttanasana   Uttanasana   Ardha Uttanasana

EXHALE   INHALE   EXHALE   INHALE

Plank

(WALK BACK)   Plank   Chaturanga   Up Dog

EXHALE   INHALE   EXHALE   INHALE

Down Dog

Chaturanga   Plank   Transition

EXHALE   INHALE   EXHALE   INHALE

Transition

(WALK UP)

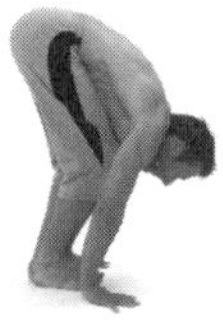

Ardha Uttanasana

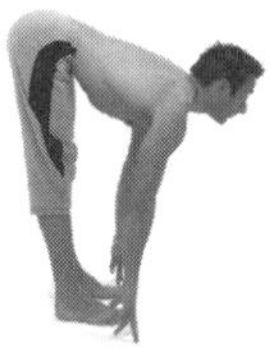

Uttanasana

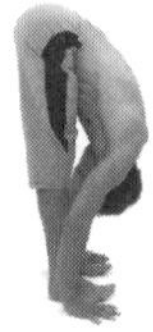

Utthita Tadasana

EXHALE

INHALE

EXHALE

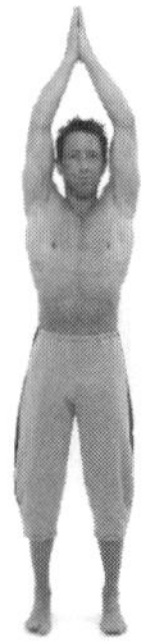

INHALE

Tadasana

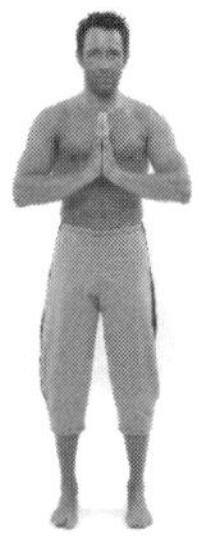

EXHALE

Tadasana

Utthita Tadasana

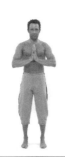

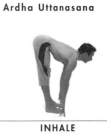

Uttanasana

Ardha Uttanasana

INHALE

EXHALE

INHALE

Chaturanga

Upward Facing Dog
(Urdhva Mukha Svanasana)

Chaturanga

Plank

(JUMP BACK)

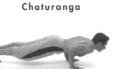

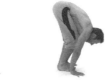

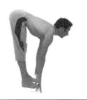

EXHALE

INHALE

EXHALE

INHALE

Transition

Downward Facing Dog

Transition

(JUMP UP)

Ardha Uttanasana

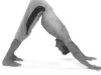

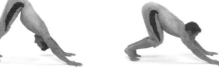

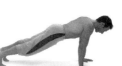

EXHALE

INHALE

EXHALE

INHALE

Utthita Tadasana

Tadasana

Uttanasana

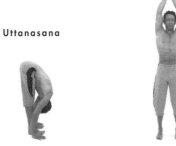

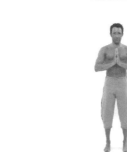

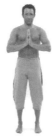

EXHALE

INHALE

EXHALE

High Performance Yoga Sun Salutations, Series B
(Circled poses can be held for several breaths to develop stamina)

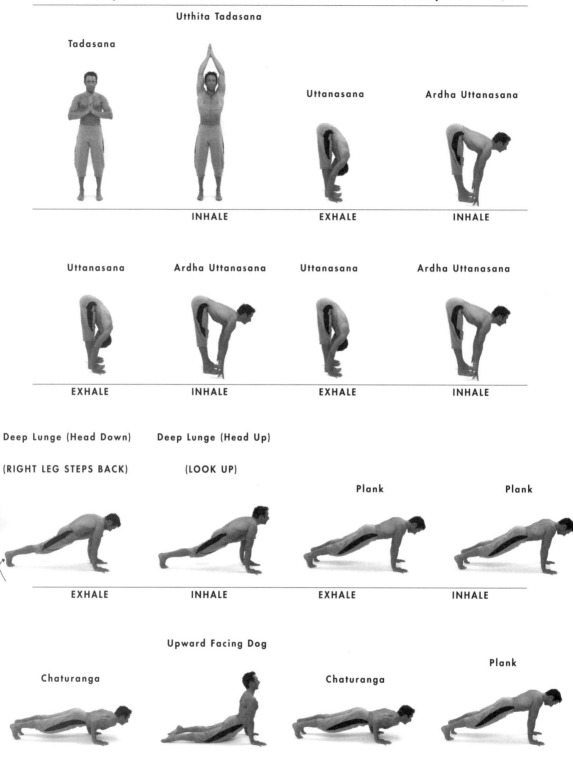

Tadasana	**Utthita Tadasana**		
		Uttanasana	**Ardha Uttanasana**
	INHALE	EXHALE	INHALE

Uttanasana	**Ardha Uttanasana**	**Uttanasana**	**Ardha Uttanasana**
EXHALE	INHALE	EXHALE	INHALE

| **Deep Lunge (Head Down)** | **Deep Lunge (Head Up)** | | |
(RIGHT LEG STEPS BACK)	**(LOOK UP)**	**Plank**	**Plank**
EXHALE	INHALE	EXHALE	INHALE

Chaturanga	**Upward Facing Dog**	**Chaturanga**	**Plank**
EXHALE	INHALE	EXHALE	INHALE

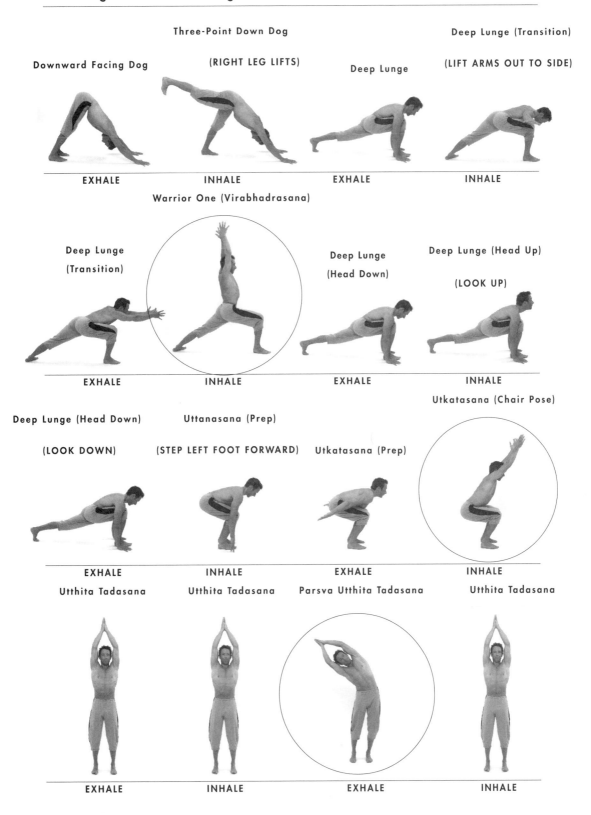

Downward Facing Dog

Three-Point Down Dog

(RIGHT LEG LIFTS)

Deep Lunge

Deep Lunge (Transition)

(LIFT ARMS OUT TO SIDE)

EXHALE   INHALE   EXHALE   INHALE

Deep Lunge (Transition)

Warrior One (Virabhadrasana)

Deep Lunge (Head Down)

Deep Lunge (Head Up)

(LOOK UP)

EXHALE   INHALE   EXHALE   INHALE

Deep Lunge (Head Down)

(LOOK DOWN)

Uttanasana (Prep)

(STEP LEFT FOOT FORWARD)

Utkatasana (Prep)

Utkatasana (Chair Pose)

EXHALE   INHALE   EXHALE   INHALE

Utthita Tadasana   Utthita Tadasana   Parsva Utthita Tadasana   Utthita Tadasana

EXHALE   INHALE   EXHALE   INHALE

Parsva Utthita Tadasana   Utthita Tadasana   Urdhva Tadasana
(Upward Facing Mountain Pose)   Utthita Tadasana

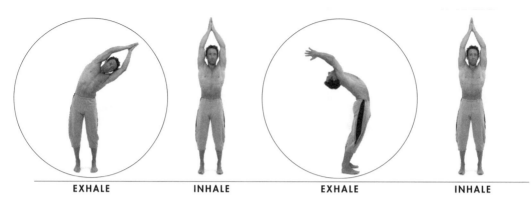

EXHALE   INHALE   EXHALE   INHALE

Tadasana

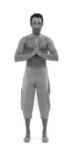

REPEAT THE SERIES USING LEFT LEG AS THE
DOMINANT LEG INSTEAD OF THE RIGHT LEG.

EXHALE . . .

High Performance Yoga Sun Salutations, Series C (Circled poses can be held for several breaths to develop stamina)

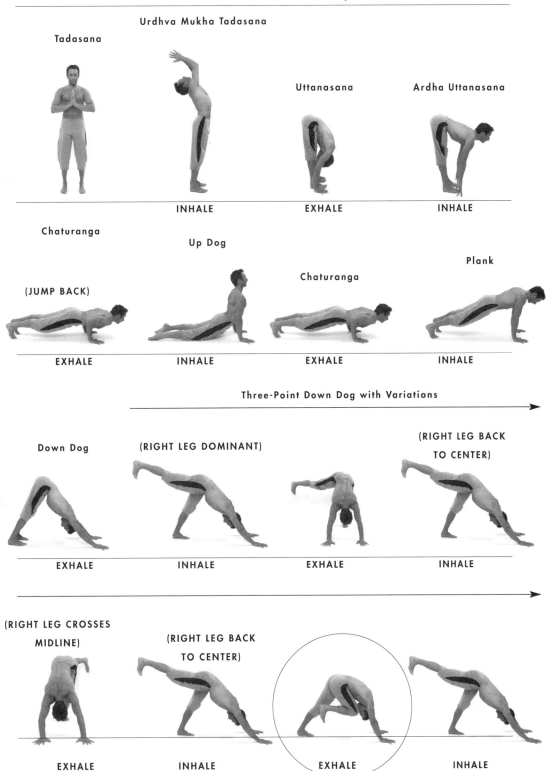

Tadasana

Urdhva Mukha Tadasana

Uttanasana

Ardha Uttanasana

INHALE — EXHALE — INHALE

Chaturanga

Up Dog

Chaturanga

Plank

(JUMP BACK)

EXHALE — INHALE — EXHALE — INHALE

Three-Point Down Dog with Variations

Down Dog

(RIGHT LEG DOMINANT)

(RIGHT LEG BACK TO CENTER)

EXHALE — INHALE — EXHALE — INHALE

(RIGHT LEG CROSSES MIDLINE)

(RIGHT LEG BACK TO CENTER)

EXHALE — INHALE — EXHALE — INHALE

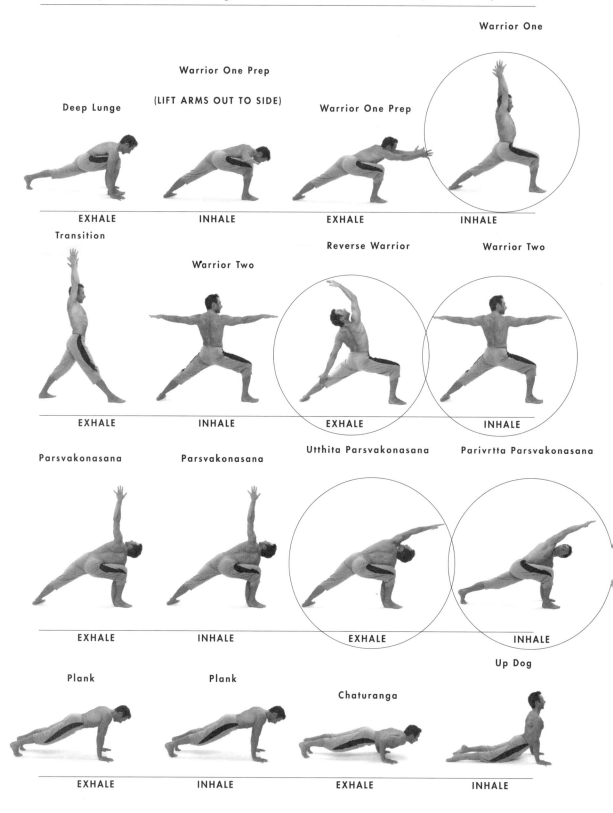

Warrior One

Warrior One Prep

(LIFT ARMS OUT TO SIDE)

Deep Lunge

Warrior One Prep

EXHALE · INHALE · EXHALE · INHALE

Transition

Reverse Warrior

Warrior Two

Warrior Two

EXHALE · INHALE · EXHALE · INHALE

Parsvakonasana

Parsvakonasana

Utthita Parsvakonasana

Parivrtta Parsvakonasana

EXHALE · INHALE · EXHALE · INHALE

Up Dog

Plank

Plank

Chaturanga

EXHALE · INHALE · EXHALE · INHALE

High Performance Yoga Sun Salutations, Series C

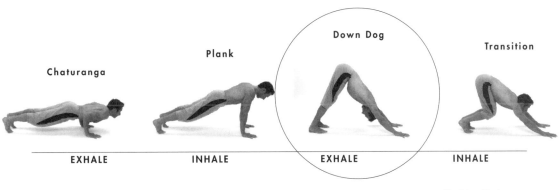

Chaturanga

EXHALE

Plank

INHALE

Down Dog

EXHALE

Transition

INHALE

Utthita Tadasana

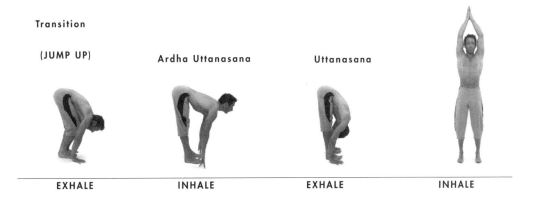

Transition

(JUMP UP)

EXHALE

Ardha Uttanasana

INHALE

Uttanasana

EXHALE

INHALE

Tadasana

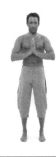

EXHALE . . .

REPEAT SERIES USING LEFT LEG AS THE
DOMINANT LEG INSTEAD OF THE RIGHT LEG.

Standing Vinyasa (Flow Sequence)

Start with right leg in active or lead position.

While you are still "fresh" I am going to challenge your extension and standing balance poses by this short sequence of poses. Hold each of the following poses for 30 to 60 seconds before moving on to the next one. After the fifth one, repeat the same five poses, but lead with your left leg.

A. Utthita Parsvakonasana (Extended Side Angle Pose)

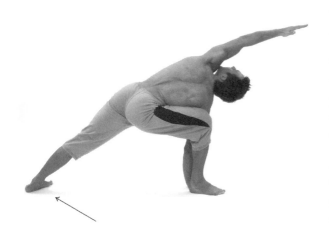

Rear foot drives the exploration of this pose.

This pose will seem familiar since you encountered it (more briefly) during Sun Salutation Series C.

Come into a deep lunge by bending your right knee until the right thigh is parallel to the ground. Extend your left leg behind you and keep it strongly extended. Your right foot points forward directly beneath the knee. Turn your left foot slightly to the right.

Place your right palm on the ground on the inside of the right foot, fingers pointing forward like the right toes. Stretch the left arm into the air as if reaching for a star. Rotate the left palm so the smallest finger is forward. Look up toward the sky under the left elbow.

Exhale and lower the left arm, reaching as far as possible to the front of you (see photo). The left side of your body should resemble a ski slope. Dance your edge here for the prescribed time and then move on to the next pose.

WHAT YOU ARE PRIMARILY WORKING: Opening of respiratory muscles, strengthening and cleansing of digestive organs, pelvic alignment.

WHOLISTIC NOTES: Stretch the entire lateral side of your body from the heel through the extended little fingers of the higher arm. Keep spinning the heart skyward. Scrape the lower buttock cheek under you.

OPTION A: Place the lower elbow on the lead knee until the palm can rest on the ground.

OPTION B: Place the lower palm on the outside, instead of the inside, of the lead foot.

B. Parsvottanasana (Side Extended Pose)

From utthita parsvakonasana (extended side angle pose, see photo, previous page), straighten your right leg and raise your torso perpendicular to the ground. Don't change foot position, but if desired you can slightly narrow your stance. Square the hips to the front as much as possible. Puff out your heart center and pull your head up.

Bring your hands into a reverse prayer gesture behind your heart. To do this, press your palms together between your shoulder blades with your smallest fingers pushing into your spine. If this is too much strain, options include interlocking the fingers, grabbing the elbows (see photo), or gripping the wrists.

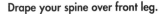
Drape your spine over front leg.

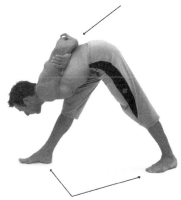

Strong roots!

Maintain a concavity to your spine and squared hips, and slowly draw your navel toward your right thigh and your chin toward your right shin. Dance your edge here for the prescribed time and then move on to the next pose.

WHAT YOU ARE PRIMARILY WORKING: Aligns pelvis, elongates spine, corrects upper body posture, enhances flexibility of hamstrings, mid back, shoulders.

WHOLISTIC NOTES: There are a hundred ways to cheat this pose. Don't. Stop descending your upper body if both knees cannot be kept strongly extended or if you begin rounding the spine. Work from the feet; root them deeply into the ground and hang in there.

C. Utthita Trikonasana (Extended Triangle Pose)

From parsvottanasana (side extended pose, see photo above), raise your torso perpendicular to the ground and untie your arms. Keeping both legs extended as if there were a small pyramid beneath them, rotate your torso to your left until your hips are now squared to the left wall. Reach both arms out to your sides so they are parallel to the ground.

Inhale your spine so that it is really elegant, then exhale and bend your torso to the right and bring your right hand onto the right ankle. Reach the left arm into the sky in line with the right arm. Maintain a concavity to your spine and keep the rear legs, rear chest, and hips in a line as if pressed up against a wall. Inhale and extend energy through each limb (see photo). Dance your edge here for the prescribed time and then move on to the next pose.

WHAT YOU ARE PRIMARILY WORKING: Because of the sequencing and the fatigue building in the legs and mind, this posture is an intensification of the effects from the prior pose; aligns pelvis from a different angle, elongates spine, corrects upper body posture, enhances flexibility of hamstrings, mid back, shoulders.

WHOLISTIC NOTES: Think of creating three triangles in order of importance: under your legs, under your lower armpit, and by the general outline of your two feet and upraised hand. Keep the spine parallel to the ground without rounding it.

OPTION A: Reach the uppermost arm forward so that it is parallel to the ground.

OPTIONS B AND C: Drop the lower palm from the shin onto the floor inside the front foot (B) or outside it (C).

D. *Ardha Chandrasana* (Half Moon Pose)

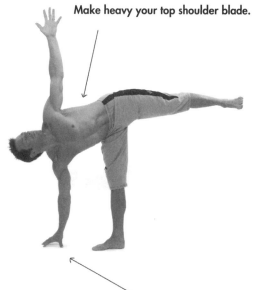

Make heavy your top shoulder blade.

Easy on the Earth!

Standing leg should remain strong and extended.

From utthita trikonasana (extended triangle pose, see photo, page 97), look down at your right foot as you bend your right knee and bring your left arm to your left hip. Come onto the ball of the left foot. Place the fingertips of your right hand about 12 inches in front of the right foot. Center yourself here for a few breaths.

Exhale completely and float the left leg away from the ground until it is parallel. Extend your right arm fully as you press the torso to parallel as well. Turn your heart center to the left and raise your left arm into the sky. Look upward until you can gaze at your left thumb. Balance (see photo) and dance your edge here for the prescribed time and then move on to the next pose.

WHAT YOU ARE PRIMARILY WORKING: Leg balance and stamina, hip opening and pelvic alignment, mental focus.

WHOLISTIC NOTES: Really pull the topmost hip joint directly over the lower hip joint. Pretend there is a softball under the palm of the lower hand. Use your inhales to "reach" your spine out of the hips.

Options include being able to gaze at the rear foot without falling and doing one-legged squats by bending and extending the lead knee.

E. Parivrtta Ardha Chandrasana (Revolved Half Moon Pose)

From ardha chandrasana (half moon pose, see photo, previous page), look down at your right foot as you bring your left finger-tips to the ground about 12 inches to the inside of the right foot. Doing this, the hips will become square to the ground. Center here for a few breaths.

Inhale and raise the right arm into the sky. Twist the lower spine to do this. Gaze at the right thumb. Balance (see photo) and dance your edge here for the prescribed time and then move on to the next pose.

WHAT YOU ARE PRIMARILY WORKING: The same effects as the prior pose (leg balance and stamina, hip opening and pelvic alignment, mental focus), plus the added benefits from a spinal twist, which cleanses and empowers the digestive and respiratory systems.

WHOLISTIC NOTES: Pretend there is a softball under the palm of the lower hand. Don't just crank the neck to look up. Allow the head to face upward as a manifestation from the lower spinal twist. Find new lines of energy on pre-fatigued thighs. Don't try harder, try softer.

Options include being able to gaze at the rear foot without falling and doing one-legged squats by bending and extending the lead knee.

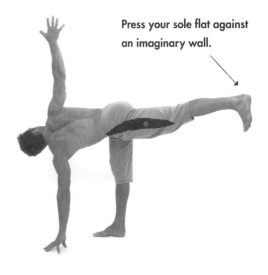

Press your sole flat against an imaginary wall.

F. Adho Mukha Svanasana (Downward Facing Dog)

From parivrtta ardha chandrasana (revolved half moon pose, see photo above), float the upraised hand and leg to the ground. Step the front foot back until your body resembles an inverted V. Feet should be hip-width apart. Hands are placed slightly wider than your shoulders. Let the spine lengthen by keeping the thighs firm, as if you are trying to lift the kneecaps up the thighs. Extend fully through arms. Turn the inner elbows toward your midline, not out to your sides (see photo).

Dance your edge here for 2 minutes and then move on to the next pose.

WHAT YOU ARE PRIMARILY WORKING: Frees restricted shoulders, lengthens the spine, stretches the Achilles tendon, hamstrings, and arm muscles. Functions physiologically like an inversion to calm the heart rate, bathes the brain stem with oxygen and nutrients.

Make your mid spine concave.

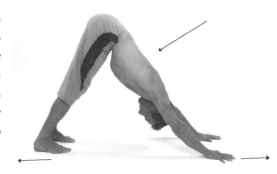

Lift your toes to lower your heels!

WHOLISTIC NOTES: You know this pose from doing it in the Sun Salutations. This pose is a bread-and-butter pose of all Power Yoga styles and is still considered a resting pose, though for the first several months it may not feel like one. Keep the heels pressed on or toward the ground as the toes point straight ahead. You should not be able to see your heels as you gaze between your feet. Spread your fingers wide. Relax your face. Your skull remains heavy and dangles like an ornament from your neck.

Repeat A through E for left leg.

Since I described the above sequence (A through E) using your right leg as the front or dominant leg, now bring your left foot between your hands and start the whole sequence again, substituting the left side for the right side in the descriptions above. When you have finished the five poses using your left leg as the dominant one, step back and assume downward facing dog.

Pacify your feet and lower back.

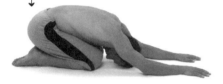

If you feel tired at this point, stay in downward facing dog (see photo, page 99) for 2 to 3 minutes. Then lower into Child's Pose (see photo here) for several recovery moments before moving on to the next poses.

Balasana (Child's Pose)

Bring yourself into a fetal position on top of your mat. Keep the ankles and knees together as much as feels comfortable. Nothing should require effort in this particular pose. Place the kneecaps and the tops of both feet on the ground. Lay your forehead on the ground and stretch your arms overhead. Let your buttocks rest on top of your heels (see photo). Breathe here for several recovery moments before moving on to the next poses.

WHAT YOU ARE PRIMARILY WORKING: During Child's Pose, your spine is flexed up to 110 degrees; the abdominal and thoracic cavities are being pressured by the thigh bones, internally massaging the organs therein; the mind is calmed due to ajna chakra or the "third eye" resting on the ground; and the heart receives a rush of nutrients, oxygen, and blood from which it greatly benefits.

WHOLISTIC NOTES: Consider this pose your main "time out" pose. Withdraw inwardly. Feel the front thighs massaging the internal organs in rhythm with your breath. Come to Child's Pose as often as you wish when your session hits those rough patches and you need a quick break. Erase any guilt about needing to take a moment to rest in Child's Pose. Just read the benefits of this posture above—you are not just schlepping about on the ground. For those with stiff ankles and feet, this is a wonderful pose to practice regularly.

The following ten poses are not done as a sequence, but individually. This means you will not have to do one leg and then the other. For each of the following poses, I've provided an option pose. Only do these poses if you felt particularly comfortable, elegant, and fluid with your breathing during standing vinyasa.

It is best to do each of the following poses at least twice if you have the time. Each pose should be held for between 30 to 60 seconds, focusing on beautiful-as-possible technical form and mindful ujjayi breathing.

Salabhasana (Locust Pose)

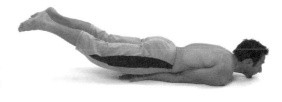

From Child's Pose (see photo, page 100), lie prone on your mat, chin resting on the mat. Stretch both arms back, with palms turned up.

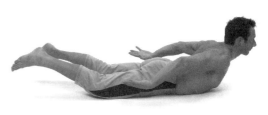

Inhale then exhale, and simultaneously raise your head, chest, arms, and legs as high as possible. Keep ankles, knees, and thighs together. Extend through the arms and legs and head. Squeeze the buttocks and keep working the posture so only the pelvis and lower abdominals are pressing into your mat (see photo). Dance your edge here for the prescribed time. Rest for a few moments by relaxing onto your mat and turning your head to one side. After doing one you may repeat the pose, do the option pose, or move on to the next main pose in the routine.

WHAT YOU ARE PRIMARILY WORKING: Back pain be gone! All areas of the spine benefit from this pose; cervical or upper spine, thoracic or middle spine, and lumbar or lower back spine. For many people, even big, strong guys, the Light of Yoga really flicks on with their initial encounter with this wonderful pose. Internal organs are greatly strengthened, especially the cleansing organs like the liver and bladder, as well as the reproductive organs.

WHOLISTIC NOTES: Press the pelvis down to elevate the chest and legs. Keep the face calm, eyes gazing at the horizon level. Stay pure and focused. Work to breathe smoothly and feel the core musculature respond with strength.

Slow-motion kicking effort here . . .

to lift here.

Option Pose: Dhanurasana (Bow Pose)

Come into salabhasana (locust pose, see photo, above). Exhale and bend the knees deeply to bring your heels toward your buttocks. Reach back with your right hand to catch the right ankle. Your knees should be about shoulder-width apart. Repeat for the left side.

Using a strong grip on the ankles, gently and gradually start "kicking" your ankles into your grip to elevate your heart rate. Keep processing your strength until only your belly rests on the floor. Gaze gently toward the sky (see photo). Breathe and dance your edge here for the prescribed time and then move on to the next pose.

WHAT YOU ARE PRIMARILY WORKING: Spinal elasticity, preparation for more advanced backbends, intensification of benefits associated with Pose #2 (locust pose).

WHOLISTIC NOTES: This is one of the main "medicines" I used to restore health to my badly injured spine and pelvis. Go slow! You should feel absolutely no compression or compaction at the lower back area.

Keep drawing the shoulder blades toward the spine and strive to create as much space as possible between your shoulders and ears.

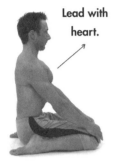

Lead with heart.

Virasana (Hero Pose)

Come into a kneeling position facing the front of your mat. Press your knees together and splay your feet apart so they rest beside the hips and you are sitting between your heels. Turn the soles of your feet to face directly behind you, and point your toes backward as well. Bring your spine beautiful and erect.

Rest your palms on top of your knees, puff out your heart center slightly, and gaze softly in front of you (see photo). Breathe and dance your edge here for the prescribed time. After doing one, you may repeat the pose, do the option pose, or move on to the next main pose in the routine.

WHAT YOU ARE PRIMARILY WORKING: Elasticity of feet, ankles, knees, and hip flexors.

WHOLISTIC NOTES: For those whose feet, ankles, knees, and hips have become weakened by furniture, cars, and all the conveniences of the modern American lifestyle, this can be a humbling pose. My personal edge still remains very close to the surface on this one. This pose is one that I call a "gateway pose"—steady effort in it will open the gateway to making other postures much more available to you. If sitting beside the feet is just too much for you, options include sitting on the heels, sitting on the inside edges of feet, or crisscrossing the feet under your buttocks.

Option Pose: Supta Virasana (Supine Hero Pose)

Soften your hands.   Knees toward midline.

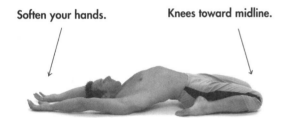

Come into virasana (hero pose, see photo above). Exhale and lower your elbows one at a time onto the floor in back of you. Allowing your breath to guide you, rest the top of your skull on your mat, then the back of the skull, then your shoulders, and finally the back of your heart.

Keep drawing the tip of your tailbone (sacrum) under you, that is, toward your groin. Eventually, stretch your arms overhead. Gaze gently toward the sky (see photo). Breathe and dance your edge here for the prescribed time and then move on to the next pose.

WHAT YOU ARE PRIMARILY WORKING: Intensification of all aspects described for virasana (hero pose, above).

WHOLISTIC NOTES: Sobering journey for many. Especially for tight athletes and others who did not do their stretching homework over the years. Very much worth the effort, as new power will start singing through the core muscles of the midsection and hips as they grow more supple. Develops a catlike kinesthetic grace.

Paschimottanasana (Western Extended Stretch)

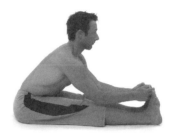

Come into a sitting position facing the front of your mat. Stretch both legs out in front of you to complete extension. Inhale and grow your spine tall and as you exhale, bend forward from the lower back to grip your two big toes with your two big fingers on both sides. This toe grip is known as the "yogic lock."

Inhale and make your back as concave as possible. Exhale and bend forward, drawing your navel toward the upper thighs, but not rounding the back. Keep repeating this process of inhaling, making your spine long and concave, and exhaling, deepening the posture by bending from the pelvis and lower back, not the upper back. Work steadily and strongly, attempting to erase the hump from the upper back.

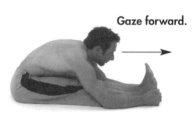

Gaze forward.

As you attain your edge, widen the elbows toward the sides of the room and finally allow the forehead to drift onto or near the knees (see photo). Breathe and dance your edge here for the prescribed time. After doing one, you may repeat the pose, do the option pose, or move on to the next main pose in the routine.

WHAT YOU ARE PRIMARILY WORKING: The entire western (or rear) spine. Another gateway pose with an incredible track record for healing everything from impotency to heart disease. One feels immediately refreshed after doing it.

WHOLISTIC NOTES: According to yogis, when you bend forward in this pose, the degree of roundedness present in your spine is a manifestation of karma, or past spiritual action meant to be overcome in this lifetime. Keep the legs highly active by flexing the toes toward your forehead and pressing the calves into the ground and lifting the kneecaps up the thighs. Options include gripping the small toes instead of the big ones and clasping the hands around the feet by interlacing the fingers.

Malasana (Garland Pose)

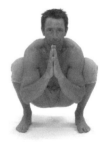

Come into a deep squatting position near the front of your mat. Over several breaths, bring the ankles close to each other but make sure both heels are flat on the ground beneath the knees. Toes can point slightly out or straight ahead depending on your hip and lower back flexibility. Drape your armpits over your kneecaps and breathe into your edge. This is the basic position known as the yogi squat.

Inhale and make your back as concave as possible. Exhale and bend forward as you reach both arms in front of you, palms turned up. Using the breath, allow the elbows to get heavier and drift closer to the earth. As your edge softens, finally reach both hands around the shins, and cup the heels in your hands. Draw your elbows toward the ground, and allow the forehead to drift onto or near the toes. Breathe and dance your edge here for the prescribed time. After doing one, you may repeat the pose, do the option pose, or move on to the next main pose in the routine.

WHAT YOU ARE PRIMARILY WORKING: Sacroiliac, lower back, hip, and ankle flexibility. Another key pose that begins to compress the abdominal viscera making the entire digestive system more productive.

WHOLISTIC NOTES: The yogi squat (*malasana*) is the best antivenom for the modern dis-eases that originate from our modern lifestyle, which refuses to use the natural squatting position to clean, wait, cook, and defecate. If you truly want better health, get rid of the furniture in your house, retrofit your modern toilet with a squatting platform (see Sources), and spend as much time as possible in the yogi squat. This pose has literally become my "wheelchair" since damaging my spine.

Option Pose: Parsva Malasana (Lateral Garland Pose)

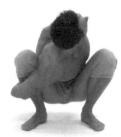

Come into malasana (garland pose, see photo, page 103). Separate the feet so that your heels are under your hip joints, but keep your palms cupping your heels. Exhale and release the right palm from under the right heel and lay it outside the right heel, palm still facing up. Then release and reach the left hand from the left heel, bringing it around the lower back toward the right heel. Lift the right hand to capture the left wrist. Bring the left hand into *jnana mudra* ("wisdom seal") by touching the index fingertip to the thumb to form a circle while extending the remaining three fingers. Softly gaze over your left shoulder (see photo). Breathe and dance your edge here for the prescribed time and then reverse for the other side before moving on to the next pose.

WHAT YOU ARE PRIMARILY WORKING: Intensification of benefits associated with malasana (garland pose), plus additional benefit from freeing up deep lumbar restriction by beginning to release tension from the short, tough pelvic girdle muscles like the quadratus lumborum and piriformis.

WHOLISTIC NOTES: Absolutely was a huge pose for helping my lower back. The position of this pose makes vulnerable the posterior longitudinal ligament, the long, tough band of connective tissue that runs along the rear spine. This is the ligament that gets totally tweaked by the concussion and compaction inherent to walking, standing, and of course, fitness activities like running, strength training, just about anything. Another, perhaps glaring, Light of the wisdom of doing Yoga will occur to many of you who try this pose on both sides and feel the difference between them. That imbalance that you feel must be ironed out and melted back into a balanced state through Yoga.

Bakasana (Crane Pose)

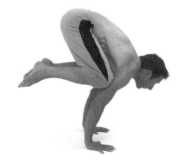

Come into a deep squatting position near the front of your mat and prepare as if you are going to do malasana (garland pose) again, but with a wider, shoulder-width stance. Keep both heels flat on the ground beneath the knees, toes pointed slightly out. Drape the armpits over the kneecaps and breathe.

Place the palms down in front of you, fingers spread wide as you lift your seat by raising the heels from the floor. Really pressure the kneecaps deeper into the armpits. Allow the elbows to bend, and if the kneecaps slide onto the triceps, try to limit that slippage. Exhale and lift first one foot off the earth and then the other. Balance on your arms and then extend your elbows to straighten your arms. Lift the head to gaze intently in front of you as you study the dynamic balancing act involved (see photo). Breathe and dance your edge here for the prescribed time. After doing one, you may repeat the pose, do the option pose, or move on to the next main pose in the routine.

WHAT YOU ARE PRIMARILY WORKING: Dynamic balance, core strength, and sacroiliac, lower back, hip, and ankle flexibility. Also improves concentration and *abhaya*, or fearlessness, due to conquering the fear of falling on your head.

WHOLISTIC NOTES: A good pose to illustrate *dharana*, or sustained concentration. Think of how your life would change if you concentrated in other aspects of your life as you are when practicing this pose. The deepening of dharana leads to meditation (*dhyana*).

Option Pose: Ekapada Bakasana (Single Leg Crane Pose)

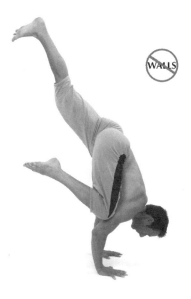

Come into bakasana (crane pose, see photo, opposite page). Exhale and extend your right leg in back of you as fully as possible. Lift your head and gaze intently before you a few feet (see photo). Play the quick edge here for the prescribed time and then lower back into bakasana (crane pose) and then repeat for the left leg. Lower into a yogi squat (page 103) before moving on to the next pose.

WHAT YOU ARE PRIMARILY WORKING: Intensification of benefits associated with bakasana (crane pose), plus muscular and mental endurance, as well as strength and balance. Improves wrist strength and shoulder girdle stabilization.

WHOLISTIC NOTES: Oooof. Wow. Good luck. Lots of core strength required for this graceful pose! Instead of just sticking the rear leg out there and hoping for the best, really radiate from your center, the navel area.

Halasana (Plow Pose)

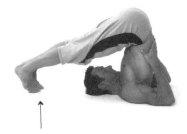

Lie supine, facing upward, on your mat, arms and legs extended. Don't get used to it, we've got work to do. Exhale and curl both knees to the chest and dome your hands so only the finger and thumb tips touch the mat. Exhale and raise first the hips and then the upper torso away from the floor until the trunk is perpendicular. The knees remain bent and both heels float near the buttocks. Quickly place both palms on the lower back to support this action by bending the elbows into your mat. Make micro adjustments to this stage until the hollow of your collarbone touches your chin. This throat lock is an important internal seal known as *jalandhara bandha*. Breathe here.

Massage the Earth with your toes.

Slightly release the throat lock by lowering the upper body just a little, then unfold both legs overhead and rest the tops of the toes on the ground behind your head. Keep both legs strongly extended. Breathe here.

Finally, remove your hands from your lower back and stretch them opposite from the legs, toward the front of your mat. Interlace your fingers and make a double fist. Over the next few breaths, "fidget" your rear shoulders under you to regain the throat lock. Gaze softly toward your navel (see photo, previous page). Breathe and dance your edge here for the prescribed time.

Release the fingers and slowly reach both arms overhead. Grip the two big toes using a Yoga lock. The Yoga lock is done by gripping your big toe with your index and middle fingers and your thumb. Moving very slowly and mindfully, begin rolling your upper spine onto your mat, then the mid spine, and finally the lower spine, all the while using the yoga lock to keep both legs close to the torso. After you have returned your entire back to the ground, curl and hug the knees against your chest. After doing one, you may repeat the pose, do the option pose, or move on to the next main pose in the routine.

WHAT YOU ARE PRIMARILY WORKING: Abdominal organ health, spinal flexibility, vascular health (particularly good for those with high blood pressure). Releases stiffness from shoulders, removes gas from the intestinal tract. The endocrine system is greatly assisted from the throat lock.

WHOLISTIC NOTES: This pose is underused by many modern teachers of Hatha Yoga. It is fantastic for the North American constitution, much better and safer than the more popular and striking shoulderstand or headstand poses, with as many if not more of the benefits. Move slowly into and from this pose as a lot is happening. Use the breath wisely to animate all actions within the pose. Breakthroughs in this pose will soon be felt in all forward folds, especially paschimottanasana (Western extended stretch, page 103).

Option Pose: Parsva Halasana *(Lateral Plow Pose)*

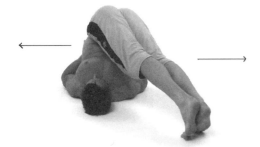

Come into halasana (plow pose, see photo, page 105). Move your palms to your lower back, near the sides of your body. Walk both legs to the right as far as possible. Gently turn your chest toward the left. Once established at your edge, tense your thighs and keep your ankles and knees together (see photo). Breathe here for the prescribed time before slowly walking both legs over to your left side and doing the same thing. Once the left side has been completed, move the legs back toward center, in line over your head, and breathe for 30 seconds or so.

Release the hands from the lower back and slowly reach both arms overhead. Grip the two big toes using a Yoga lock (see above). Moving very slowly and mindfully, begin rolling your upper spine onto your mat, then the mid spine, and finally the lower spine, all the while using the Yoga lock to keep both legs close to the torso. After you have returned your entire body to the ground, curl and hug the knees against your chest. Move on to the next main pose in the routine.

WHAT YOU ARE PRIMARILY WORKING: Intensification of benefits associated with halasana (plow pose), plus more spinal elasticity and colonic cleansing from the spinal twist. Many dis-eases stem from an accumulation of encrusted matter throughout the intestines and colon.

WHOLISTIC NOTES: This pose returns digestive and elimination prowess to your system. It's like doing internal housecleaning. Also, lateral flexibility to the spine is the first thing that goes when we grow older. This greatly underused pose retards old age by keeping the spine supple and the internal organs functioning with lots of digestive firepower.

Navasana/Ardha Navasana (Boat/Half Boat Pose)

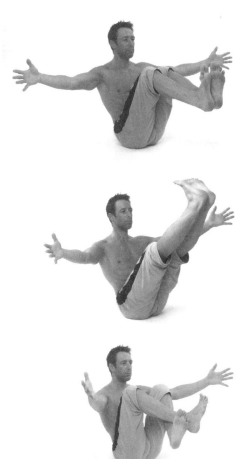

Come into a sitting position facing the front of your mat. Stretch both legs out in front of you to complete extension. Raise both arms, fingers outstretched and palms facing each other, parallel to the ground. Inhale and grow your spine tall, and as you exhale, lean the upper torso away from your feet while you raise both legs from the floor until both feet are at your eye level. Spread the toes and draw them and the inner arches of the feet toward you and press the balls of the feet into the air. Balance on your sacrum and experience the burn of the abominals. This is ardha navasana, or half boat pose (see photo). Breathe into your edge here for a few moments.

Inhale and draw both legs higher while simultaneously raising your heart center toward the knees, still balancing on the sacrum. Keep raising the legs until the feet are higher or at least even with the top of your head. Try to make your back as concave as possible and move your navel toward the upper thighs, but without rounding the back. This is paripurna navasana, or full boat pose (see photo). Breathe into your edge here for a few moments.

Grand finale: Inhale, crisscross your feet (see photo), bend your knees, bring the feet close to the upper torso. Exhale, uncross your feet, and extend them back into half boat pose (see photo). Inhale, crisscross your feet (opposite the way you just did), and bring the feet close to the upper torso. Exhale, uncross your feet and extend them back into full boat pose (see photo), and keep repeating until your form becomes too inelegant to bear.

WHAT YOU ARE PRIMARILY WORKING: Abdominal muscles (both upper and lower plates), upper and lower gastrointestinal tract, core strength, core balance, mental focus. Stimulates root chakra (muladhara).

WHOLISTIC NOTES: Killer, I know. It's great. Kinda makes the expensive abdominal and fitness machines seem ridiculous. They are. Just do your best until the strength comes on line, which happens remarkably quickly. Don't grit. Priority is being elegant through the difficulty and moving fluidly, if not poetically.

Savasana (Corpse Pose)

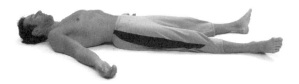

Lie supine, facing upward, on your mat. Stretch both legs out in front of you to complete extension. Feet should be placed hip- and shoulder-width apart. Heels in, feet fall out to the sides like an open book. Stretch both arms, fingers outstretched and palms facing upward to your sides. A grapefruit-sized space separates your upper arm from your ribs.

Inhale and raise your chin to your chest. Take one last loving look at your body that served you so well during this difficult practice session. Thank it. With a feeling of gratitude for your courage, perseverance, and willingness to accept and to go Higher, close your eyes and gently lay your skull down on your mat (see photo).

WHAT YOU ARE PRIMARILY WORKING: The letting-go muscle. The body/mind can only heal when it is calm. Savasana calms both body and mind so the spirit can dance. This pose calms the inner war and balances the whole.

WHOLISTIC NOTES: Technically the easiest asana of all. But spiritually the most difficult, for savasana asks us not only to give death to the body, but also to the mind. A fragile truth arises from the recalcitrant mental whispers of savasana; letting go of the fear of letting go is more difficult than the actual letting go. How elegantly will you be able to ultimately let go?

HP YOGA: THE GREEN TARA PRACTICE

Begin by engaging ujjayi breathing and don't stop ujjayi until the final pose.

> 3 x Ardha Surya Namaskar (Half Sun Salutation)
> 2 x Series A Modified
> 1 x Series B (both legs = 1 set)
> 1 x Series C (both legs = 1 set)
> 5 x Series A

Then do these movements, holding each for 30 to 60 seconds. Focus the mind with ujjayi breathing and the ego with honoring your edge.

1. Standing Vinyasa (flow sequence). Start with right leg in lead position.
   A. Utthita Parsvakonasana (Extended Side Angle Pose, page 96)
   B. Parsvottanasana (Side Extended Pose, page 97)

C. Utthita Trikonasana (Extended Triangle Pose, page 97)

D. Ardha Chandrasana (Half Moon Pose, page 98)

E. Parivrtta Ardha Chandrasana (Revolved Half Moon Pose, page 99)

F. Step back into Downward Facing Dog (Adho Mukha Svanasana, page 99)

Repeat A–F for left leg.

2. Salabhasana (Locust Pose, page 101)

Option Pose: Dhanurasana (Bow Pose, page 101)

3. Virasana (Hero Pose, page 102)

Option Pose: Supta Virasana (Supine Hero Pose, page 102)

4. Paschimottanasana (Western Extended Stretch, page 103)

5. Malasana (Garland Pose, page 103)

Option Pose: Parsva Malasana (Lateral Garland Pose, page 104)

6. Bakasana (Crane Pose, page 104)

Option Pose: Ekapada Bakasana (Single Leg Crane Pose, page 105)

7. Halasana (Plow Pose, page 105)

Option Pose: Parsva Halasana (Lateral Plow Pose, page 106)

8. Navasana/Ardha Navasana (Boat/Half Boat Pose, page 107)

9. Savasana (Corpse Pose, page 108)

Now, just let go.

Release any judgment as to how "good" or "bad" you may feel about this session.

It's over, so let it be over.

Find your muscles with your awareness, then, using a sighing exhale, let them go.

Just let them melt right off their bones and into the earth.

Find your organs with your awareness, then, using a sighing exhale, let them go.

Just let them vaporize right into empty air. Poof!

On your next exhale, let the body idea go.

No-body remains.

There is nowhere to go.

Find your mind, then let it go, too.

Poof!

No more mental activity.

No more physical activity.

Just . . . space.

Surrender fully into this spaciousness for several minutes.

Slowly bring consciousness back to the physical body. Feel the presence of your weight resting upon an ever nurturing Mother Earth. Wiggle your fingers and toes beneath the infinite Father Sky whose smiles bring you sunshine and whose laughter gives you rain. Slowly arrange yourself into an easy fetal position, hands sandwiched between your knees. Rock yourself ever so gently, like a baby in a cradle. Feel good about what you just did. Feel at one with the universe around you. You are yogi now, no longer separate from the difficulties or the joys that make up the moments of your life. Feel at one with it all.

Until your next HP Yoga session, may you walk with the rhythm of your breath, and dance with the many delights of your own unique, precious, and Sacred Journey . . .

In India, instead of saying good-bye they say *Namasté*. It means the sacred space inside of me recognizes and honors the sacred space inside of you. In this sacred space, we are one.

I bow to you, Noble Wholistic Fitness Warrior. *Namasté!*

CHAPTER 4

Meditation

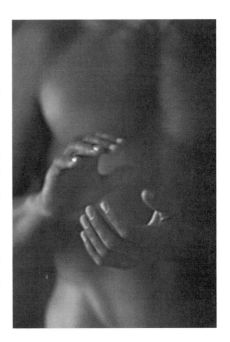

NOW COME THE TOOLS YOU will need to perform your Meditation assignments found in your Daily Practice, Chapter 6. Your short-term goal in this discipline is just to do it!

Even small volumes of prescribed Meditations will cause your ego to rationalize not doing it.

Meditation is one of those things that many people blow off, as if it were somehow less important to personal fitness training than Strength or Cardio workouts. But it's not. In fact, if you blow off Meditation, my program is not going to gel for you. Wholistic Fitness will escape you if you disregard Meditation. It's like chopping off one of your legs and wondering why you have trouble balancing. It's very hard to explain the impact of Meditation upon one's life, which accounts for a lot of people never doing it. But trust me, Meditation will bring you much more than just a new perspective to your workouts. It might just illumine your entire being.

The longer term goal through Meditation is to quiet and better control the mind. To achieve this the space between your thoughts must lengthen, or increase. Yogis call the constant arising of thoughts *vrtti*. Fundamental to the practice of yoga is stopping the unending whirls of thought. A busy mind creates a busy body, that is, your cells are kept in a continually agitated state. A calm, controllable mind creates a much happier, relaxed, and more comfortable body.

> *Life is not busy. It's your mind that is busy.*
> —COACH ILG

One way to illustrate how our accumulated thoughts affect the vibratory state of our cells is to imagine placing a shallow saucer of water on top of a quality stereo speaker. With no music from the speaker, the water is peaceful and calm. This is the state of your mind during Meditation.

Now crank some heavy metal rock and the water jumps as if boiling. This turbulence is due to molecular agitation and is similar to the state of your mind when you let yourself become stressed. Which do you think is a more healthy state for your body/mind to be in each day? Over a year? How about a decade? Meditation helps stabilize the body/mind with a serene but adaptable amenity. Stress and worry contracts your mind. Meditation expands it.

Now I'm going to show you some Meditation techniques based on several different traditions. I've backed these up with some of my own methods that I find especially effective in achieving body/mind serenity and management.

BEEPER GURU: BREATH AND POSTURE

I have created several nonformal Meditation techniques within my WF system using something that most people wear every day: a watch. The trick is, you need a watch with an alarm that goes *beep!* or something like a *beep!*

You may not even need a watch to do this. If you work at a computer, you can set the computer to beep at you. Some cell phones also have alarms that can be programmed. I had one student, an accountant, who used a cooking timer at her desk. Be creative.

Set the alarm to beep every hour. Really dedicated warriors can set it to go off every fifteen minutes. But don't do any more than once every fifteen minutes or the exercise loses potency.

Upon hearing the beep, notice where your

- breath
- posture
- thought

was in the moment that the alarm went *beep*.

Posture

As the exercise continues over the course of the day, begin to notice how often the Beeper Guru catches you out of posture. Adjust yourself using my postural awareness guidelines on page 29. Don't get angry with yourself, a fierce teacher is the Beeper Guru. Remember you are trying to restore consciousness to something (poor posture) that has been unconscious perhaps for decades. Be easy but firm with yourself. Elegant posture equates to a calmer nervous system and a more relaxed cellular state.

Breath

Notice if the Beeper Guru caught you with your breath high, shallow, or unconscious. Adjust your breath to a healthier state by taking a few ujjayi breaths as I taught you in Chapter 3, then ask yourself the following three questions:

1. *Was the thought positive or negative?* Or, put another way, was the thought fear-based or love-based? Were you happy when it went off? Depressed? Anxious? This shines a light on how much time we spend in pessimism or optimism. You might be surprised.

2. *Was the thought helpful or harmful?* Put another way, was the thought egocentric or compassionate? When most of our thought energy is concerned with protecting the "I" or clinging to thoughts of "me" or "mine," the cells of our body remain tense. This degenerates your cellular health. Holy people have halos because they have learned how to take themselves Lightly. Chronic egocentric thinking creates density to our energy and sparks the host of psychologic dis-orders and syndromes we see today. Shifting the majority of your thoughts to cheerful, helpful, and compassionate ones reduces tension and anxiety. Swami Rama teaches, "The mind is a reservoir for numerous powers. By utilizing the resources which are hidden within it, one can attain any height of success in the world. If the mind is trained, made one-pointed and inward, it also has the power to penetrate into the deeper levels of our being. It is the finest instrument that a human being can ever have." You do not need antidepressant pills to become happy. The same mental power that habitually flows toward negative thoughts such as, "I am not pretty enough," or "I can't do this; it's too hard," or "Screw it, I'll go back on my diet and exercise program tomorrow," can also be directed in a more positive groove. Knowing how to steady your mind must occur before you can expect any results from visualizations, prayers, affirmations, quests, or resolutions. Most people never experience a successful internal world because they have not done the work of disciplining and purifying their mind. A WF student learns how to concentrate their mind first of all. Knowing how to concentrate makes your mind far more manageable and user-friendly.

3. *Was the thought appropriate to the action being performed?* This relates to WF Lifestyle Principle 3: Appropriate Action. If the Beeper Guru keeps catching you not being present with what you are doing, then your body and mind are chronically out of sync. If you are folding clothes, think about folding clothes. How elegantly can you fold the clothes, or how fast, or with how much appreciation for the

clothes? Appropriate thinking and action is really fun. Being present with what is instead of focusing on what things "should be" is a major stress reliever.

ZAZEN

Zazen, which means "just sitting," is a staple discipline of Zen Buddhism and will be your only formal style of Meditation during your Green Tara program. Sitting zazen is essentially "just sitting" cross-legged and keeping your mind concentrated upon two things: (1) maintaining an upright and stable sitting posture, and (2) observing your breath.

To prepare for a prescribed zazen session, find or create a space where you can sit in solitude and not be interrupted for a few minutes. Anywhere will do. I had to do my zazen sessions at 4 A.M. in the bathroom while living with college roommates.

I've also sat zazen just beside my bed at various times during my life. When there is a genuine will to rise higher, you will find the time and space to meditate.

Optimally, a Meditation space is made more special by including a small puja table (tiny altar) with any or all of the following: a candle, a picture of a teacher who was or is important to your personal or spiritual growth, and incense. Music, if used, should be very, very subtle. Today there are many choices of Zen music, traditionally shakuhachi flute music.

Returning to this special place every session creates an appropriate vibratory level for deeper Meditation experiences.

As mentioned above, finding a time to sit can be a considerable challenge. Dawn and dusk are supposedly the most powerful times for Meditation. Indian yoga gurus say that *brahamuhurta*—between 4 and 6 A.M.—is best for Meditation because the outer world is still asleep and your mind is immersed with peacefulness and goodness. I think that is contingent upon one's constitution, but you should give several times a good try before settling on one. I find the early morning is better for the mind, because it is calmer, but the body is cold and often rebels at the zazen posture described below. In the evening, the mind is busier, but the body is more supple.

But the important thing is to sit when the chances are less likely that you will be interrupted. For family warriors, this can be daunting. I have faith in you, however. When there is a will . . .

I'll begin by teaching you the correct body position, then the mental posture, and finally offer some hints on handling a rebellious ego.

The Body During Zazen

1. Sit elegantly on the ground in a cross-legged position. Turning those ten words into your reality might be the work of ten years, so relax. Getting the zazen sitting posture is, for some of us, a task of Herculean proportions while for others, it's no big deal. Chalk it up to karma.

   Fold your legs into a cross-legged position and place your sit bones on the edge—not the middle—of a zafu, or sitting cushion. Sitting on the edge of the zafu will help decrease shearing torque at the ankles, knees, and hips, and it will help keep the spine in the optimal position until you can do your zazen sessions comfortably in Padmasana (full lotus posture, page 116) without a pillow.

   For those with knee and hip issues, consider a small bench upon which you half-sit, half-kneel, which the Japanese Zen people popularized. This bench relieves lateral pressure on the knees and hips. It is known as a seiza bench.

   However, if you are not under medical supervision for your knees or hips, try to deal with attaining the traditional cross-legged sitting position.

2. Hold your spine erect, but not stiff. Shoulders should be in line with the ears. There should be slight tension throughout the upper body; this helps focus a wandering mind. Consciously relaxing your legs if they begin to hurt will help. Elegance and steadfastness are your top priorities here. Do your best to sit magnificently.

3. Position your hands in front of the navel, left over right, palms upward, thumb tips barely touching. Align the middle crease of your left index finger on top of and with the middle crease of your right index finger. Do not rest your elbows on your thighs.

4. Draw your shoulders in line with your ears. The upper arm should hover a few inches opposite your upper ribs. The image and degree of tension should be as if an egg were sandwiched between the inside of your upper arm and the upper ribs. Don't let the egg drop, but don't smash it either.

5. Lengthen the back of your neck by drifting your chin toward the notch in your collarbone, but not on it. Keep your eyes half shut and softly gaze beyond a point about two or three feet in front of you. Allow a half-smile to emerge.

A common household pillow will do for a zafu, or sitting cushion. Sofa pillows are better than sleeping pillows because they are firmer. I still use an old, simple zafu that looks like something even the dog wouldn't bother with. I must admit, however, the new generation of V-shaped, buckwheat-filled, paisley-print zafus in the New Age catalogs and bookstores are quite fetching for the spiritual materialist!

COACH'S CLUE ON SITTING MAGNIFICENTLY

I like to pattern my zazen posture after one of the beautiful mountains I've climbed. I do my best to sit like a mountain that remains magnificent through winter storms and summer heat. Keeping my body like a mountain, I imagine my breath passing into and from my body like an autumn breeze brushing the golden leaves of aspen trees. Body like mountain, breath like wind.

The Mind During Zazen

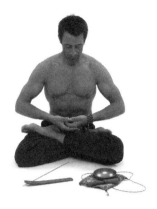

Coach Ilg in zazen posture.
Full lotus.

First, concentrate on the passage of air at the nostrils. Do not manipulate the breath in any way. This is more tricky than you may suspect. Just let the breath be.

Second, watch it like a hawk. Just observe.

Third, start focusing your mind by counting the inhales and the exhales. Number them in your mind, from 1 to 10 as they pass through the nostrils.

Count each breath like this:

inhale, count as **1**

exhale, count as **2**

inhale, count as **3**

exhale, count as **4**

> Think about your zazen posture in this way: If someone unfamiliar with zazen observed you during your session, how would they describe you? You would want them to think, "Wow, I would like to do what that person is doing. They look so peaceful and serene."

And so on. If you can reach 10 without one random thought intervening, you must be a reincarnated Buddha. Most of us poor schmucks can barely get to 3 before some stupid thought rudely interrupts the simplistic counting.

For those of you who are not Buddhas, welcome to the most frustrating fitness experience you'll ever have—zazen! Competing in a World Championship? Easy when compared to zazen. Very important to keep a lightheartedness about this stuff. When your counting does get interrupted by a random thought, resume counting at the number your mind was on when the thought-interruption occurred.

If you ever reach the number 10 without a random thought interrupting your counting, begin again at number 1 and repeat for the prescribed amount of zazen time.

If your mind is especially distracted during a given day, try counting your breaths backward from 100 to 0. Doing this improves concentration and is good for novice sitters.

The Ego During Zazen

The ego is that part of our consciousness that is identified with and is all very concerned with the self as apart from others. The ego protects the "I," as in "I am walking the dog." It is the nature of the ego to desire mental entertainment. In fact, I see many people walking their dogs outside my home. But very few of them are actually "walking their dogs"—do you see what I mean? Most of them are talking on cell phones, or have their foreheads wrinkled up with some thought. That's the ego at work. The ego gets bored walking the dog. It's somehow not enough to just merge into the dog world and be content with the trees and birds and the other million delights that make up reality. So, the ego starts its clamoring—it wants to talk on the cell phone, rush home to the football game and chips, or fantasize about that cute coworker. Always pulling you out of the present, that's the ego.

Since zazen effectively shuts off all mental activity save for counting of breaths, you can imagine how bored and crabby your ego will become. Talk about temper tantrums. This constant reaching out for some form of mental entertainment for the ego has long been recognized as an initial hurdle to be overcome by many spiritual traditions. But why is unbridled thought so "bad"? Why must we overcome it?

Have you ever tried to cross a busy freeway at rush hour? I hope not. You probably would not be reading this book if you had. You would have been hit and killed because of the high volume and speed of the traffic.

> This technique—not restarting the breath counting at number 1 after a random thought interruption—is not traditional. It is my experience, however, that it gets too damned depressing for most students to keep returning to the number 1 over and over again. After two years of daily zazen, I was still unable to pass 8 before a thought interrupted my breath counting. To make matters worse, the closer I got to 8, the more likely it became that my mind would get distracted by the likelihood of a new "personal record." It was crazy. Finally, my master allowed me to restart my breath counting at the number upon which I had gotten distracted instead of restarting on number 1. Shortly after my master's leniency, I experienced *satori* (a moment of spiritual awakening).

You have mental traffic too, in the form of thoughts. What you may have never been told, however, is that you alone are in charge of how congested and how fast you want your mental traffic to be. Your thoughts can create a busy, polluted freeway at the mercy of other busy-minded people or a peaceful country road where you are in control. By which would you choose to travel?

When you spend too much time in egocentric thinking—thoughts revolving about your personal preferences, comforts, desires, and dramas—you are creating more and faster mental traffic. In the same way you would find it hard to hear and see a friend across a freeway shouting at you above the din of the traffic, a busy mind limits what you hear and see in life. It is hard to see things from a higher perspective when you remain caught in the thick of traffic.

Zazen is like the traffic helicopter that shows you images of your mind, as if it were a busy freeway or a country road. It can be a bit depressing at first to see how busy the traffic is, but with practice, the traffic can be reduced or even suspended. Silence! Peacefulness! Ah! Om! Zazen can transform the freeway into a wilderness preserve in the flicker of an instant. How valuable would that be to you?

During zazen you will notice sensations coming and going. Some are nice. Many are annoying or unpleasant, especially the longer you try to sit still, doing nothing. You will probably want the nice and pleasant sensations to hang around and the uncomfortable, annoying ones to leave you alone. See the attachment to nonreality? The reality is that pleasurable moments will come and go and painful moments will come and go. But your ego wants something different from that reality; it wants to keep the pleasurable and get rid of the painful. So, you start clinging to your desire for pleasure instead of experiencing reality. Right there is the root of all human suffering; wanting things to be other than the way they truly are.

Let me approach this in another, less urban, way. Zazen can pull out mental dis-ease by its root. It works something like this: You sit down and fold your legs into a cross-legged position and adjust your upper body into your best zazen posture. You start witnessing and then counting the breaths. Soon, a thought comes along like, "This is stupid." See? Right there! That was your ego. Or, "Sitting like this hurts my knee and lower back." Or, "Gee, check this shit out, I'm actually meditating! This is cool, I feel peaceful." Or a classic one, "I wonder how much longer I have to go." Those are all ego dramas, thoughts concerned with the "I" or "mine" or "my." During zazen, such thoughts should be scooped aside so you can resume counting the breaths.

You see, it is only possible to get *up*set if you are *set* on something in the first place, right? Zazen helps unsettle you so it will become impossible for you to ever become upset. How valuable would that quality be to you?

The Process of Optimal Zazen Posture

You can tell a lot about a person just by watching them trying to sit still in a room for a while. Sitting still in the classic zazen posture may at first be like riding a bucking bronco. Restrictions in hip and leg flexibility make the zazen posture absolutely terrifying for some. Stick with it anyway. Staying faithful to your yoga routine will really help you gain comfort for your zazen sessions.

Gaining a beautiful and comfy zazen posture will be like doing downward facing dog (adho mukha svanasana) in Yoga. When you did your first down dog and the teacher told you that was actually a "resting pose," you probably wanted to slap some sense into the teacher. A resting pose! Your arms were shaking with fatigue, your Achilles tendon was aquiver with tension—this was no "resting pose"! But what happened? With practice, you found that down dog can be relaxed into. Zazen is just the same.

Leg position in zazen is of utmost consequence. The purpose of the proper leg position is to ground three main chakra or energy centers as close to the earth as possible: the root of the spine and the outside (lateral aspect) of your knees. This facilitates not only the subtle energy system but equates to the integrity of the spine, which has seven other energy centers or chakras.

Commit to a high personal standard of postural elegance during zazen. Doing so helps develop inner character.

Here are the leg positions listed in progressive fashion.

Novice: Burmese Style

Sit on the edge of the zafu (cushion). Bring the left heel close to perineum. Place the right foot in front of the left foot, heels in line, no bones crossing. Heels turned up slightly. Sit upright.

Intermediate: Siddhasana

Sit on the edge of the zafu, place the left heel near the perineum and rest the sole of the left foot against the right inner thigh. Place the right foot over the left ankle, keeping the right heel near the pubic bone. Place the sole of the right foot between the inner thigh and calf of the left leg.

Advanced Intermediate: Ardha Padmasana (Half Lotus)

Consultation with a yoga teacher is suggested at this stage. Sit on the edge of the zafu, and draw the left heel close to the perineum. Bend the right knee and place the right foot on the top of the left thigh so that the right heel presses into the lower left intestines. *Do not* "sickle" the right ankle to make it fit onto the left thigh. The right ankle bone, not the right foot, should be resting upon the left thigh. The right foot should be nearly off the side of the left thigh.

Advanced: Padmasana (Full Lotus)

Consultation with a yoga teacher is suggested at this stage. From Half Lotus, lift the left foot with the hands and place it on the top of the right thigh. Both heels should press into the intestines. Turn the soles of both feet upward (see photo, page 116).

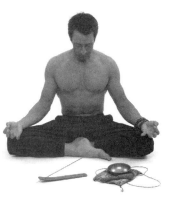

Burmese

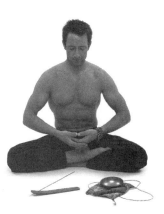

Siddhasana

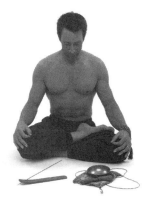

Half Lotus

Early Morning Zazen

When this is prescribed for you, plan ahead. Know what time in the morning will be quiet enough for you to have 10 to 20 minutes to yourself. Do not compromise. Do the following:

- wake up;
- mindfully go to the bathroom, use mouthwash if desired, but do not brush your teeth (it takes too much time and the ego starts chirping);

- sit zazen using the posture and breath counting techniques as described above;

- halfway through your allotted sitting time, mindfully switch leg position;

- sit zazen;

- close your formal session of zazen. Begin your day by brushing your teeth with zazen mind, which means begin your regular "worldly duties" consciously instead of mindlessly!

OTHER MEDITATIONS DURING GREEN TARA

The following nonformal Meditation assignments appear in your Green Tara program. Let's take a look at them.

Periodic Renunciations

This assignment, a longtime WF standard, is a practice of nonattachment and also supports the yogic tenet of *aparigraha*, or nonhoarding. It will help declutter your home and mind. Simplification is high on the WF checklist of Things to Master.

1. Get a heavy-duty plastic bag, like a trash liner. With a firm mind, go to your closet and open it. Look at your wealth of clothes.

2. Close your eyes. Imagine the poor, the hungry, the ill, and the unclothed. Breathe gratitude for your blessings of abundance. Open your eyes.

3. Using your zazen-developed concentration and a compassionate heart, place into the bag any item that you have not used or appreciated in the past eight months.

4. Do the same thing in as many rooms of the house as possible. Note: Just do one room per session. WF is not trying to change your entire life all at once. Take your time!

5. Take the items to Goodwill or a similar charity. Do not sell the items!

Barefoot Yoga Rule

This rule triggers many insights that will dovetail into other WF work later on. This rule provides a natural way of transforming brittle and overly sensitive soles, arches, and ankles into supple, strong, and fit feet. It also neurally stimulates acupressure points on the feet, which benefits the major organ systems in the body. It is a very helpful, grounding practice for uptight and stressed people who may have strayed too far from their natural way of ease and being.

1. Hold a "family" meeting.

2. Introduce a new house rule: Only bare feet in the house. No shoes allowed!

CHAPTER 5

Nutrition

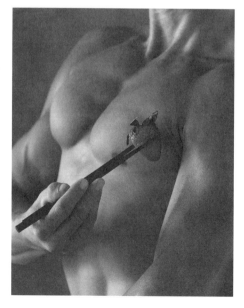

IN THIS CHAPTER, YOU'LL LEARN how encompassing Nutrition can really be and you will be offered specific and practical guidelines for experiencing healthy, joyful Nutrition.

According to WF philosophy, you experience Nutrition through your environment, occupation, relationships, posture, breath, hobbies, thoughts, fitness training, sleep, and awareness. How you read this very sentence—your breath and posture right now—is a more potent form of long-term Nutrition than what you ate for lunch yesterday. There is no off switch to your real diet because there is no off switch to your life. The constantly shifting things happening to you, within you, and on you, are what truly feed—or starve—you.

I consider Nutrition to be like the sun of WF. It radiates outward, giving life, energy, and illumination to my other four

Fitness Disciplines. Perhaps you could use some of this luminosity, especially if you are confused about what you should be eating and when and how much. If you are, that does not surprise me. In fact, I get more questions about Nutrition than I do about any other component of fitness. At the beginning of this millennium, nearly half of all Americans complained about being overweight and confused about what and how much to eat. I might add that the confusion didn't stop us from spending nearly $300 billion eating out and an average of $2 billion on "fat burning" supplements.

In some ways, I think the "experts" are to blame for the bewilderment. The amount of hype and input from nutritional experts, dietitians, and health supplement marketers has effectively drained the fun, the beauty, and certainly the sacredness out of eating. No wonder why everybody is so confused—one week low-carbohydrate diets are "good" for you, the next they are the work of the devil. Any given nutrient, food, fad, or eating philosophy can be "clinically found to cause" anything from increased sex drive to coronary heart disease depending upon who profits from the "clinical studies." Authors and corporations also exploit the snarl about Nutrition for monetary gain.

It's a shame, all this confusion and aberrant eating behavior, because if anything can sabotage a personal fitness program, it is poor Nutrition. I don't have my own line of herbs or nutritional supplements to sell you. I have no investment in anything but a desire to have you experience what I and my students enjoy: a path of clarity when it comes to Nutrition.

So what is my clear answer to "good nutrition?"

I've kept ten long-standing WF Nutritional Guidelines through the years. They are easy to live by and have withstood the weathering of dozens of FDA changes to personal nutritional standards. Like all my other WF disciplines, these ten basic guidelines have helped thousands of my students across the world for twenty years. They are simple tokens of "hip pocket" nutritional wisdom intended to guide you effectively in your food choices:

1. Take a sacred pause before eating.

2. Eat mainly raw, whole foods.

3. Eat several servings of fruit and vegetables per day.

4. Limit fat intake; eat moderate amounts of protein and carbohydrates.

5. Consider nutrition in both physical and spiritual ways.

6. Half of effective nutrition is about cleansing and elimination.

7. Reduce dairy and meat to nominal levels.

8. Eat high-fiber foods.

9. Generally, your stomach contents should be one-third food, one-third fluid, one-third air.

10. Your diet keyword is: Moderation.

1. TAKE A SACRED PAUSE

Begin each meal with a moment of grateful silence or, if you prefer, a moment of prayer. I don't care if you are eating alone at home or with your friends at a restaurant, do it. During this sacred pause, feel gratitude for all the people who helped create, package, and deliver that food to your mouth.

> Your physiological facts are cause for contemplation: In less than one year, you will replace 98 percent of your atoms. You will regenerate an entirely new skin this month, as well as assemble a new skeleton. This week you will regenerate a fresh stomach lining, and your liver will renew itself every six weeks. Your body is a master of regeneration, yet how often do you dwell on how quickly you age? How often do most of us appreciate this regenerative miracle of our bodies?

In this day and age especially, Nutrition should be a simple and joyful affair. You no longer have to hunt game, gather herbs and roots, fast during famine, or walk several miles every day for drinking water. Access to refrigeration; year-round produce; premium-quality grains, fish, meat; and drinkable water is better now than ever before in human history.

Don't turn eating into an obsession. Keep it as it was intended, as a source of regular joy. I've made it a point in my own life not to stray so far from hands-on herb picking, crop harvesting, and fishing that my respect and appreciation for my food becomes lost. Don't allow your natural, nourishing wisdom to vanish. So many people come to me seeking to regain common dietary sense from a quagmire of useless diet plans and products, digestive aids, and even psychological counseling for eating disorders.

Although fitness experts propose all sorts of nutrients, diets, and "revolutionary" nutritional products, seldom are these things successfully used for longer than a few months, let alone a lifetime. Here is what those experts miss: Most diets only separate us from the divine joy of Nutrition. Learning to take a sacred pause before putting anything into your mouth helps restore appreciation and connection with the beauty and joy of eating.

Whole foods and herbs are living organisms the natural molecular makeup of which has not been modified. Eating natural whole foods and herbs means that you are eating things that still tingle and vibrate with life force (pran). Life begets life. Due to this simple fact and the nature of our digestion and elimination systems, WF embraces a vegetarian-based approach to daily food intake. That doesn't mean you "can't" eat meat or fish or poultry occasionally—the operative word being "occasionally."

Just as life begets life, so too does death beget death. Let's be honest; eating a lot of flesh foods, like hamburgers, hot dogs, meat, chicken, means that you are eating a lot of decaying and putrefying substances. I know it's hard for our generation to equate a rotting carcass with a burger, but that is the truth of the situation. Such foods leave many more toxic metabolites in us that stress our physiology than does, say, fruit.

Now, the yogis would go one step further. They would say that the energetics of chronically eating corpses that have suffered inhumane slaughter imprints and degrades a yogi's psychologic and spiritual health. You don't need to agree or disagree with this. But I do know that once Meditation skills have increased in my students, their changes in dietary choices usually involve eating less food overall and making fewer meat-based choices. I think this happens because a more conscious fitness athlete can more accurately feel the energetic influence of various foods in their body.

> Some people wonder if I am a vegetarian. No. Although I haven't personally eaten meat for about fifteen years, Kathy and I eat fish maybe once or twice a week on average. Neither of us is attracted to poultry, save for the occasional use of egg whites. But that is Kathy and me. You are you. Most students find that by following my ten guidelines, attractions to denser forms of foods, like flesh foods, usually begin to naturally fall away while an attraction toward raw and whole foods, like fruits, vegetables, and herbs, increases.

Sometimes these dietary changes are small, like the enjoyment of cleansing teas at night instead of something less nutritious. But sometimes dramatic dietary shifts occur in other students. This happened to my wife, Kathy, when we first lived together. Although she had no big issue with eating meat, when she moved in with me she felt just fine eating tofu and soy-based foods instead of meat. I did not push her at all. It "just felt right to my body," she said of the switch. Certainly, our physiology and psychology is equipped to enjoy occasional eating of flesh foods. Again, the key word is "occasional."

The natural integrity of junk, or processed, foods, on the other hand, has been genetically modified or otherwise molecularly engineered. These substances, as well as any foods that have preservatives (which do just that—they are embalming agents), contain isolated nutrients that do not serve the natural cellular regeneration and support. WF is not big on this "engineered food." We prefer *real* food.

3. EAT SEVERAL SERVINGS OF FRUIT AND VEGETABLES PER DAY

Eat lots of produce for a healthy digestion and elimination, not to mention a host of vitamins, minerals, amino acids, and enzymes not found in other food groups. Think fiber—roughage, as your mom may have called it. Gotta have it, and it's becoming more and more of a rarity in today's overly processed food supply.

One of the best things about living in Southern California are the year-round farmers' markets, found in any number of towns on any given weekend. When I lived high in the Rocky Mountains, such deliciously sweet and lusciously seductive fruits and vegetables just weren't available. So I now know what a blessing it is to have such great access to organically grown fruits and vegetables. The second-best option is to shop at a natural foods grocery store. The more we fitness warriors support their efforts, the less "steroid produce" we have to eat from the larger commercial chains.

Here is why it's important to eat the natural stuff. When you isolate a nutrient, like taking the vitamin C out of an orange and processing it into a vitamin pill, that nutrient has become inert. It has no synergy, no life force to it. When you eat an isolated nutrient, your body expends its own energy to make it into some type of recognizable whole again. Your body tries to transform junk food into wholesome food. This junk food eating forces a complex, taxing, and bizarrely unnatural physiologic procedure that drains your energy and produces a toxicity within your cells. The effect of eating too much of these isolated nutrients is an inefficient assimilation process that interferes with nutrient transfer and metabolism. Your body starts sending signals that it needs more nutrients, so you eat more. But you don't need more food, you need better assimilation of incoming nutrients. You've unwittingly created your own unique metabolic disorder caused by not eating whole foods in the first place.

4. LIMIT FAT INTAKE; EAT MODERATE AMOUNTS OF PROTEIN AND CARBOHYDRATES

I know you are sick of food statistics, such as how many calories of this you are supposed to have in relation to that. So forget all that. Instead, just do this: Look at your meal before you eat it. Keep each meal one part fat, two parts protein, and three parts carbohydrate.

Here is how this might translate into each meal:

Breakfast: Two scrambled egg whites on an English muffin with fruit jam and a banana. (Note: Yolks are only eaten in a 1:2 ratio with egg whites in WF. This is because yolks contain LDL cholesterol and the yolks are denser vibrationally, not good for yogis.)

Lunch: Rice and tuna with a small side salad.

Dinner: Sautéed veggies over a bed of Basmati rice with soy-braised tofu cubes.

Not confusing at all, is it? In other words, don't sweat the ratios, use your intuition and enjoy your meal. That is most important of all.

5. CONSIDER NUTRITION IN BOTH PHYSICAL AND SPIRITUAL WAYS

From now on, consider Nutrition as coming to you in three ways: what you physically put into and on yourself (physical nutrition), and what you put around you (spiritual nutrition).

Physical nutrition is what most dietitians and nutritionists consider as the only form of nutrition: foods and beverages and drugs that can be counted in terms of calories, grams, ounces, milligrams, etc. This form of nutrition is very beautiful and needed, but is also the most "dense" and least important in the long term.

But physical nutrition is also what you put on yourself, such as lotions, sunscreens, the type of lighting you work under, antiperspirants, perfumes, shampoos, conditioners, hair treatments, clothes, all of the things that should be supporting the regenerative quality of your body/mind. A WF lifestyle includes an awareness and optimal choices for all these things.

Spiritual nutrition is what you put around you and relates to your mental health and spiritual nourishment. Take your occupation for instance. Are you doing what you cherish doing? Or do you hate your boss and count down to the weekend? It requires no great feat of psychology to realize the foolishness of eating a beautiful and healthy breakfast and then climbing into your car for an hour or two of road rage before having to endure another day of internal hell by working at a job you hate. You think your job is *not* a form of Nutrition?

How about your relationship with your spouse, girlfriend, boss? Is it nourishing or stressing you?

Do your entertainment choices harm or help your hormones and mental peace?

Was your last conversation true, helpful, and kind, or was it gossip-based?

Is your home environment conducive to a vibrant calm? Is your home clutter-free or messy?

A big part of WF nutritional work requires looking at the feng shui of your life. In other words, instead of asking yourself, "What did I have for dinner?" you can ask yourself, "What surrounded me for dinner?" Did it include uplifting conversation or watching TV? Crazy wis-

MOVEMENT IS NUTRITION!

Our addiction to comfort and laziness is beginning earlier than ever before. According to the National Longitudinal Survey of Youth, our children are getting fatter at an alarming rate. Throughout the 1990s, the percentage of significantly overweight Hispanic and black children ages four to twelve doubled. Caucasian children fared only slightly better, showing a 12 percent increase over the same period. Combine those stats with these facts: Our leading toy manufacturers steadily increase their production of motorized toy cars for toddlers and decrease the production of toddler tricycles that are pedal-powered.

Is it really wise to encourage our already over-fat and under-strong kids to become psychologically dependent upon motorized instead of self-propelled movement so early? We are getting fatter and more unhealthy with each passing year. Clearly, just moving our body is a valid and important form of Nutrition and accounts for a huge difference between physiologic and chronologic age. Lawrence Golding, a professor at the University of Nevada who has spent decades studying the links between aging and exercise, says, "The absence of physical activity, and not age, accounts for most of the deterioration in physical fitness and body composition."

dom, I know. But how you place things around you matters greatly to your health. For that reason, in WF, anything that surrounds you must be considered a form of Nutrition.

6. HALF OF EFFECTIVE NUTRITION IS ABOUT CLEANSING AND ELIMINATION

Foods that gently strengthen and cleanse the colonic system as well as the cellular body need to be eaten regularly. These foods (and drinks) enhance tissue exchange or the transfer of nutrients across the cell membranes, which improves metabolism. Most people do not think about this of course, unless I say the word "prunes" or "bran"! But I'll touch on this digestive aspect more below.

On a more subtle cellular level, a whole host of foods can help keep the "skin" of your cells as healthy as the skin of your body—soft, elastic, and effective at "breathing." Foods such as bok choy and kale, nutrients such as lecithin and garlic, and teas such as ginger and chamomile are particularly good. I am particularly fond of Calli Beverage as my main cell cleanser (see Sources, under Sunrider). Calli is an ancient Chinese herbal beverage that is prepared and drunk like hot tea.

7. REDUCE DAIRY AND MEAT TO NOMINAL LEVELS

I've already asked you to shift away from meat, but what the hell is wrong with dairy for crying out loud? Am I telling you, no milk? No cheese?

Of course you can have some milk and cheese now and then, as well as some eggs occasionally. Moderation, remember? Certainly, cultural conditioning can play a role in your metabolism of dairy products, but for most fitness-conscious Americans it's best to keep the dairy in the cow, or you might start looking like one. The large number of lactose intolerant people in this country confirms this. Believe me, this whole not-eating-cheese thing hurts me as much as you—I'm German and cheese is to Germans what cell phones are to Los Angelenos!

Eating a lot of dairy, besides being inhumane and high-impact on Mother Earth (please visit a commercial dairy farm at least once in your life), contributes too much dampness, cold, mucus, and phlegm to the body. There is also a lot of fat in dairy products. Nothing gives me a "thick skin" and an extra pinch of fat around my waist faster than eating dairy. Still, that doesn't always stop me from having a slice of havarti cheese on a cracker with a glass of red wine—thank goodness! Balance in life works best.

DAIRY IS FROM COWS, EGGS ARE FROM CHICKENS

Some people wonder where eating eggs falls into the WF nutritional approach. Eating eggs is okay, but practice the "M" word: moderation. I usually eat only egg whites or egg substitutes like Egg Beaters, but no more than a couple of times per week. If you do eat eggs and are not into the egg substitutes, try eating one whole egg to every two egg whites.

8. EAT HIGH-FIBER FOODS

Low-fiber and meat-based diets can contribute to stool that is as much as 75 percent bacteria. Honestly, people are less "full of shit" than they are full of bacteria. It ain't healthy. This much bacteria in the body encrusts digestive and elimination organs, rendering them hard and ineffective. The stagnate bacteria also create a veritable internal swamp that fosters common problems like constipation, varicose veins, wrinkled skin, low back pain, belching, heartburn, indigestion, appendicitis, and obesity through malnutrition. Using laxatives only compounds the problem by weakening elimination organs through substituting strength, not developing it.

9. GENERALLY, YOUR STOMACH CONTENTS SHOULD BE ONE-THIRD FULL OF FOOD, ONE-THIRD FLUID, AND ONE-THIRD AIR

It's easy to eat from ego, instead of true physiologic hunger. Sensei Kishiyama told me to observe wild animals to know the flow of wise Nutrition. So I did. Wild animals are not overweight, do not read diet books, do not consult with nutritionists, eat only when hungry, and appear to be immersed in various states of rapture when they do eat.

We should be so wise as the wild animals. Overeating issues kill more people in our country than any other disease. Not surprisingly, it is an untrained mind and undisciplined ego that again lies at the root of this, our self-written tragedy. Staying just a little bit hungry throughout the day is wise. It's great and even vital to feel "light" instead of "thick," "agile and alert" instead of "heavy and lethargic." Eating to your heart's content is not contentment for long. Eating as an application of Appropriate Action to your efforts in self-cultivation, on the other hand, will keep your energy humming beautifully throughout the day. What feeds you most valuably begins not with your tongue, but with your mental discipline.

10. YOUR DIET KEYWORD IS MODERATION!

Long ago, the Buddha put forward a Path of Moderation. There is no better path to take in regard to Nutrition than that one. Worrying about food and what it may or may not do to your body only leaches minerals from your cells and retains fluid. The thing is, no clear answer can come from me, or any other advice or external counsel. The only clear answer comes from knowing that Nutrition is a highly individual process. It, like everything in your life, is a dance. Your nutritional needs, temperament, and assimilation capacities will change over the course of your life. That is a good thing. This variety makes the dance fun.

When to Eat

Eat when it feels appropriate. Five words. But it will probably take a while for you to master them.

It is high spiritual progress to eat, not according to convention or condition, but appropriately to your physiologic hunger. I think the best I can do here is share with you my own experience from which you can draw your own interpretation in support of your unique dietary and lifestyle needs.

Eat to Live, Don't Live to Eat

Personally, and this should be no measure of your own intuitive wisdom, I dig Mexican food and the Mexican "siesta" lifestyle. My attraction toward this lifestyle arose from my years as a sponsored athlete. My ideal day is like this: Wake up early and do pranayama or meditation before eating a very light breakfast of rice or oatmeal. While digesting, I work in my home office. After Nature has called, I'm empty and primed to crank off a good Cardio workout like a mountain bike ride. After a shower, I enjoy my largest meal of the day, say, Huevos Rancheros or a potato and egg burrito (egg substitute, of course!). Then a nap. After more office work and another bowel movement, I still have time for cross training if needed, maybe yoga or a gym workout. A late—but light—dinner of veggies and tofu with a salad and herbal "night" tea finishes me off. Many days are not conducive to this ideal, but note how my diet and daily activities are centered around my training and physiologic needs. Hey, if you can't live your days like this, I tell you what, next election you guys vote "Ilg for President" and I will make two things imperative: (1) WF will become the National Fitness System, and (2) a "siesta lifestyle" and a four-day work week will become mandatory.

But seriously, be wary of eating a large midday meal, because unless you can afford to siesta, doing so is sure to bring on a postprandial dip. This dip is a physiologic slowdown due to increased blood flow to the gut to aid digestion after eating. It is what invites the afternoon energy slump and is the reason behind the increased surge of soda sales and other forms of pick-me-ups—that don't do anything but add more useless calories to your day (and waist)—in the afternoon.

If you can't have a siesta, it is best to eat two to three light meals a day, known also as "grazing." Fruits and raw veggies like carrot or celery sticks are examples of grazing options. A healthy energy bar is also an option. I use either an herbal whole food bar called a Sunbar or sometimes a PowerBar (see Sources).

SEVEN NATURAL WONDERS

Working in unison with the ten WF Nutritional Guidelines are seven supplemental guidelines that I call the Seven Natural Wonders of Nutritional Awareness. When practiced faithfully, they lead to a nutritional awakening and make it virtually impossible for you to ever overeat again. Take your time getting to know them. Practice them as often as possible for fastest results.

Seven Natural Wonders of Nutritional Awareness

1. Prepare (or at least eat) your food mindfully.

2. Do not talk while chewing.

3. Use chopsticks.

4. Chew thoroughly.

5. Eat with beautiful posture (preferably seated cross-legged upon the earth in a quiet environment).

6. Don't lunge for your food. Lift the food like the gift that it is toward your mouth.

7. Feed the needs of the body, not the wants or desires of the ego. When hunger arises, ask yourself, "Is this a physiologic hunger, or is it just psychologic hunger? Do I really need to eat or snack right now or maybe just breathe through this impulse for a few minutes?"

OTHER STUFF

Here are some miscellaneous items about my approach to Nutrition that will help you adapt to my program over the next few months.

- If you must drink coffee, limit your intake to one to two cups in the morning. Better idea: Replace with a nourishing tea such as Calli Beverage (see Sources).

- Reduce foods that are made mainly from sugars. Aliases of sugar include: sucrose, fructose, corn syrup, high fructose corn syrup, modified corn starch, brown sugar, and maltodextrin.

- Don't consume too many starchy foods, particularly white starches that are not naturally white: wheat, flour, sugars, etc.

- Keep intake levels of saturated fats and hydrogenated oils low. Hydrogenation destroys the nutritional value of the oil; margarine is an example. Try to stay away from those oils that tend to harden at room temperature, like animal fats, palm oil, and coconut oil. Examples of "good" oils are olive, safflower, sunflower, sesame, canola, and corn oils.

- If you are interested, you can use the same whole food herbs that I've used personally and professionally for twenty years. I've included the contact for these herbs in the Sources section.

DRUGS AND ALCOHOL: A WF PERSPECTIVE

WF does not pass judgment if you drink alcohol or get stoned. I know my encounters with drugs have made me a more understanding, compassionate teacher and coach and family man.

We use recreational drugs to get a "hit" of an enlightened state. Can't blame people for wanting that! Just remember that drug use weakens your life force. Wish it could be different, but that is the way the game is played. Everything about spiritual awakening is about looking inside, not outside, yourself.

If you drink or use drugs, use them less than usual from now on. If you can't seem to be able to do that, contact me through wholisticfitness.com. I'll do my best in whatever way I can for you.

If you use on the weekend, make it every other weekend. If you use every day, try to make it every other day. Get friends to help you. We're all just here, doing our best given the tools we've been handed. Don't feel ashamed, embarrassed, or scared. The WF warrior way through drug use is like everything else we do in spiritual work: First we accept it, then we honor it as a teacher. With time, you'll hopefully see the folly of regular drug use when compared to the joy of becoming clear, healthy, and full of pran (life force). Working out WF style increases pran; drugs deplete it.

I remember really having to hunt to find good sources of protein foods to supplement my vegetarian-style diet. The only tofu available back in the early 1980s, for instance, was the wet, sloppy, slushy Chinese style. Couldn't do a damn thing with it. It is crazy easy these days—given the new generation of soy products, rice products, and tofu products—to eat vegetarian versions of sausage, hamburgers, chicken, bacon, ice cream, and even cheesecake. Many of these can be found at your local grocery market, natural food store, or via the Internet.

CHAPTER 6

Daily Practice

THE TIME HAS ARRIVED FOR me to show you how to pull the preceding five chapters together and choreograph a day-by-day personal fitness practice. This will be your first taste of Wholistic Fitness.

Four weeks from now, if you follow the program below, you'll see and feel why WF is unlike any other personal fitness system in the world.

You can cross-reference all the following workouts in the appropriate chapters we've just covered. For example, any Strength Training movement can be found listed in the order it appears in your workout in Chapter 1 of this part. Any Strength Training technique, such as the 3-Stage Technique, can be found at the end of that same chapter. I've put page numbers next to each movement and technique for easy, fast cross-referencing.

Don't stress if you are unable to do all the workouts for that day. Just pick the priority one(s) and do your warrior best. If you know that you are more stiff than you are strong, make sure you prioritize Yoga during your training week. If you are trying to lose body fat as your main goal, then prioritize Cardio training and follow through on the Nutrition guidelines I've set in Chapter 5.

Don't try to make up missed workouts by cramming several workouts into the next day. Instead, just keep flowing through the week. Never stress. You've got your whole life to become wholistically fit. Doing too much too soon is not going to help.

I've choreographed the fitness disciplines in the order that provides the optimal training effect. However, if you need to switch the order, you can. Consistency comes first.

Good luck, Noble Warrior! May your Daily Practice be strong and sincere.

Please remember to take your time. I'll say it again. This Green Tara program will be the most difficult because we are biting off the biggest chunk of the WF pie. A lot of new techniques and adjustments will need to be "chewed" over these next four weeks. The next programs, covered in Parts Two and Three, will be a lot easier to slide into once your groove has been set by this program.

THE GREEN TARA DAILY PRACTICE

Wholistic Fitness Training Precepts

1. Be prepared

2. Be on time

3. Give 110 percent

Monday. Recovery and Scheduling Weekly Workouts

Mondays are traditional WF recovery days. You don't need to do any physical workouts today. None. You'll know why a week from now.

Mondays are busy for many people and after six days of high-quality workouts, you will need this day to focus on your work while giving your body time to prepare for another six days of workouts.

Even if you don't feel like taking this day off from training, I want you to anyway. Ned Overend, the great mountain bike and Terra-X champion, told me that most athletes "train too easy on their hard days and too hard on their easy days." So, if you keep hitting your Monday recovery days with a lot of energy, chances are likely you are not putting 110 percent of your effort into each workout during the training week.

What I do want you to do each Monday (or on Sunday evening) is to go to your schedule book and block out the time needed to do your workouts each day. Then, use Mondays to mentally rehearse your performances in each of the Five Fitness Disciplines and Four Lifestyle

Principles. Where could you have been more noble? How are you going to do better this week? Visualize yourself doing the upcoming workouts in a strong, elegant, and focused manner.

Some WF students enjoy receiving bodywork (massage) on Mondays. Not a bad idea.

Tuesday. Leg Day in the Gym

Meditation: Beeper Guru: Breath and Posture (page 112).

Cardio: None or Cardio Commute (see page 76).

Yoga: None or flow through a few rounds of one or more HP Yoga Sun Salutations as a warmup before your Strength Training workout.

Strength: Do the Green Tara lower body workout. This is your main workout of today. Feared by the novice, cherished by those who've climbed her summit.

Prescription Notes

- All sets to momentary failure, unless otherwise noted.

- Recovery phase: 30 to 45 seconds unless otherwise noted.

- Active warmup: Perform a few minutes of Cardio to raise the body temperature.

Stiff Leg Deadlifts (page 47)

Do 2 sets of 4 repetitions.

Do not use heavy weights or go to momentary muscular failure. Just focus on executing the movement with a beautiful, flat back and poetic flow.

Leg Extensions (page 48)

Do 3 sets of Staccato Technique: Hold the top position for 10 seconds, then do the exercise for 10 seconds, repeat that stick-and-go sequence until the 1-minute mark is reached. Recover for 1 minute. That is one set.

Leg Curls (page 48)

Do 3 sets of 6 to 8 repetitions.

Upper body stays quiet, pinch the glutes continuously.

Superset: Go from A to B without resting for 2 sets.

A. Back Squats (page 49)

Do 10 repetitions.

Then, without allowing your ego to rebel, head over to the leg press apparatus and immediately do:

B. Leg Press (page 50)

Crank it, baby, for 1 minute!

After you've reached the 1-minute mark, you can get out of the leg press machine and stagger about for a minute, but use the first 30 seconds of your recovery interval to adjust any weight on your leg press or back squat bar (less is more, remember!) and with zazen mind, walk over to the squat rack and get ready to do your next set of back squats within 1 minute. After doing two Supersets like this, move on to the next Superset.

Superset: Go from A to B without resting for 2 sets.

A. Back Squats (page 49)

Do 10 repetitions.

Then, without allowing your ego to rebel, step back away from the squat rack, give yourself some room, forget about anybody in the gym (this is to diminish your ego) and immediately do:

B. Jump Squats (page 50)

Crank 'em, baby, for 1 minute!

After you've reached the 1-minute mark, you can stagger about for a minute, but use your recovery interval to adjust any weight on your squat bar (less is more, remember) and with zazen mind focused on being more strong, more beautiful in your next set, do another Superset within 1 minute. After doing two Supersets like this, move on to the next movement. Keep your workout flowing from start to finish.

Leg Extensions (page 48)

Yes, we get to revisit your throne here just to make sure your training effect is up to WF standards by doing another set of Staccato Technique: Hold the

> Potential Warrior Students should do 2 sets of leg extensions. Potential Master Students need to crank off 3 sets.

top position for 10 seconds, then do the exercise for 10 seconds, repeat that stick-and-go sequence until the 1-minute mark is reached. Recover for 1 minute. That is one set.

<table>
<tr><td>

Potential Warrior Students should do a total of 3 sets. Potential Master Students need to crank off 4 sets.

</td><td>

Standing or Seated Calf Raises (page 51)

Do 2 sets of Staccato Technique: Hold the top position for 10 seconds, then do the exercise for 10 seconds, repeat that stick-and-go sequence until the 1-minute mark is reached. Recover for 1 minute. That is one set. You can change from standing to seated calf raises (or vice versa) after the first set, if desired.

</td></tr>
</table>

Abdominal Superset: Go from A to B without resting for 2 sets.

A. Oblique Twists (page 55)

Do 1 minute.

<table>
<tr><td>

Potential Warrior Students should do a total of 3 Supersets. Potential Master Students need to crank off 4 Supersets.

</td><td>

B. Medicine Ball Crunches (page 53)

Do 1 minute.

Congratulations on completing your WF leg day! Thanks for playing. May your recovery be quick for Thursday's workout!

</td></tr>
</table>

Wednesday. HP Yoga

Meditation: Early Morning Zazen (page 119). Sit zazen for 20 minutes, switching legs after 10 minutes.

Cardio: None or Cardio Commute (page 76).

Yoga: Do the High Performance Yoga Green Tara practice.

Begin by engaging ujjayi (page 83) breathing and don't stop ujjayi until the final pose.

3 x Ardha Surya Namaskar (Half Sun Salutation) (page 86)

2 x Series A Modified (page 87)

1 x Series B (both legs = 1 set) (page 90)

1 x Series C (both legs = 1 set) (page 93)

5 x Series A (page 89)

Do these movements, holding *each* for 30 to 60 seconds. Focus the mind with ujjayi breathing and the ego with honoring your edge.

1. Standing Vinyasa (flow sequence). Start with right leg in lead position.

   - Utthita Parsvakonasana (Extended Side Angle Pose, page 96) exhale into

   - Parsvottanasana (Side Extended Pose, page 97) into

   - Utthita Trikonasana (Extended Triangle Pose, page 97) into

   - Ardha Chandrasana (Half Moon Pose, page 98) into

   - Parivrtta Ardha Chandrasana (Revolved Half Moon Pose, page 99)

   - step back into Downward Facing Dog (Adho Mukha Svanasana, page 99).

   Repeat for left leg.

2. Salabhasana (Locust Pose, page 101)
   Option Pose: Dhanurasana (Bow Pose, page 101)

3. Virasana (Hero Pose, page 102)
   Option Pose: Supta Virasana (Supine Hero Pose, page 102)

4. Paschimottanasana (Western Extended Stretch, page 103)

5. Malasana (Garland Pose, page 103)
   Option Pose: Parsva Malasana (Lateral Garland Pose, page 103)

6. Bakasana (Crane Pose, page 104)
   Option Pose: Ekapada Bakasana (Single Leg Crane Pose, page 105)

7. Halasana (Plow Pose, page 105)
   Option Pose: Parsva Halasana (Lateral Plow Pose, page 106)

8. Navasana/Ardha Navasana (Boat/Half Boat Pose, page 107)

9. Savasana (Corpse Pose, page 108)

Beautiful work, I am very proud of you! Now, bring your Yoga off your mat and into your life!

Thursday. Upper Body in the Gym

Meditation: Beeper Guru: Breath and Posture (page 112).

Cardio: None or Cardio Commute (page 76).

Yoga: None or flow through a few rounds of one or more HP Yoga Sun Salutations (page 86) as a warmup before your Strength Training workout.

Strength: Do the Green Tara Upper Body Workout. This is your main workout of today. Not as demanding as was Tuesday's leg day, but do not arrive at the gym underfocused. There is plenty of WF adventure in this workout.

> Potential Warrior Students should do one more set than is called for. Think you want to become a Master Student? Do 2 extra sets then.

Prescription Notes

- All sets to momentary failure, unless otherwise noted.

- Recovery Phase: 30 to 45 seconds unless otherwise noted.

- Active Warmup: Perform a few minutes of Cardio to raise the body temperature.

Pull-ups (page 57)

Do 2 sets of however many or few you can. It's not the amount of repetitions I want from you, it's your best effort that matters. Just pull. No machines allowed! Just you and your inner spirit!

V-Handle Pulldowns (page 57)

Do 2 sets of 10 to 12 repetitions.

> Can you say, "forearm pump"? Now you can see why I created this particular technique to improve my rock-climbing endurance.

V-Handle Pulldowns

Do 3 sets of 10 repetitions using a Ku Bottom Form Technique as your "recovery" between sets. Welcome to the world of Coach Ilg: Instead of taking a break between sets, draw the bar as close as possible to your chest and hold it there for 5 ujjayi breaths, then begin the next set. Your hands will never leave the V-Handle until the entire three sets are done.

Hang Cleans (page 58)

Do 3 sets of 8 repetitions.

Lots of technique to learn here and only four weeks to learn it. Go!

Dips (page 59)

Do 2 sets of however many or few you can! It's not the amount of repetitions, it's your best effort that matters. No machines allowed! Just you and your inner spirit.

Superset: Go from A to B without resting for 2 sets.

A. Dumbbell Flyes (page 60)

Do 10 repetitions.

Then, using the same pair of dumbbells, switch your hand and arm position and get ready to pump.

B. Dumbbell Bench Presses (page 60)

Do 15 to 20 of them . . . yeah, baby! I want high-frequency repetitions—pretty speedy tempo here. Keep the form, but go fast. After doing 15 to 20 reps, recover for 30 to 45 seconds. That is one Superset.

Bench Press (page 60)

Do 2 sets of 15 repetitions.

Use ujjayi breathing only. Strict form.

Seated Dumbbell Lateral Raises (page 62)

Do 3 sets of 10 to 12 repetitions.

Barbell Curls (page 63)

Time to learn my infamous "Envelope Technique":

Open your "envelope" by doing the movement for 1 minute. Inside your envelope, there are 2 more sets of 6 to 8 repetitions, so you will have to add more weight on the barbell. Then, I want you to close your envelope with a fourth and final set of 1 minute. Recovery between all sets should be limited to 30 seconds. Essentially, sets 1 and 4 are endurance tests, while sets 2 and 3 develop your deep fiber power. Here is the quick-glance choreography for doing Envelope Technique:

Set 1: Do the movement for 1 minute

Sets 2 and 3: Do the movement for 6 to 8 repetitions

Set 4: Do the movement for 1 minute

Two-Bench Triceps (page 64)

Do 2 sets of 1 minute.

Use escape plans (page 64) if needed, but never quit.

Abdominal Superset: Go from A to B without rest for 2 sets.

A. Medicine Ball Crunches (page 53)

Do 1 minute.

B. Suspended Leg Raises (page 54)

Do 1 minute.

Congratulations on completing your WF upper body day! May your recovery be quick for Saturday's EEE-GAD workout. (I didn't call it "EEE-GAD" for nothing!)

Friday. Intervals, Intervals, Intervals!

Meditation: Early Morning Zazen (page 119). Sit zazen for 20 minutes, switching legs at 10 minutes.

Cardio: Here you go. Be brave, Noble Warrior! Be brave.

Cardio of Choice

Assigned Intervals (page 73)

20 minutes @ Zones 1 & 2

5 sets x 1-minute intervals @ Zone 4 w/1-minute RI

5-minute RP

3 sets x 3-minute intervals @ high Zone 3 w/2-minute RI

20 minutes @ Zones 1 & 2

Saturday. EEE-GAD in the Gym and HP Yoga!

Note: If you're feeling tired, select whichever discipline you need more work in, Strength Training or Yoga. Then do that program. You can also alternate these workouts each week instead of doing both of them on the same day. But for the optimal WF training effect, do them both!

> Potential Warrior Students should do one more set than is called for. Want to go for Master Student quality? Do two more sets. Remember, there is no dishonor in throwing up. There is dishonor, however, in not finishing something you've begun. WF Warriors never give up.

Yoga: High-Performance Yoga, the Green Tara practice. Follow the same routine as was prescribed for Wednesday.

Strength: Do the EEE-GAD workout below using all the same exercises and techniques you learned during the weekday workouts on Tuesday and Thursday. There is one new movement that comes with a new technique: Overhead DB press, which comes nicely gift wrapped with my dastardly 3-Stage Technique (page 65).

> The name says it all. The EEE-GAD full-body workouts were finalized in 1986 and have been serving our students across the nation very well ever since. The real trick is to master the entire workout from start to finish with unwavering attention to posture and lifting tempo.

Prescription Notes

- All sets to momentary failure, unless otherwise noted.

- Recovery Phase: 30 to 45 seconds unless otherwise noted.

- Active Warmup: Perform a few minutes of Cardio to raise the body temperature.

Pull-ups (page 57)

Do 2 sets of however many you can do. Develop upper "surge."

V-Handle Pulldowns (page 57)

Use the Envelope Technique:

Set 1: Do the movement for 1 minute

Sets 2 and 3: Do the movement for 6 to 8 repetitions

Set 4: Do the movement for 1 minute

Superset: Go from A into B without resting for 3 sets.

A. Dumbbell Flyes (page 60) for 10 reps.

B. Dumbbell Bench Presses (page 60) for 20 reps at a high frequency.

Superset: Go from A into B without resting for 3 sets.

A. Back Squats (page 49) for 10 reps.

B. Leg Extensions (page 48) using the Staccato Technique (page 137). Hold the top position for 10 seconds, then do the exercise for 10 seconds, repeat that stick-and-go sequence until the 1-minute mark is reached. Recover for 1 minute. That is one set of Staccato Technique.

Seated Dumbbell Press (page 62)

Do 2 sets of 3-Stage Technique (page 65).

Quick Glance Choreography for the 3-Stage Technique:

1–20 seconds: Do only the top half of the movement

21–40 seconds: Do only the bottom half of the moment (at quicker tempo)

41–60 seconds: Drive hard for the finish line by doing the full range of the movement in as strong a form as possible!

The entire set lasts 1 minute.

Two-Bench Triceps (page 64)

Do 2 sets of 1 minute.

Barbell Curls (page 63)

Use the Envelope Technique.

Set 1: Do the movement for 1 minute

Sets 2 and 3: Do the movement for 6 to 8 repetitions

Set 4: Do the movement for 1 minute

Abdominal Superset: Go from A to B without resting for 2 sets.

A. Medicine Ball Crunches (page 53)

Do 1 minute.

B. Suspended Leg Raises (page 54)

Do 1 minute.

Congratulations . . . EEE-GAD!

Sunday. Cardio!

Cardio: Do Cardio of Choice (page 74) for 1 to 3 hours. Stay within Zones 1 and 2, and at the lower end of Zone 3—no higher intensity than that! See Table 2.1, Cardio Zones (page 75).

Yoga: If you did not do either the HP Yoga, Green Tara routine, or the EEE-GAD workout on Saturday, if you're feeling up to it, knock it out today. But don't push yourself if your body is feeling really sore (that is, "feeling well trained" in WF parlance). Better to just get in the Cardio and mellow out. Remember, tomorrow is Monday, your "off day" from training.

You did it! A week of WF workouts! Your ability to link together four of these weeks is going to transform your body/mind and spirit into unprecedented levels of fitness. There ain't nothing like Wholistic Fitness.

Stay sincere—your spirit is nurtured by your sweat.

CHAPTER 7

Cycle Summation

UPON YOUR COMPLETION OF FOUR consistent weeks on my Green Tara program, take seven days off from training. If desired, you can continue doing Yoga every other day.

Limit Cardio to three 30- to 60-minute workouts done on nonconsecutive days and at an intensity level no higher than Zone 2 (see Table 2.1, page 75).

You may practice Meditation as desired.

No Strength Training should be done during this week.

Use the extra time normally spent training to share with family, friends, or to be by yourself.

At some point, read the next chapter to prepare psychologically for your next program. It will push you in as many ways as the Green Tara did. Get ready for it.

And if your arms are not too well trained to pick up a pencil, you may wish to answer the following questions regarding your performance during the Green Tara program:

Green Tara Cycle Summation

Date started:

Date finished:

Today's date:

Finish this sentence:
The Green Tara program has given me a renewed sense of . . .

Strength Training

1. Note your consistency during this discipline.
2. How did the upper and lower body workouts go?
3. And the EEE-GAD workout?
4. Which gym movements seem harder than others? Why?
5. Which seemed easier? Why?
6. Any changes in physique?
7. Think you have what it takes to ever become a WF Master Student? If yes, what qualities will you have to develop to get you to such a high level of body/mind and spiritual fitness?

Cardio

1. Any standout reactions in this discipline?
2. How did the assigned intervals go? Did you have any physical or emotional resistance?
3. Were you able to do any Cardio Commutes? If not, why not?
4. What was your weekly average in terms of Cardio hours logged?

Yoga

1. What is your first reaction to the word "Yoga" these days? How has it changed from four weeks ago?
2. How did the HP Green Tara practice go?
3. Were you able to maintain ujjayi breathing through the forms?
4. Name the three poses that you find most difficult. Note any commonality among them. (Coach's Note: These three poses hold your Highest teachings. Dive deep into them.)
5. Finish this sentence: My first excursion into HP Yoga made me realize . . .

Meditation

1. How did the zazen sessions go?
2. The primary lesson I learned from the Breath and Posture Beeper Guru was:
3. Note how you felt after taking your items to charity after your Periodic Renunciation.
4. What do you think about being in bare feet?

Nutrition

1. Did you notice any changes in your dietary attractions during this cycle?
2. Describe *exactly* what you ate and drank yesterday and the manner in which you consumed it. Include supplements, drugs, everything.
3. Did you adjust your diet in any way? If so, how?

Number the WF disciplines below from 1 to 5, starting with the one you really need to focus on during the next program.

Strength Training

Cardio

Yoga

Meditation

Nutrition

What do you do with these answers? Well, I've kind of tricked you into becoming your own personal trainer! I use information gathered from my students' Cycle Summations to more accurately design their next training program. I want you to do the same based on your own answers. Which fitness disciplines do you shy away from? Which are you best at? How consistently are you drawing your fitness endeavors into your daily life? Use the answers above to motivate yourself: Make a promise to strengthen your weaker areas in the next program. This is the type of gumption that is required from a WF Warrior! The pursuit of balance is a constantly evolving process of self-understanding. Go for the wholeness.

Hey, I think I hear something . . . could it possibly be Cosmic Yang calling you to play?

THE INTERMEDIATE PROGRAM: THE COSMIC YANG PROGRAM

The personality of my Cosmic Yang program comes with a mandatory but not always so charming quality of intensity. This program delivers quite a punch. The Strength and Cardio elements along this part of your WF journey are in explosive contrast to the cycles that surround them. It is said that "in skating over thin ice, our safety is in our speed." Your journey into Cosmic Yang transforms the strength and spirit developed in the Green Tara program into a deeply functional and athletic caliber of fitness that will never leave you. Train hard, but relax into the intensity of the utterly classic Cosmic Yang.

Cosmic Yang is a challenging, physiologically diverse program that increases high-end fitness transfer.

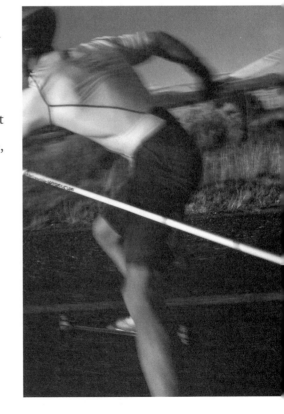

Often, these teachings yield a lifelong sense of self-confidence. I designed the Cosmic Yang to intensify the life force of a Wholistic Fitness student. I think too many people schlep around in their lives, never pursuing their goals and dreams with what yogis know as *tapas*, or inner fire, inner desire! The next four weeks is guaranteed to ignite your *tapas*, using the "gym temple" and intervals during Cardio to achieve much of this inner fire. I want this rekindled inner fire to burn away all that stuff that is holding you back from your highest dreams.

Get ready—the spiritual energy that is gained from the simple concentrated effort required by this program will rock you. An established classic since 1988, Cosmic Yang is not soon forgotten by those who have journeyed her world of pain and pleasure.

Cosmic	=	**Universal**
Yang	=	**Light, Creative, Explosive, Masculine, Fire, Active**

I trust you will authenticate this classic Wholistic Fitness teaching to the best of your ability. Zero timidity—take charge and go.

Let's get Cosmic . . .

Fluid power is the absence of drama.
—COACH ILG

CHAPTER 8

Strength Training

Learning to become fast takes time.
—COACH ILG

NOW THAT YOU'VE DEVELOPED YOUR BODY'S structural integrity through Green Tara's Strength Training workouts, it's time to dig into a new avenue of strength. That avenue is speed-strength, more popularly known as power.

Experientially, I developed my most explosive power as a Nordic ski jumper and as a boulderer (climbing up boulders using a gymnast's powerful moves and ballet-like balance sequences). Pure dynamic power was needed in both those sports. Academically, I learned a lot about power training when I helped create and edit *Plyometrics: Explosive Power Training for Athletes* by James Radcliffe and my former boss, Bob Farentinos, Ph.D. If the training movements in this program excite you and you are a glutton for more fast-twitch punishment, get that book (see Sources). For now, I want you to think about three basic but wonderful aspects to power development: physiologic power, practical or applied power, and inner or spiritual power.

PHYSIOLOGIC POWER

From a physiologic perspective, power is the ability to move the greatest amount of resistance in the shortest possible time. To accomplish such a task, your body is equipped with fast-twitch muscle fibers. These fast-twitch fibers are the same kind that a 100-meter sprinter uses. Marathon runners, on the other hand, rely mostly on slow-twitch fibers. I like developing the fast-twitch fiber fitness of my students because I have found that developing just a little bit of speed within muscles carries over tremendously into overall strength. You'll see. Power training is fun to learn and well worth the effort in the long term. I can always tell a power-trained athlete from a conventionally trained one. There is a special glimmer in their eye and a particular vibrancy in their presence. Besides, no WF student ever gets through my basic studies without knowing by direct experience the difference between regular strength and explosive power.

The upcoming power movements can be tricky to learn. Cosmic Yang workouts will impart a degree of explosiveness and kinesthesia to your fitness that you probably have not yet tapped. It won't necessarily be how strong you are that will account for your success in this cycle, but how fast you are. Learning to become fast takes time. Be patient. Once your nervous system makes the necessary adaptation, power movements (such as the classic Hang Clean on page 58 or Jump Squats on page 50) are exceedingly rewarding. Power movements tend to turn heads in the gym, since 99 percent of conventional Strength Training exercises are not power related. By the end of these four weeks, you'll command a far more coordinated sense of power than you have right now.

APPLIED POWER

I've lost count of how many times the speed strength I acquired through Cosmic Yang has made all the difference in my athletic endeavors. The faster I got in the gym, the more confident I became in my races and in my extreme sport performances. Surprising myself and most of my competitors in endurance sports, I found year after year of harnessing power in the gym during my off seasons did wonders for my endurance sports. Power training delayed my slow-twitch fibers from fatiguing. In mountain and road cycling races over three hours, for instance, I found that as the race wore on, I could repeatedly attack with greater speed than my non–power trained competitors, especially up steep mountains. I liked that! If the race

The letter on page 153 was sent to me by Noble WF Warrior Student Joe Gutcher, a wrestler, husband, father. Joe's letter is the epitome of the three aspects of power training that are so transformational.

Coach Ilg,

I'm writing to express some overdue gratitude for what you and WF have done for me. A month ago, at the end of my Power Training phase, I received a call from a coach in Bismarck, N.D., at the University of Mary. I was asked to come out and practice with their wrestling team while they prepared for Nationals, with a possible chance of earning a scholarship. So after much debate I quit my job, borrowed money for airline tickets, and flew my wife and myself out there (my daughter stayed with grandparents).

The weekend went well! By the time I was flying back home, I'd beaten their guy in a match 12–2 (he was ranked fifth in the nation) and was offered a full ride! They were impressed that I could keep the pace of their practices even though I hadn't competed in over two years. I don't have to tell you why I was able to perform so well, because you know why.

That brings me to why I have written you. First, I would have never made the trip if it hadn't been for WF, I would have been too scared. Second, my mind/body just wouldn't have made it through workouts designed for college athletes peaking for Nationals. Basically my skills would never have shone through.

For those two things my undying gratitude is yours.

Thanks,

Joe Gutcher

P.S. I gave up the coffee! I was like a cocaine addict with that stuff.

---

came down to a some sort of a mad sprint for the finish, I carried a lot of confidence to the line because I knew I had done a helluva lot more Jump Squats and Power Cleans than anybody else during the off season.

Applied power also has more subtle qualities. You might, for instance, notice that your "Chaturangas" during Yoga come easier, or that holding the deep Warrior postures is not as taxing. These are positive training effects stemming from power training. Best of all, perhaps, is the energy you'll save from having a quicker step throughout your workday. Many students have reported gaining much more energy from their Cosmic Yang experiences. They allude to having more pep at the end of a workday to play with their kids or do fun things because they are not as tired.

INNER POWER

Even more important than the physical and practical qualities of power training is its spiritual benefit. The more powerful you become in the gym, the more powerfully you'll take hold of your life. In my own experience, duplicated by numerous WF students like Joe Gutcher (see sidebar), I found I was less hesitant to jump on opportunities as they arose in daily life during my power training cycles. I learned that power training had a lasting transpersonal effect that "powered" me out of a funky mood or out of my comfy bed early in the morning to go meditate or run. Power training helped me accelerate over the obstacles in my life with the grace and efficiency of a cheetah. I would go that extra step out of my comfort zone and accomplish things more powerfully. It felt good.

GO FOR IT!

Over the next four weeks, I really want you to go for it in the gym! I've intentionally juxtaposed the explosive nature of Cosmic Yang with the precise-form-is-everything attitude of Green Tara. I've done this so you know right away that WF ain't about eating granola and being all nitpicky in the gym. It's about ditching that timid streak inside of you that might be keeping you from reaching your greatest dreams. Step on the throttle, baby, and have some explosive fun!

FOR OPTIMAL TRAINING

Here are three considerations to get the most from your upcoming Cosmic Yang gym workouts.

1. Train with a Partner

Though most of these movements will be the same as in Green Tara, some of them, such as Gunther Hops (see page 155), are new and can be quite kinesthetically challenging. Until you learn to coordinate your body/mind in sync with their technique, be prepared to have your ego humbled once again. A training partner can help spot technique flaws and keep you confident. He or she can also spot you on the heavier sets, and you can help each other fine-tune the nuances of these beautiful movements.

2. Emphasize the Yang

In Green Tara you learned that every repetition in the gym should express three distinct qualities: yin (female, slower, lengthening of muscle fibers), yang (male, explosive, shortening of muscle fibers), and neutral (transition). During Cosmic Yang Strength Training get mentally geared for cranking out a strong yang, or explosive, phase. Remember, it is the phase that occurs on the concentric contraction—the muscle fibers shorten as they contract—it's what happens when a barbell is lifted toward the chest during a barbell curl.

3. Merge into Your Exhales

Exhales are everything during Cosmic Yang. You will learn the spiritual dimension of all this later on. For now, really make an audible exhale as you blow the weight as you exert. This audible exhale also helps blow away self-doubt as you begin an intimidating set.

You are now ready to enter the hallowed chambers of Cosmic Yang! Here are the new Strength Training exercises that you will encounter in Chapter 13, the daily practice of your new program. I am now adding new ingredients to the basic recipe. Study well!

As in Chapter 1, I'll begin with the lower body, then the midsection, and finally the upper body exercises.

> Our deepest fears are like dragons guarding our deepest treasures.
> —RAINER MARIA RILKE

COSMIC YANG STRENGTH TRAINING

PHYSICAL BENEFITS

number of cells at the moment of contraction is improved

maximum contraction capability is improved

peripheral circulation is increased

ability to handle blood pressure spikes is increased

TRANSPERSONAL BENEFITS

develops a "go for it" attitude

LOWER BODY STRENGTH TRAINING

Gunther Hops

Assume a standing position (no weight is used with this movement) with your hands held in a prayer position near the heart. Lower into a quarter squat by bending your right knee beneath you. Extend your left leg directly out to the side of you. Keeping your spine flat and with your eyes gazing toward the horizon, explode up into the air by forcefully extending your right knee.

As your body reaches its maximum height, draw the left leg under you so that both legs are extended directly beneath you.

As your body starts coming back down, laterally extend your right leg off to the side. Ideally, as you impact the ground, both feet hit simultaneously. Drop into a deep knee bend on your left knee, which should be directly under you.

Now, explode up and off the left knee by extending it, and repeat this leg switch for the prescribed time or reps.

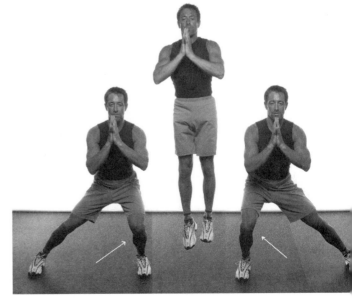

YIN PHASE: Attenuating the impact of your feet hitting the ground.

YANG PHASE: Exploding away from the ground.

WHAT YOU ARE PRIMARILY WORKING: Explosive power, midsection transfer strength, skill coordination, threshold Cardio fitness.

WHOLISTIC NOTES: A classic Nordic ski racing movement straight from Norway. Another Old World Viking torture test. Who needs fancy equipment? This plyometric (speed-strength) movement inspires tremendous lower body power while enhancing lateral mobility. As fatigue sets in, the upper body will tend to collapse forward. Counter this apologetic posture by keeping your heart center pulled up. Mental tenacity and inner conviction are the spiritual qualities associated with "Lord Gunther." Focus on height, not frequency. Be noble in your effort here. Do your best.

Knee Tuck Jumps

Assume upright stance. Tuck your thumbs under your armpits and raise your arms parallel to the ground. Keep your elbows high. Bend both knees slightly and flatten your spine into an elegant posture. Look straight ahead.

Rapidly dip into a quarter squat by bending both knees at the same time and then, using that recoiled energy of your thighs, jump upward and drive your kneecaps to the elbows by doing a type of midair abdominal crunch.

The instant your feet land back onto the ground, explode them back up again, driving the kneecaps to the elbows. Repeat as fast as possible for required reps. Keep your head as still as possible.

YIN PHASE: Attenuating the impact of your feet hitting the ground.

YANG PHASE: Exploding away from the ground.

WHAT YOU ARE PRIMARILY WORKING: Explosive power, leg speed, midsection transfer strength, skill coordination, threshold Cardio fitness.

WHOLISTIC NOTES: Get the hell outa Dodge, cowboy! Knee tuck jumps improve not only vertical jump but leg speed as well. This is accomplished through a decreased reaction time; so *react*. Explode off the ground in the same instant you impact it. Go! The transpersonal aspects of this exercise loosen insecurity of self. So, if you are feeling insecure about the direction of your life, do this movement and it will help you jump forward into the next phase of your life.

Hook thumbs under armpits.

Drive knee to elbows.

Ab Wheel

Grasp both ends of an Ab Wheel (see Sources), with your palms facing down. Assume a kneeling position on the ground. Place and hold the Ab Wheel on the ground as if you were in a hands-and-knees position. Bring your ankles together. Flex your knees so you bring both feet into the air behind you. Look down at the Ab Wheel beneath your face.

Roll the Ab Wheel slowly out in front of you, controlling its speed by contracting your abdominal muscles in an eccentric (lengthening) manner. Stop the rolling about halfway out, then roll it back to your starting position, again using your abdominals, this time using concentric (shortening) action. Repeat as prescribed.

> As you advance into your body/mind fitness training, your midsection work improves the processing of your reality—your "gut check," your "gut reaction." Do you have the "guts" to meet and walk your dragons?

YIN PHASE: **Rolling the wheel away from you.**

YANG PHASE: **Rolling the wheel toward you.**

WHAT YOU ARE PRIMARILY WORKING: **Your "core" muscles of the abdominals, obliques, spinal stabilizers, and pelvic girdle stabilizers.**

WHOLISTIC NOTES: **All those fancy-schmancy abdominal machines and knock off abdominal training gizmos and here I am telling you that nothing beats a stupid little $10 wheel that's been around forever. But it's true. This little dandy is core training at its purest. I want you to progressively flirt with a fuller range of motion as your abdominals and lower back muscles strengthen. This movement will quickly sharpen all athletic activity and postural presence by producing Herculean midsection strength and power. Having trouble with those Chatarungas in the HP Yoga routines? You won't after doing these!**

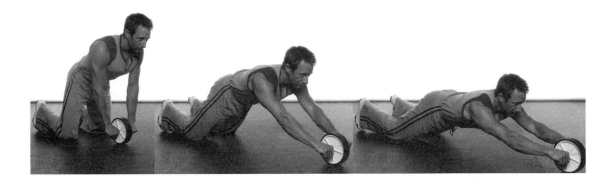

Dumbbell Arm Swings

Stand upright with a light dumbbell in each hand. Bend both knees into a quarter squat position with hips squared and feet shoulder-width apart. Hold the dumbbells beside each hip so their handles are perpendicular to the ground and your palms face each other. Keep your head straight, eyes at horizon level. Tilt the shoulders slightly forward.

Start making like you are Michael Johnson and start moving your arms like a sprinter dashing for the finish line, powerfully and quickly driving one arm forward and up above the head while punching the opposite elbow backward. Then switch as fast as possible. Repeat this high speed, alternating sequence for the prescribed time or reps.

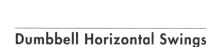

Knees slightly bent

YIN PHASE: None.

YANG PHASE: As your arms drive your hands up, down, backward, and frontward.

WHAT YOU ARE PRIMARILY WORKING: Upper body power, arm drive, core power.

WHOLISTIC NOTES: Do this movement before a mirror to check for postural beauty and speed. Be very yang; get aggro! Meditate upon speed, speed, and more speed for fast arm turnover. What inner weakness must be overcome before your arm turnover can increase? Drive with force into your goals and dreams.

Dumbbell Horizontal Swings

Stand with a light dumbbell clasped by both hands. Interlock your fingers around the dumbbell handle. Bend your knees and lower into a quarter squat position with feet shoulder-width apart. Square your hips to the wall in front of you. Look straight ahead.

Extend your arms so that you are holding the dumbbell at chest level in front of the body. Flex your elbows slightly but keep both elbows high. Imagine hugging a beach ball.

Initiate a torquing motion by pulling the dumbbell to your right until your left shoulder is near your chin. Keep looking straight ahead.

As your left shoulder comes under your chin, dynamically twist your torso in the opposite direction, toward the left, as if you are at bat trying to hit a home run.

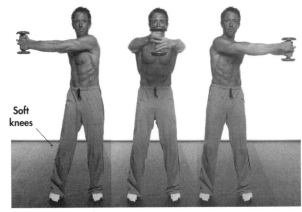

Soft knees

Continue the swing until your right shoulder comes under your chin, then repeat this swinging side-to-side motion. Increase your speed, faster and faster. Repeat this alternating sequence for the prescribed time or reps.

YIN PHASE: None.

YANG PHASE: The entire side-to-side swinging motion of the arms.

WHAT YOU ARE PRIMARILY WORKING: Transverse obliques, rectus abdominus, lower back muscles, shoulders, arms, pelvic girdle stabilizers, upper body power.

WHOLISTIC NOTES: The speed work issues from the shoulders and arms; limit all hip and leg involvement to stabilizing the dynamics of the upper torso. This is a really fast exercise, so don't lose your grip on the dumbbells. The meditation here is pure velocity! Fiery midsection training like this enhances intuitive wisdom for knowing what is most appropriate to our highest truth.

UPPER BODY STRENGTH TRAINING

Bent Arm Dumbbell Pullovers

Place a moderate-weight dumbbell perpendicular on a flat bench. Position yourself at a perpendicular angle to the bench. Rest your head on the far edge of the bench. Your shoulders should be resting comfortably on the bench. Suspend your hips below the level of the bench. Use a hip-wide foot stance to stabilize your body.

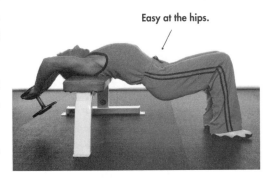

Easy at the hips.

Reach over, cup the inside top plate of the dumbbell by pressing your palms against the inmost top plate, and bring it overhead. Slightly flex your elbows. This is your start (top) position.

Lower the dumbbell in back of your head during a nasal inhale. Feel the stretch to your rib cage. Don't allow your hips to rise.

Once the dumbbell reaches parallel to the ground in back of your head, quickly raise it to top position with an exhale. Repeat and establish a strong groove.

YIN PHASE: Lower the dumbbell toward the ground.

YANG PHASE: Raising the dumbbell away from the ground.

WHAT YOU ARE PRIMARILY WORKING: Elasticity of the rib cage/chest fascia, external obliques, respiratory diaphragm muscles, pectoral muscles, core balance.

WHOLISTIC NOTES: Your hips are your guru here. Your entire pelvis must remain soft. Getting into and out of this exercise requires awareness. Feel the tightness dissolve in the upper torso.

Repetition Jerks

Stand upright holding a moderately weighted Olympic barbell across your upper chest in front of your neck. Grip the barbell with hands slightly farther apart than your shoulders with your palms facing the sky.

Squat down a few inches to store energy in the legs, then jerk the barbell overhead as fast as possible in a fast-twitch movement. Do not push or press the barbell. Jerk it directly overhead to catch it again at arm's length, still overhead.

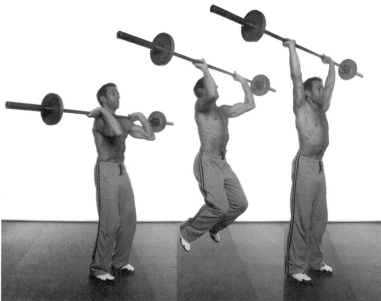

Hold the barbell overhead for a moment before lowering it slowly onto the upper chest again. Repeat for prescribed amount of reps.

YIN PHASE: Lowering the barbell from the overhead position to the chest.

YANG PHASE: Exploding the barbell overhead from the chest.

WHAT YOU ARE PRIMARILY WORKING: Fast-twitch fibers throughout your shoulders and arms, neuromuscular coordination; develops mental pre-play abilities.

WHOLISTIC NOTES: This is a full-body expression through the shoulders, a powerful transpersonal exercise grossly underused by the mainstream. Taking leadership of your life requires strong, powerful shoulders. This leadership is not a right; it is a responsibility that you must develop.

Concentration Curl

Sit on the edge of a flat bench. Let's train the right arm first. The left arm is the passive arm; its elbow rests on the left knee. The left palm is placed on the inside of the right knee, creating a nesting place into which the lower tricep/elbow of the right arm is placed. Keeping the back flat, reach down and grasp a dumbbell with the right hand. Use an underhand grip. Keep your shoulders squared.

Begin with an explosive curling movement by bending the right elbow and curling the dumbbell toward your chin. Once the dumbbell reaches your chin, slowly lower it back to the starting position described above. Repeat for prescribed reps. Switch to the other arm.

YIN PHASE: Lowering the dumbbell toward the ground.

YANG PHASE: Raising the dumbbell toward your chin.

WHAT YOU ARE PRIMARILY WORK- ING: Biceps and mental concentration.

WHOLISTIC NOTES: Strive for smooth as silk transitions. Curl the pinkie finger toward the shoulder as you raise the dumbbell. Listen inwardly to your biceps; many subtle teachings are arising. Greatness lies not in being strong, but in the right use of strength.

Lying Triceps Extensions

Lie supine (face up) either on the ground or on top of a flat bench. Hold a barbell at arm's length overhead using an overhand, false grip (thumbs on the same side of the barbell as your fingers). Place your hands no wider than your shoulders. Position your upper arms so they are perpendicular to the ground throughout the entire exercise.

Inhale as you bend your elbows, slowly lowering the barbell to your forehead. Keep your elbows in line with your armpits as you do this.

Smoothly exhale and extend the elbows and press the barbell overhead again to the start position. Repeat for the required amount of repetitions.

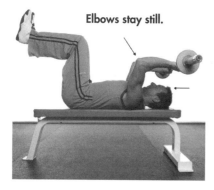

Elbows stay still.

YIN PHASE: Lowering the barbell toward your forehead.

YANG PHASE: Raising the barbell away from your forehead.

WHAT YOU ARE PRIMARILY WORKING: Triceps, neural skill control, and mental concentration.

WHOLISTIC NOTES: Simplicity and purity. Repetition and perseverance of mind. Fine-tunes inner listening skills to hear the fabulous details of how breath affects form. Lower back will want to arch. Use the ultra yin foot position (page 60) to counteract this inferior form.

Power Cleans

Note: Power Cleans are actually Hang Cleans (see page 58), except that you begin the movement with the barbell on the floor.

Stand over a weighted Olympic barbell. Bend at your knees and grip the bar with palms facing you, about shoulder width apart. Bend your knees deeper so that your hips are set low and your shins are close to the barbell. Make your back as flat as possible. Look forward, not down. Arms are extended.

Phase One: The Slow Pull

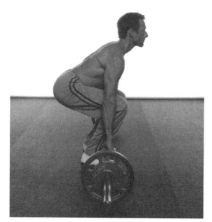

Exhale and slowly pull the barbell away from the ground by extending your knees. Do not jerk the barbell up (see photo).

Phase Two: The Jump Phase (see Hang Cleans, page 58)

Once the barbell passes your knees, pull the barbell explosively toward your chest by doing three things simultaneously: (1) shrug your shoulders toward your ears, (2) jump your feet off the ground by extending your hips (thrusting them forward), and (3) point your elbows toward the sky.

Phase Three: The Catch Phase (see Hang Cleans, page 58)

As the barbell reaches its maximum height from Phase Two, bend your knees and quickly squat under the barbell so you can catch the barbell across your upper chest. Stand up. Your palms will now face toward the sky, and your upper bones should be parallel to the ground. Pause here.

To return the barbell to the ground, jerk both your elbows backward, let the barbell "fall" until you catch it at arm's length near your hips. Then, bend your knees and lower the barbell slowly to the ground. Repeat for prescribed amount of repetitions.

YIN PHASE: Lowering the barbell to the ground.

YANG PHASE: Raising the barbell to your chest.

WHAT YOU ARE PRIMARILY WORKING: Everything.

WHOLISTIC NOTES: A key lift to enhance all athletic performance. There is not any aspect of the physical or mental bodies that are not challenged by this wonderful, classic movement. You must really visualize and practice to get this one. There is no machine in the world that comes close to duplicating the intricate, dynamic power of this beautiful lift.

CHAPTER 9

Cardio

The arrow had best not be loosely shot.

—HENRY DAVID THOREAU

COSMIC YANG NOT ONLY BUILDS power for you in the gym, it does the same in its Cardio component as well. To impart power into your Cardio fitness during this cycle, you will be doing my classic "Minutes Are Forever" interval workout, which I'll detail below. The next four weeks contain quite a few moments of high-intensity hurtin' during both your gym and Cardio workouts. Because of that, I want to make sure you know the WF warrior's way to cope with high-intensity workouts.

NATIVE ZEN

I once described Cardio training to a New Age magazine interviewer as "a form of native Zen." Why? Because the initial meditation instructions given by any good Zen teacher to new students is to have them pay attention to their breath and to their posture. Their instruction would continue along lines like this, "When random thoughts intrude upon your meditation on breath and posture, pull your attention back to the breath."

Does this sound familiar? It should. Breath and posture is the first Wholistic Fitness Lifestyle Principle (see page 27).

No better coaching counsel could be given for doing Cardio workouts as well. One moment of awareness is one moment of purity. The more consciously you follow your breath and pay attention to your posture, the more awareness you begin to live with. More awareness during Cardio workouts brings more and deeper meaning into other aspects of your life. You don't need to "do" anything extra to become more conscious. Just bring awareness to whatever you are already doing, especially during Cardio workouts.

Do you see how all increased fitness always returns, over and over again, to the shining basics? Do you understand why coaches are driven nuts when their athletes don't pay attention to "fundamentals"? What good is a fast midfielder in soccer if he or she can't control the ball? None. What good is it to become cardiovascularly fit if it doesn't make your life more meaningful and rich? None. So what if doing Cardio makes you live longer if you are just surviving instead of thriving?

The effort inherent in any Cardio workout turns into suffering only when your ego pulls you away from conscious attention to the moment. Return your awareness to the breath, for example, and suffering dissipates. The ego, which likes to attach to discomfort and drama, drowns in breath and posture awareness. Purity, perspective (which includes performance strategy), and most of all, peacefulness, thrives in it.

A few millennia ago Kottitha wrote:

> . . . *mind unruffled*
> *shaking distractions away*
> *like the wind-god*
> *scatters a few*
> *forest leaves.*

I've worked with a lot of elite Cardio athletes. Most are surprised, if not stunned, by my "unplugged," low-tech, Zen-based teachings. Here are well-known professional or Olympic-class athletes and I am adjusting their foot position as we stand in line together at the grocery market. I guess they think how they stand in line in the grocery store somehow doesn't count as a valid part of their training regime like, say, a Max VO2 (maximal oxygen consumption) test in the human performance lab. In Wholistic Fitness it sure does. How you do anything is how you do everything!

COACH ILG ON OBEDIENCE TRAINING

Paying attention to our breath and posture during Cardio workouts is at first like training a puppy. We must sharply yank the leash to bring an undisciplined, frolicking dog to heel. After enough yanks, the dog eventually understands it is better just to do what we want. Once the dog becomes disciplined, we no longer need the leash. We trust that our dog will come when commanded. The dog is now free to run and be "free" while other, less disciplined dogs must remain tethered to their leashes.

Trust and freedom can only be achieved through steady discipline and a wise, caring master. Do you have the self-discipline to become free? What is the leash that you use to discipline the unruly mind? In WF, we use Lifestyle Principle 1: Breath and Posture.

You only have one new Cardio workout in your Cosmic Yang training cycle. But it's a beauty. It's simple and powerful. I call it the "Minutes Are Forever" interval workout. Here is how you do it.

Pick any Cardio activity of choice. Then,

- Warm up for 10 to 20 minutes at Zone 1–2
    a. Go hard for 1 minute (Zone 3–4)
    b. Recovery pace for 1 minute
    c. Keep it up for 10 minutes: 1 minute "hard" followed by 1 minute "easy."
- After your tenth "hard" interval, recover for 10 minutes at Zone 1. Then, buckle up your warrior belt and
- Repeat A through C
- Cool down for 10 to 20 minutes at Zone 1.

CHAPTER 10

High Performance Yoga

I'VE DESIGNED A BEAUTIFUL HIGH Performance Yoga program for you to practice the next four weeks. It takes less time than the Green Tara, but packs a wallop of body/mind benefits. Before taking a look at your new Yoga poses for this cycle, I want to show you how to handle an issue that accompanies most people's experience with Yoga: emotional fallout.

TACTICAL IGNORANCE

Have you become an expert at shelving your doubt, anxiety, and confusion?

Do you have heartburn or stress that troubles you at night? Where do you think that stress goes? Do you think taking a sleeping or antidepressant pill magically erases the root of your anxiety?

Do you begin each day using a push-button program to override the residual stress? Wake up. Coffee. Shower. Bite to eat. Kids. Commute. Go through the motions at work. Maybe you find some relief to the automotion in your workout or Yoga class? If this sounds like you, don't feel bad. You are not alone.

These push-button programs that you play throughout the day are known in spiritual work as *tactical ignorance*. Like the word processing program in a computer, you become so entrenched in dealing with what Steven Covey calls "the thick of thin things," that you fail to appreciate the process of your life. Sometimes a crisis has to occur as a spiritual wake-up call to freeze your program, forcing you to reboot and find a fresh perspective.

Yoga heads off this eventual fallout by encouraging a slow but steady stream of released emotions from within the hidden tissues of your body.

EMOTIONAL FALLOUT

Don't be surprised if you find yourself "getting emotional" during these Yoga routines. It's a natural side effect from releasing the tension in your tissues. As you bravely breathe into all those nooks and crannies of your body, a whole new inner dialogue speaks up. This melting away of restricted muscles is what allows your hidden emotions to surface. I've cried, laughed, cursed, moaned, gasped, hyperventilated, astral-traveled, and slept during Yoga. I want you to welcome all emotions, but treat them like raindrops—let them fall upon you, but roll right off.

The manner in which Yoga filets your emotions may feel very raw at first. It's like, "Uh-oh, I don't want to go there!" as you lean into a hamstring stretch. But if you are willing enough not to run away from the pose and continue to relax into the stretch, a whole bunch of pent-up feelings may start coursing through you. Some of these feelings are frisky and seem excited to be set free. Other feelings are more recalcitrant and you need to breathe even more deeply into their release. Sometimes when tissue-stored emotions are granted liberty from whichever body part they've been hiding in, the intensity of their release is shocking. Sadness, annoyance, grief, fear, the smell of your grandparents' house—it's crazy what lies within. That is why the Yoga Masters teach us that the inner body is a microcosm of the entire universe. It's all right there, hidden in the stringy tautness of your illiotibial band or there, in the deep tendril of your adductor magnus. One of my favorite poems springs to mind, "The Clay Jug," from Kabir:

Inside this clay jug there are canyons and pine mountains,
and the maker of canyons and pine mountains!
All seven oceans are inside,
and hundreds of millions of stars.
The acid that tests gold is there,

and the one who judges jewels.
And the music from the strings that no one touches,
and the source of all water.

If you want the truth, I will tell you the truth:
Friend, listen: the God whom I love is inside.

—translated by Robert Bly

Mature Yoga practice requires resolution in a game of clever hide-and-seek played with the hidden knots and bands of tension in your body. Keep it a game. Never be ashamed of turbulent feelings that arise during a Yoga session. If doing a pose produces tears, there is no need to look around, feeling guilty and self-conscious, hoping nobody sees your emotional fallout. Your Yoga sessions are a haven for self-healing. In fact, feeling ashamed might well be what put tension there in the first place. Spiritual breakthroughs happen when you quit living your life based on the opinions of others. Consistent, high-quality Yoga practice helps teach you how to be true to yourself.

GETTING TO KNOW THE POSES

Here is your High Performance Yoga: Cosmic Yang practice. Any new postures that I did not cover in Chapter 3, Green Tara, are described here. Note how I have changed the choreography of your warmup (Sun Salutations). You are using the same series as in Chapter 3, but in a different format.

YOGA: THE COSMIC YANG PRACTICE

Begin by engaging ujjayi breathing (see page 83) and Mula Bandha. You can first gain access to Mula Bandha by contracting the urogenital muscles as if attempting to hold your bladder. Draw that contraction energy up and into the space between your hip bones. Holding that energy, relax any clutching of the gluteal muscles. This is tricky stuff and demands utmost concentration in the early years. Don't stop engaging these two "faithful companions"—ujjayi breathing and Mula Bandha—until Savasana, the final pose.

Begin by doing three rounds of the Half Sun Salutation, followed by two rounds of Series A Modified, followed by three rounds of Series A, followed by one round of Series B, followed by one round of Series C and then five rounds of Series A. You should have broken sweat and be totally focused by the end of this warmup.

Sun Salutation Warmup

> 3 x Ardha Surya Namaskar (Half Sun Salutation)
>
> 2 x Series A Modified
>
> 3 x Series A
>
> 1 x Series B (both legs = 1 set)
>
> 1 x Series C (both legs = 1 set)
>
> 5 x Series A

Then do these movements, holding each for 30 to 60 seconds. Focus the mind on ujjayi breathing and the root lock, Mula Bandha. As in the Green Tara, option poses are provided for you to grow into!

Adho Mukha Svanasana (Downward Facing Dog)

See Green Tara (page 99). You also do this pose in your Sun Salutations.

Option Pose: Vasisthasana (Name of a Sage)

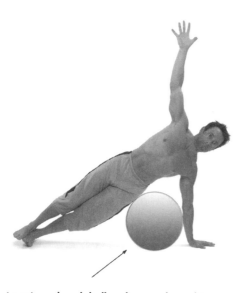

Imagine a beach ball under your lower hip.

It is best to come into this challenging one-arm, one-leg balancing pose by maintaining the strength of the legs in downward facing dog. Exhale and turn the feet, legs, and torso 90 degrees to the right. Stack the left foot, ankle, knee, and hip directly over the right foot, ankle, knee, and hip. Stretch your right arm along the right edge of your body. Breathe here.

Completely exhale, and bend your right leg. Capture the big toe with a yogic lock (see page 103). Breathe here.

Completely exhale and extend the right leg and right arm simultaneously. Breathe here.

Repeat for the other side.

WHAT YOU ARE PRIMARILY WORKING: Core strength and balance; hip flexibility; mental concentration; shoulder, arm, and hand strength.

WHOLISTIC NOTES: Imagine there is a big beach ball under your lowermost hip. Keep the torso lifting forward and the elevated leg should be lifted from the buttock. Don't be attached to the goal. Failure or success should never disturb the mind that is fluid with the process of life.

Malasana (Garland Pose)

Option Pose: Parsva Malasana (Lateral Garland Pose)

See Green Tara (page 104).

Utthita Hasta Padangusthasana (Extended Hand–Big Toe Pose)

Option Pose: One-Legged Squat

This is a fun standing balance pose with a challenging functional squat as an option. Stand in Tadasana (Mountain Pose, page 86). Exhale and come into a standing forward fold similar to Uttanasana (Extended Stretch Pose, see page 86). Move your left hand onto the left hip and catch the right big toe with a yogic lock (see page 103). Breathe here.

Inhale and raise your upper torso to perpendicular and simultaneously lift your right leg out in front of you, still using the yogic lock. Breathe here.

Exhale and turn your right leg out the side. This is Utthita Hasta Padangusthasana.

To do the one-legged squat option pose, exhale and draw the right leg back to center. The right foot is flexed 90 degrees and is still caught in the yogic lock. Reach your left arm out to the side for balance. Breathe here.

Exhale and bend your left left leg as deeply as you can, attempting to come into malasana (garland pose, see page 103) with your right leg extended in front of you. Stay in this "bottom pose" for several breaths.

Exhale and "blow yourself back up" until your left leg has become straight and extended once again. Release the yogic lock and allow the right leg to return to the ground.

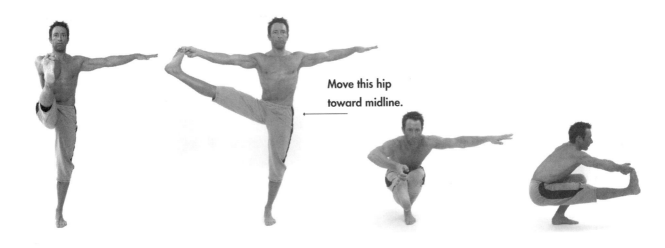

Move this hip
toward midline.

Repeat for other leg.

WHAT YOU ARE PRIMARILY WORKING: Leg and lower back strength, hip flexibility, and dynamic balance.

WHOLISTIC NOTES: This is a good pose to entice your friends into doing Yoga. When taking your captured (nonstanding) leg out to the side, roll its thigh bone outward. Keep your supporting foot soft, but strong. Keep your upper torso pulled upright but keep softening throughout the hips and waist.

Padangusthasana (Foot and Big Toe Pose)

Spread hip joints laterally.

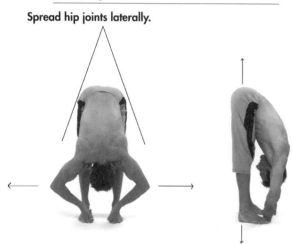

Stand in Tadasana (Mountain Pose, page 86), then exhale and bend forward from your lower back. Catch both big toes with your thumbs and first two fingers (this is the yogic lock, see page 103). Your palms face each other. Get a good grip and breathe here.

Inhale and reach your chest forward and up to make your back as concave as possible. Look gently about four feet in front of you. Keep your thighs strong and the legs extended.

Exhale, send your elbows out to the sides and pull your navel between your upper thighs. Use your arm strength and let your biceps bulge with the effort of pulling the crown of your head toward the ground between your feet. Breathe here for the required time, but keep the pose engaged the whole time.

WHAT YOU ARE PRIMARILY WORKING: Toning of the abdominal organs, stimulation of the digestive organs, hamstrings and lower back flexibility.

WHOLISTIC NOTES: This pose can really gain some needed "real estate" in your hamstrings and lower back. A wonderful way to treat lower back pain. But you must really prioritize getting that initial concavity to your spine before the exhale into the finish position. To create this concavity, stretch from your pelvis to reach the spine out of the hips.

Prasarita Padottanasana (Extended Foot Pose)

Assume a wide-legged stance, about 4½ or 5 feet wide, facing the long, left edge of your practice mat. Place your hands on your hips. Flex your thighs so your legs feel strongly connected to the ground. Make your spine as concave as possible.

Exhale, bend forward, and reach your hands under your legs with your palms on the floor, fingers facing the same direction as your toes.

Inhale, raise your chest, look forward, and make your spine as concave as possible.

Exhale and bend your elbows and reach them further in back of your legs than previously. Draw the crown of your head onto the ground. Breathe here for the required time.

WHAT YOU ARE PRIMARILY WORKING: Abductor muscles, hamstrings, and some of the benefits associated with Sirsasana (Headstand Pose, page 175).

WHOLISTIC NOTES: Keep pressuring the outer edges of your feet into the ground and don't allow the knees to bend. Keep lifting the kneecaps up your thighs. Work inwardly to "spread" each buttock away from the other to increase sacroiliac space.

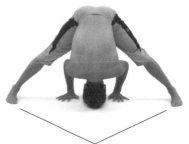

Turn toes in.

Fold from your hips.

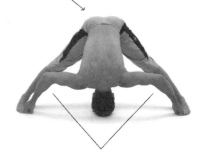

Pull up on big toes.

Utthita Trikonasana (Extended Triangle)

You did this pose in your Green Tara practice (see page 97). Remember to do both sides.

Parivrtta Trikonasana (Revolved Triangle Pose)

Assume the pose Utthita Trikonasana (Extended Triangle) with your right leg in front. Turn your trunk 180 degrees backward by drawing your left hip and left ribs forward to rest the left hand onto the ground beside the outer edge of your right foot. Extend the right arm into the air directly in line with the left arm. Face the palm of the right hand forward and gaze at your right thumb. Do both sides.

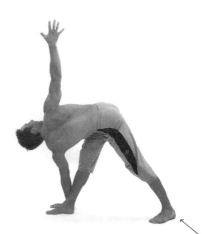

Find outer edge of this foot.

WHAT YOU ARE PRIMARILY WORKING: Balance, coordination, strengthening of hip and pelvic muscles, elongation of lumbar muscles; increases space and suppleness to the rib cage, rinses cleansing organs of toxins, deepens focus.

WHOLISTIC NOTES: Use the extended arm to create room for the ribcage to revolve toward the sky. Keep both feet firmly planted and use the rear foot to ignite lengthening throughout the spine. If the lower hand doesn't reach the ground beside the lead foot, place it on the ankle and use it to accentuate the spinal twist.

Adho Mukha Svanasana (Downward Facing Dog)

Step back to down dog for 2 minutes. (Down Dog is a commonly used abbreviation for Downward Facing Dog, page 99), which you are familiar with from the Sun Salutations. Here, however, you have two minutes to really use this pose as a recovery pose and to explore the pose more fully.

Dolphin Pose

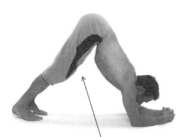

Keep thighs firm.

From downward facing dog, bend both elbows and lower onto your elbows and forearms. Your heels will elevate off the ground, which is fine, but keep your heels hidden behind your second toes. Then, interlace all your fingers except for the two smallest fingers, which should lie parallel to each other and pressed into your mat. Do not bring the wrists together. Do not allow the elbows to wander wide; instead, keep them securely positioned under your shoulders. Breathe here for the required time or do the options.

WHAT YOU ARE PRIMARILY WORKING: Central back strengthening; scapular flexibility; shoulder, arm, and hand strength and alignment; leg flexibility; endocrine system and cardiac health.

WHOLISTIC NOTES: This striking pose is really a preparatory posture for developing specific strength and balance for Sirsasana (Headstand Pose, see page 175). Instead of using wall and props to learn Sirsasana, it is best to develop the root strength and core balance by doing Dolphin Pose. Keep working the shoulders down the spine and maintain a soft facial expression.

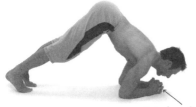

Interlace fingers.

Option Pose: Dolphin Levers

Not a classic yoga posture, but a superb strength and endurance builder for Sirsasana (see next option). From Dolphin Pose, inhale and "lever" your chin forward and beyond your hands.

Exhale, pressure your elbows into the ground to help draw your head back to standard Dolphin Pose.

Repeat this cycle of inhale-lever-out, exhale-return-to-Dolphin-Pose 15 times.

WHAT YOU ARE PRIMARILY WORKING: Same as Dolphin Pose, with an added dimension of strength endurance.

WHOLISTIC NOTES: Trust the breath and flow, baby! This is a wonderful movement for females who might be lacking upper body strength endurance and a great movement for males who might be really restricted throughout the shoulders and upper back.

Option pose: *Sirsasana* (Headstand Pose)

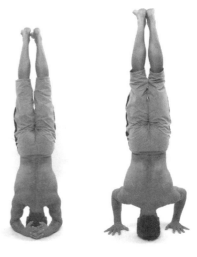

Caution: Do not attempt Sirsasana until you can comfortably perform Halasana (Plow Pose, see page 105) for at least 5 minutes and feel comfortable with both Dolphin Pose and Dolphin Levers. If you get dizzy or see spots while attempting Sirsasana, come down and try again another day. If the dizziness or spots continue, contact an experienced Yoga teacher or other health counsel.

From Dolphin Pose, position the crown of your head into the cradle of space created between your hands. Walk your feet toward your face until your trunk is nearly perpendicular to the ground. If there is a growing amount of uncomfortable pressure on your neck or head, do not continue. Keep pressing the outer edges of your forearms down to alleviate any pressure on your neck. Breathe here. Hanging out in this phase could require several months.

Inhale, activate Mula Bandha, and lift the legs up to vertical. Create space between your shoulders and ears by depressing your shoulder blades. Relax your face. Press the balls of your feet toward the sky and spread your toes. Breathe here evenly for the required time.

WHAT YOU ARE PRIMARILY WORKING: Everything, which is exactly why Sirsasana is known as the king of all asanas. Stimulation of the brain cells, pituitary and pineal glands begin to bring balance to mental and emotional activity while improving the quality of sleep. Respiratory fitness and immunity is increased and the awakening of Ajna and Sahasrara chakras restores intuitive wisdom, clear thinking, and higher intelligence.

WHOLISTIC NOTES: Steady the head and arms with smooth ujjayi breathing. The integrity of this pose should reflect the same qualities as in Tadasana (Mountain Pose, see page 86). Stretch the sides of the body upward to create lightness and balance.

Plank Pose

You have become quite familiar with Plank Pose (page 87) from your Series A Modified Sun Salutations. Do for 10 breaths.

Option pose: "Ilgaranda" Push-ups

I'll describe this in four stages.

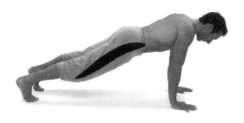

Stage 1: Plank Pose to Chaturanga.

Exhale and lower your torso down to the floor from plank pose by bending both elbows. As you lower yourself toward the ground, draw your elbows back and in, that is, toward your feet and ribs. Stop lowering once your upper arm bones are parallel to the ground. This is the popular version of Chaturanga Dandasana, the Four-Limbed Staff Pose (see photo).

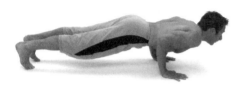

Stage 2: Lever Out

Inhale and while holding Chaturanga position, lever out onto your tippy toes (see photo).

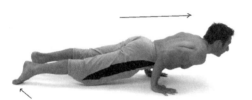

Stage 3: Scoot Back

Exhale and while still holding the Chaturanga position, scoot back onto the balls of both feet and return to the stationary Chaturanga Dandasana Position (see photo). (Note: This levering out and scooting back is the traditional Chaturanga.)

Ooooh!

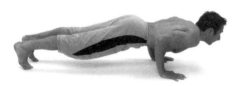

Stage 4: Push to Plank

Inhale and push yourself up to plank pose. Repeat Stages 1–4 as prescribed.

I refer to doing Stages 1 through 4 as "Ilgarandas"—actually my yoga students came up with the name and it seems to have stuck.

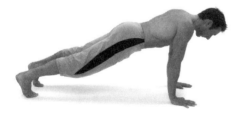

WHAT YOU ARE PRIMARILY WORKING: Strength endurance and pain threshold.

WHOLISTIC NOTES: I use this a lot in my classes as a prefatigue movement so that the ego gets tired and quits being so boisterous. After doing a few of them, you will know what I mean. Important to go with the flow and focus on keeping the elbows tight to the sides of your body.

Option Pose: Pincha Mayurasana (Peacock Pose)

Assume the Dolphin Pose (page 174). Unlock your fingers and press your palms into your mat. Spread your fingers wide to increase your support base for the pose. Make sure your hands are in line with your elbows and your elbows are no wider than your shoulders. Walk your feet toward your elbows until your torso is nearly perpendicular to the ground. Breathe here.

Exhale and lift or kick gently your right leg overhead, followed quickly by your left. Stabilize. Don't be too quick to move the ankles and knees together. Press the balls of both feet toward the sky. Create space between the shoulders and ears by depressing your shoulder blades down the spine. Gaze steadily between your forearms.

Spread fingers wide.

WHAT YOU ARE PRIMARILY WORKING: Strengthens the shoulders and arms, stretches the respiratory diaphragm and intercostal muscles. Elongates the abdominal connective tissue to prepare for advanced back-bending postures. Centers and calms chattering minds. Develops core strength and balance. Overcomes doubt and depression.

WHOLISTIC NOTES: Curl the tip of your sacrum toward your groin once you are balanced. Never stop pressing the forearms down to lift the upper arms and shoulders. Let the power of your feet pull you into lightness and steadiness.

> Before moving on to the final four postures, do Series A for 3 to 5 rounds then drop into Child's Pose for 1 minute. This strong flow sequence is placed here to regain some internal heat. I doubt that you have forgotten what Child's Pose is, but if needed refer to page 100.

Paschimottanasana (Intense Western Stretch)

You have done this pose in Green Tara's yoga routine (page 103). Do it now for 2 minutes, which will allow you to merge deeply into yourself.

Arkana Dhanurasana (Shooting Bow Pose)

From a sitting position with both legs extended in front and being held with a yogic lock (page 103), exhale and draw the right toe toward the right ear by bending the right elbow. Keep extending the left leg down into your mat. Breathe here (see photo).

Exhale and extend the right leg as vertically as you are able (see photo). Keep breathing and making the right leg more vertical during the required time before lowering it to the ground. Repeat for other leg.

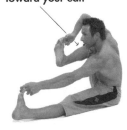

Draw big toe toward your ear.

Spin your heart skyward.

WHAT YOU ARE PRIMARILY WORKING: Pelvic alignment, hip flexibility, leg suppleness, abdominal strength, lower back tonality.

WHOLISTIC NOTES: This pose was a breakthrough for me in overcoming my spinal injury. I recall the morning well. I was fooling around with it while in the hot tub of my California condominium, which was a necessary practice just to alleviate the pain in those days (not too long ago). The heated waters mixed with my steady years of limited asana practice and was topped off by doing this pose in that heated water. As I held the pose on my right side, breathing, listening, playing my edge, suddenly pop! A huge adjustment deep within my lower back occurred. I saw stars, man. A rush of cerebral spinal fluid and some prana charged up my spine. Since that morning, my chronic back pain from my spine injury has steadily decreased. After that day, I've no longer needed any aspirin or ibuprofen and certainly no lower back surgery. Arkana Dhanurasana shot a healing arrow right into my lower back pain and the Light of Yoga was illuminated for me in a very beautiful and significant way.

Option Pose: Eka Hasta Bhujasana (One-Handed Arm Pose)

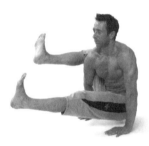

From a sitting position with both legs extended in front, exhale and bend your right knee. Using your arms to help the process, tuck your right shoulder under your right knee. Once the right knee is situated high on the right shoulder, place your palms down on the ground beside each hip. Breathe here.

Exhale and lift your whole body off the ground and balance. Breathe here. This is Eka Hasta Bhujasana. Repeat for other leg.

WHAT YOU ARE PRIMARILY WORKING: Shoulder, arm, and abdominal (core) strength.

WHOLISTIC NOTES: Flex the ankles to draw your toes toward you; this helps activate Mula Bandha and brings your center of gravity closer to the midline, allowing the balance issue to become a little easier.

Marichyasana I (Seated Sage Twist 1)

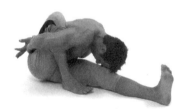

Sit on the ground with your legs extended in front of you. Bend your right knee, bring your right heel close to your groin and plant all four corners of your right foot on your mat. The shin of the right leg should be perpendicular to the ground. Stiffen your left leg and make your mid spine concave.

Exhale and turn your right arm around the right shin as you hook your right forearm against your middle back with your right palm facing backward. Bring your left hand behind your back and capture the right hand with the left. Breathe here as you finagle your grip.

Inhale and stretch your spine upward. Exhale and twist your spine to the right, gazing at your left leg. Breathe here.

Find an easy exhale and bend forward from the lower spine to rest your nose and chin on the shin of the left leg. Pressure the back of the left leg down by firmly flexing the left foot toward your head. Keep your shoulders square and breathe smoothly. Hold for prescribed time then repeat for other side.

WHAT YOU ARE PRIMARILY WORKING: Grip strength, better blood circulation to the abdominal organs, hip and shoulder flexibility.

WHOLISTIC NOTES: Don't rebel, accept your inner tension by relaxing. Roll the shoulders back. Move your upper torso and head forward.

Option Pose: Marichyasana III (Seated Sage Twist 3)

This dastardly spinal twist tends to entwine more than just your spine—it entwines your mind as well.

First, establish the twist: Sit on the ground with your legs extended in front of you. Bend your right knee, bring your right heel close to your groin and plant all four corners of your right foot on your mat. The shin of the right leg should be perpendicular to the ground. Stiffen your left leg and make your mid spine concave.

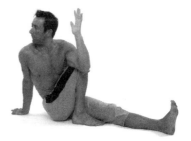

Exhale and turn your left elbow in front of your right knee, keeping your left forearm perpendicular to the ground as if you were making a salute (see photo). Work the left elbow against the right knee to act as a lever to deepen the twist to your internal organs. Press your right fingers into the ground to accentuate the twist. If you are getting tense or a lot of a sensation here, then stay here. If you are relaxed and breathing smoothly, proceed.

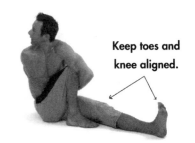

Keep toes and knee aligned.

Now, exhale and bend the left arm around the right shin in an inward rotation of the left humerus (upper arm bone). This may be quite a moment for some of you, as it was (still is) for me. Keep inwardly rotating your left upper arm bone as you reach your right arm behind your back by bending the right elbow and capturing the gamely struggling left hand.

Turn your head and gaze over your right shoulder with soft eyes. To intensify the twist, move your hands away from your spine.

WHAT YOU ARE PRIMARILY WORKING: Big-time squeezing and thus detoxification of the liver, intestines, kidneys, and spleen. Lower back pain will be greatly reduced if not erased once this pose is accomplished. Shoulders become free and the size of the abdominal cavity is reduced.

WHOLISTIC NOTES: This pose was a real button pusher for me. Iyengar, the most prolific modern Hatha Yoga Master, promised freedom from "splitting backaches, lumbago and pain in the hips" if I did this pose. Sign me up, I thought. It took me one year to do this pose, practicing it at least two times per week. Iyengar's promise was not broken. This pose, difficult as it was for me, greatly eased my chronic back pain and proved to be yet another gateway into more seductive, advanced poses.

Salamba Sarvangasana (Supported All-Parts Pose)

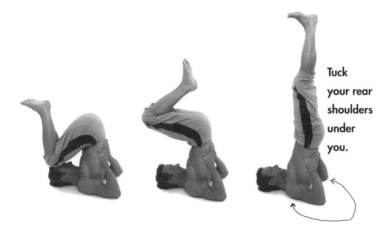

Tuck your rear shoulders under you.

An important, highly medicinal pose that must be executed safely. Let's take it in three specific stages, and I'll omit the wholistic notes in exchange for this specificity.

Stage 1: Liftoff

Assume a supine position on the ground and extend your arms beside you, at your sides, palms facing down. Bend your knees to draw both heels close to your buttocks. Exhale, press your fingertips against the ground, and raise your torso and legs simultaneously. Keep your knees bent and aim them for a spot over your forehead. Quickly bring your palms onto your lower back to support your legs and torso overhead (see photo).

Stage 2: Stabilization

With your knees still bent, raise your torso and hips closer to your chin. Keep the chin slightly away from your collarbone. Work your hands downward, closer to your armpits. Increase the pressure of your elbows against your mat. Your thumbs should be placed on the side ribs, and your fingers press the back ribs toward the spine (see photo). Breathe here.

Caution: If you start experiencing any pressure in the neck, head, ears, eyes, or throat, come down and try again another day. If these symptoms persist, spend some extra time refining your Adho Mukha Svanasana (Downward Facing Dog, see page 99) until your body adapts to this pose.

Stage 3: Extending the Legs

Exhale and straighten your legs toward the sky until they are vertical. Press your hands deeper into your back as you move your sternum toward the chin. Relax your face and work on steadying your entire body (see photo).

When you have completed your prescribed time in the pose, slowly bend your knees toward your forehead. Exhale and straighten both legs and reach your toes to the ground behind your head as in Halasana (Plow Pose, page 105). Breathe here.

Exhale and take your hands from your lower back and clasp your two fingers around your two big toes using a yogic lock (page 103). Slowly, and keeping your legs straight, roll your upper spine down onto the ground, then the middle spine, and finally the lower spine, all the while keeping your legs close to your torso.

Exhale and squeeze both knees into your chest with your hands. Breathe here before finally relaxing and extending your legs to lie in a supine position.

WHAT YOU ARE PRIMARILY WORKING: Nearly all the benefits of Sirsasana (Headstand, page 175) with even more beneficial influence upon the glands of the thyroid and parathyroid. Blood flow to the heart, neck, and skull is increased, and as a result, headaches, insomnia, mood swings, depression, irregular heartbeats, and hypertension disappear. Since your abdominal organs are inverted, their attachments grow stronger, enhancing their function, so that digestion and elimination problems evaporate. These are but a few of the curative effects from learning this pose, but you can see why the ancient Masters referred to this nurturing, soothing posture as the "Mother of All Asana." Its name means "All Parts" because the pose heals "all parts" of the body.

Option Pose: Eka Pada Sarvangasana *(One-Legged All-Parts Pose)*

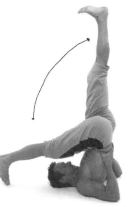

From Salamba Sarvangasana, exhale and float your right leg down to the ground until all five toes of your right foot touch the ground behind your head. Keep both legs strongly extended. Reach the left heel away from the right to ensure maximum height and length of the left leg. Breathe here for prescribed time.

Exhale and raise your right leg to meet the left one overhead. Breathe here, and then repeat for other leg.

When both legs have been trained and brought together overhead, slowly bend your knees toward your forehead. Exhale and straighten both legs and reach your toes to the ground behind your head as in Halasana (Plow Pose, page 105). Breathe here.

Exhale and take your hands from your lower back and clasp your two fingers around your two big toes using a yogic lock (page 103). Slowly, and keeping your legs straight, roll your upper spine down onto the ground, then the middle spine, and finally the lower spine, all the while keeping your legs close to your torso.

Exhale and squeeze both knees into your chest with your hands. Breathe here before finally relaxing and extending your legs to lie in a supine position.

WHAT YOU ARE PRIMARILY WORKING: All the benefits of the preceding pose, Salamba Sarvangasana, with more direct work on the digestive organs and kidneys. More skill coordination is required as well.

WHOLISTIC NOTES: Keep both thighs firm and extend your hips. The leg that is held perpendicular should maintain a clean, vertical line. Press the ball of the foot of the higher leg into the sky.

Savasana (Corpse Pose)

Do this pose from the finish of the Green Tara program (see page 108) for 5 to 20 minutes.

YOGA: THE COSMIC YANG PRACTICE

Begin by engaging ujjayi breathing (see page 83) and don't stop ujjayi until savasana, at the end of the session.

2 x Series A Modified

3 x Series A

1 x Series B (both legs = 1 set)

1 x Series C

5 x Series A

Then do these movements, holding each for 30 to 60 seconds. Focus the mind on ujjayi breathing and Mula Bandha (see page 169).

1. Adho Mukha Svanasana (Downward Facing Dog, page 99)
   Option Pose: Vasisthasana (page 170)

2. Jump into Malasana (Garland Pose, page 103)
   Option Pose: Parsva Malasana (page 104)

3. Utthita Hasta Padangusthasana (Extended Hand–Big Toe Pose, page 171)
   Option Pose: One-Legged Squat (page 171)

4. Padangusthasana (Foot and Big Toe Pose, page 172)

5. Prasarita Padottanasana (Extended Foot Pose, page 173)

6. Utthita Trikonasana (Extended Triangle, page 97)

7. Parivrtta Trikonasana (Revolved Triangle Pose, page 173)

8. Down Dog (page 99)

9. Dolphin Pose (page 174)
   Option Pose: 15 Dolphin Levers (page 174)
   Option Pose: Sirsasana (Headstand Pose, page 175)

10. Plank Pose (page 87)

   Option Pose: 5 Ilgaranda Push-ups (page 176)

   Option Pose: Pincha Mayurasana (Peacock Pose, page 177)

11. Series A and Child's Pose (page 100)

12. Paschimottanasana (Western Extended Stretch, page 103)

13. Arkana Dhanurasana (Shooting Bow Pose, page 177)

   Option Pose: Eka Hasta Bhujasana (One-Hand Arm Pose, page 178)

14. Marichyasana I (Seated Sage Twist 1, page 178)

   Option Pose: Marichyasana III (Seated Sage Twist 3, page 179)

15. Salamba Sarvangasana (Supported All-Parts Pose, page 180)

   Option Pose: Eka Pada Sarvangasana (One-Legged All-Parts Pose, page 181)

16. Savasana (Corpse Pose, page 108)

CHAPTER 11

Meditation

THE COSMIC YANG PHASE BRINGS three new Meditation practices: Rasa Eating Exercise; Beeper Guru: Smiling; and Early Morning Cleaning Ritual. The combined impact of these specific meditations at this point in your training will empower your self-realization like never before.

Coming into this phase, your mental training has begun to mature through your zazen sessions. You've had four weeks of realizing the difference paying attention can make—to anything! Cosmic Yang Yoga, Strength, and Cardio workouts are designed to dwindle your ego away, thus clearing verbal and symbolic thinking enough so that a ripeness for spiritual experience is at hand.

Before I describe your specific Meditation practices for this cycle, I want to congratulate you for doing this Meditation stuff. Of all my WF disciplines, getting people to slow down their minds—even for a few minutes each day—represents high challenge for me as a body/mind teacher. For those of you who have now been sitting the zazen, studying your mind, you know how apparent the busyness of your mind actually is. Some of you may have also realized that you pay attention much less than you think. Phillip Kapleau, author of the classic book *The Three Pillars of Zen,* comments that, "For the ordinary man, whose mind is a checkerboard of crisscrossing reflections, opinions, and prejudices, bare attention is virtually impossible; his life is thus centered not on reality itself but in his ideas about it." When Kapleau used the phrase "bare attention," he was using it in its Buddhist sense, which means training yourself to pay attention to what is. I remember reading that the actress Goldie Hawn said that to keep her personal and family life centered in such a chaotic occupation she had to stay focused on enjoying the smaller things in life because "Tiny moments are everything."

In this cycle, you will be doing Meditation assignments that can transform mundane duties—cooking, cleaning, eating—into forms of inner guidance. Your tiny moments will become clearer and sharper, and at the same time each of those tiny moments may seem to expand. If I can get you to expand your moments, I will have set you free to create more spaciousness within. From that inner spaciousness your clouds of hectic thinking will disappear and the cornerstone of your spiritual life, awareness, will be established.

Over the next four weeks, I would like you to work on accepting everyone and every circumstance as your guru. See what each person or situation is trying to teach you in terms of sensitivity and mindfulness. Wholistic Fitness means using your exercise as a vehicle for spiritual growth, and cultivating mindfulness keeps us from being swept away by thoughts, emotions, fantasies, reactions. Those who do not work on themselves long for escape from being human, that is, feeling pain, dealing with dragons, fully experiencing simple joys, tiny moments. Cosmic Yang teaches you to go into your humanity to become more whole and more awake human beings—instead of human doings.

BEEPER GURU: SMILING

Last cycle, I introduced you to the Beeper Guru to help you pay attention to your Breath and Posture. This cycle will have you work with the Beeper Guru in another, even more simple, manner—smiling!

Thich Nhat Hanh, the Dalai Lama, Christian mystics, Sufi teachers, modern psychologists, physicians—you name the Master and the prescription is sincere and well proven: Just smiling more often bestows a surfeit of transpersonal growth, physiologic health, and spiritual progress. Smiling is one of the most effective ways to return to the body from the compulsive mind and overactive egocentric behavior.

Be not afraid, Noble Warrior, to smile more often and for no good reason! A tremendous ally will be found in the smile that too frequently remains chained in tension from the deluded ego mind. Here is how to do the Beeper Guru Smiling assignment.

Beeper Guru: Smiling

(a nonformal Meditation aid)

As in the earlier Beeper Guru (page 112), set an alarm to *Beep* every hour. Really dedicated warriors can set it to go off every fifteen minutes. But don't do any more than once every fifteen minutes or the exercise loses potency.

Upon hearing the beeper (or realizing the trigger) do this: *Smile!*

Early Morning Cleaning Ritual

(a formal Meditation assignment)

1. Wake up, relieve yourself.

2. Sit zazen for 25 conscious breaths. Switch leg position and sit zazen for another 25 conscious breaths.

3. Taking zazen mind with you, sweep the floor of a chosen room or area (kitchen, patio, hallway). Then, holding two wet cloths, assume a yoga squat (like malasana, page xxx) and clean the floor with them. Keep your mind with the cleaning. When attention wanders from the cleaning, bring it back to it. See page 272 for an "action shot" of me doing this ritual.

4. Carefully rinse out the cloths, and place them in your laundry hamper to end your session.

After this assignment, reflect on how blessed you are at having shelter, water to clean with, and floors to walk on. Appreciate everything that usually goes unappreciated. This ritual should take no longer than fifteen minutes; move mindfully.

THE RASA EATING EXERCISE

In Indian philosophy there is a wonderful word that is rich with complex meanings. The word is "rasa" and from what I gather, the closest translation would be "taste," as in "Can you taste of the essence of an ocean breeze?" However, a better, more fundamental interpretation of this word might be "juice" or "marrow" or "sap." Rasa is the quality that defines a thing's most essential nature. When you comprehend the rasa of food, for example, you experience the intricacies of sweetness, or astringency, or saltiness. To reach this deeper understanding, one must remain present and conscious while eating; then a connection can be made with the marrow of any food in the present moment.

Discovering rasa is cultivating the art of finding the "juice" of everything. Think here of holding and breathing into a yoga pose, for example. Discovering the rasa of a yoga pose is to savor its vital sap as you unlock the keys toward balance and counterbalance, between extension and flexion.

The Rasa Eating Exercise is best done during one meal where you are alone and not likely to be interrupted, at least for several minutes.

1. Before eating a meal, take a quiet moment to look at the food. Close your eyes and clear your mind. Open your eyes and take in the sight before you. Feel a moment of intense gratefulness for another amazing meal that has been provided just for you by the complex efforts and energies of countless works of nature and humans. If you are consuming a flesh food at this meal, give an extra amount of appreciation for the being that gave its entire life to fuel your own life for just a few more hours.

2. Pick up the food with your hands or eating utensil and pay attention to the touching of the food. As the food passes your lips, practice eating quietly, noting the food's texture, firmness, temperature, smell, and moisture.

3. Listen to the food as you chew. Are the sounds soft, crunchy, rhythmic, slurping? Note if you have a tendency to lunge or suck at the food.

4. Experiment with slowing down or chewing more thoroughly. While slowing down your eating, fully engage your sense of taste. Seek the various flavors: sour, sweet, spicy, pungent, aromatic, astringent. Discover which tastes dominate and which psychological sensations arise as you chew.

5. After a few more moments of this exercise, resume your normal eating pattern. You may find that you enjoy this notion of slowing down and mindfully appreciating your food. And as you tune up your rasa cultivation, you may discover that what you thought you were hungry for wasn't really hunger at all, but rather an addictive characteristic or emotional craving.

When you start maturing your connection with Rasa Eating Exercise, you may find yourself making changes in your eating behavior without special effort or force. Just bringing awareness to what we do often gives birth to a natural process of transformation.

At higher levels of WF studies, the WF master student uses eating awareness to remain clear and present within all of the senses. This simple exercise imparts two teachings, the wonderful rediscovery of the depths of nutrition by all our senses and the idea of eating consciously. Rasa Eating Exercise is a practice of mindfulness and appreciation.

Nutrition

D URING THE GREEN TARA PROGRAM, one of the things I asked you to work on in your Nutrition understanding was to consider Nutrition in two forms: physical and spiritual. I told you that Nutrition nourishes you in three ways: what you put into and on yourself (physical nutrition), and what you put around you (spiritual nutrition). According to this WF perspective, you know now that your thoughts, hobbies, occupation, entertainment, relationships, and your skin care are all forms of Nutrition. I've broadened your perspective of Nutrition from things that can only be measured in grams and ounces to an all-inclusive acceptance of everything under the sun. Your highest workout in Nutrition, therefore, is to continuously scan your internal and external environment and ask, "How is this nourishing me?"

During Cosmic Yang, I want you to keep learning and practicing all the tools I gave you in Green Tara. It is important to stabilize the more yin elements of WF training quickly. That is, I want your Nutrition and Meditation disciplines to reach a base pattern of consistency as soon as possible. I am not to changing any of the diet guidelines given in Chapter 5.

Philosophically, however, I want to prepare you to deal with some emotional fallout from my program that usually starts right about now, when students enter my second training cycle. WF starts pushing emotional buttons when it comes to Nutrition because although mine is not a hard-core vegan approach, it is a vegetarian-based one. In other words, eating WF style means making a conscious effort to eat raw, whole, and plant foods over dairy, flesh, and engineered or processed (junk) foods. For optimal training, go back and reread Chapter 5. This will reinforce and provide more depth to the material below.

TEN VIRTUES OF THAT WHICH NOURISHES

It is said that knowledge is power. In regard to our national obsession with junk food and weight-loss diets, it is marketing, not self-knowledge, that is holding highest power. Using enough glitzy advertising, a cleverly spun book or celebrity-endorsed infomercial, and an entrepreneur can make millions out of a relatively insignificant micro nutrient or some strange diet plan. It happens all the time. A miracle diet or an energy supplement, when enthusiastically embraced by a celebrity, is an easy sell compared to cultivation of conscious awareness. It's a reflection of our materialistic mentality that we only associate "good" Nutrition with tangible things like pills and powders.

How then do you learn to limit inaccurate, degenerative Nutrition and emphasize accurate, regenerative Nutrition? By listening to your food choices and seeing if they match up with the following ten virtues of Wholistic Fitness Nutrition.

Each time you make a choice in Nutrition, be it food, drink, or vibration (music, media, self-talk, word choice, skin care), see if it has these qualities. I will give an example of each, but there are many other examples that each virtue commands, so use your creativity as you contemplate the list.

> ### YOGA OF NUTRITION
>
> From B.K.S. Iyengar's introduction in his book, *Light on Yoga:*
> "Character is moulded by the type of food we take and by how we eat it. Men are the only creatures that eat when not hungry and generally live to eat rather than eat to live. If we eat for flavours of the tongue, we over-eat and so suffer from digestive disorders which throw our systems out of gear. The yogi believes in harmony, so he eats for the sake of sustenance only. He does not eat too much or too little. He looks upon his body as the rest-house of his spirit and guards himself against over-indulgence."

TEN VIRTUES OF WHOLISTIC FITNESS NUTRITION

1. If Used Regularly, It Does No Harm

I am going to use herbs to illustrate this virtue. In ancient China, herbs came classified in three categories: utility, royal, and toxic. Utility herbs are associated with the spices with which we are familiar: dill, sage, paprika, etc. They have little nutritive value but add taste to certain foods. Eating too much of them would make you sick, however. Toxic or medicinal herbs are those herbs intended to be consumed acutely for a short period of time to help balance an imbalance or illness in the body. These herbs, such as guarana, are commonly found in many inferior herbal "pep pills." Derivatives of toxic herbs are also used in prescription and illegal drugs. Such herbs were never intended be eaten regularly.

In between the utility and toxic herbs are the royal herbs, so called because temple physicians of ancient China fed the emperor large amounts of such herbs every day to ensure his longevity and energy. If you have ever wondered why the Chinese know so much about herbs, it goes back several thousand years to these imperial herbologists whose heads would be lost if the emperor got sick. Keeping him as healthy as possible was their only job and life security. You can imagine how well they did their research! Royal herbs, also known as "food grade" herbs, are the only herbs that should be eaten daily.

2. It Feels Better the Longer It Is Used

Like your favorite pair of jeans, good Nutrition choices should only feel better and better as the years go by. Whole foods and herbs are intended to saturate the body over a period of months and even years in order to affect health and balance in your organ systems. An example that comes to my mind is rice, particularly Basmati rice. The smooth, rich, woody aroma of Basmati cooking in my rice cooker during the day fills my home and soul with appreciation and joy. I never tire of combining Basmati with other food; it enhances and elevates the taste and nutrition of so many of my favorite dishes.

3. When It Is Limited in Supply, It Still Pleases a Lot

Think here of springtime flowers in a high alpine meadow. You know that the summers up here are brief, which makes the dancing hummingbirds and explosion of high country color all the more poignant. So nourishing has such nature been to me, I feel such an image might be my dying thought. What do think will be yours? What has nourished you deeply in your life, although its supply was limited?

4. When It Is Abundant, One Never Tires of It

Your loved one. Sun. Showers. Flush toilets. Money. Health. Peace. Presence of God/Good.

5. When Chaotic, It Brings Calmness

6. When Lethargic, It Brings Energy

Wholesome Nutrition—things like whole foods, herbs, breathing, meditation, and exercise—are adaptogenic. If you are stressed, wholesome Nutrition calms you. If you are lethargic, wholesome Nutrition gives you energy. If your nervous system is agitated, an herbal tea such as chamomile, a few moments of breathing or meditation, or going out for a run will soothe and calm you. The glands responsible for pumping stress hormones such as adrenaline are countered through the adaptogenic qualities of wholesome Nutrition. Amazingly, if you are feeling lethargic and you take those same forms of Nutrition, you feel more energetic. Unwholesome Nutrition, on the other hand—such as sodas, meat, fatty foods, processed foods, lack of conscious breathing, tension, and lack of exercise—does not have adaptogenic qualities.

7. It Is Refreshing to Body and Mind

8. In Solitude, It Is an Uplifting Companion

Consider: A candlelit hot bath. A cup of tea. A good book. A fresh salad. A walk.
Now consider: A fast-food burger. A soda. A bag of chips. Watching TV.

9. It Removes Unwholesomeness

Do you remember in Chapter 5 when I taught you about how certain cleansing foods help remove bacteria and sluggishness from the digestive system? Nature intended to support wholesomeness. Nature knows that "united we stand, divided we fall." So why choose Nutrition that is divided, isolated, and unwhole? Eating wholesome foods and choosing wholesome spiritual Nutrition eventually purges the unnatural urges and cravings that you have for unnatural and unwholesome things. I remember quite vividly how eating concentrated herbal whole foods gradually erased my lifelong addiction to Diet Coke. My compulsion to drink that stuff gradually eased out of my mind as I kept eating the herbs. Within a few weeks, I lost the addiction. I have seen the same shift occur in dozens of my students. Cigarettes? Gone. Coffee? Gone. Doughnuts, cakes, beer—I have seen them all fall away from students' lifestyles when they just fed their body/mind wholesome forms of Nutrition.

10. It Encourages Spiritual Appreciation

Last night Kathy made a beautiful organic salad, baked salmon with rice, and steamed vegetables. We sipped Australian merlot as I joined her in the kitchen to chat about our day and remark on how beautiful the meal was becoming. I admired her sexy, fit body as she swayed to and fro cutting, slicing, chopping, and stirring. In her slight movements there was great poetry, in her lean muscles were years of self-respect, and seeing this I fell in love with her all over again. The sounds of cooking interrupted my reverie and with them arrived scents of garlic, onion, and gomasio. Soon, we carried the steaming dishes to our low mealtime table. I exchanged our wine for tea and lit a few more candles. Seated cross-legged before the wood table, we looked into each other's eyes, then around our peaceful home, and joined hands for our sacred pause. I asked aloud, "Could this moment be any more wealthy?" Making wise Nutrition choices, physical and nonphysical, invites many such simple but powerful moments of spiritual appreciation. Once Nutrition is truly mastered, prayer is no longer obligatory, it is just natural.

LIGHTNESS

Read through the ten virtues again:

1. If used regularly, it does no harm.

2. It feels better the longer it is used.

3. When it is limited in supply, it still pleases a lot.

4. When it is abundant, one never tires of it.

5. When chaotic, it brings calmness.

6. When lethargic, it brings energy.

7. It is refreshing to body and mind.

8. In solitude, it is an uplifting companion.

9. It removes unwholesomeness.

10. It encourages spiritual appreciation.

Whole foods meet these criteria. So do forms of spiritual Nutrition such as mantra, positive self-talk, politeness, meditation, volunteering, and fitness workouts.

Can you say the same about degenerative, processed foods such as fast foods, cigarettes, or energy pills? Does gossip, car addiction, television, rudeness, or a sedentary lifestyle meet these virtues? Anything that does not meet these virtues should be considered medicinal, or toxic (same thing), and as such should be used only acutely, not chronically.

WF is not an omnipotent, strict presence scowling over your shoulder to see if you are being "bad." WF is not about counting your fat points with your carbohydrate points or whether or not you are eating in some mathematically calibrated "zone." Don't drain the spiritual beauty from Nutrition. That's what screwed you up in the first place. You got lost in the muck of too much input.

During this cycle, I want you to get Real with your Nutrition again. Feel the beauty of your foods. Nutrition is your lifelong companion and guide. Your Nutrition provides Lightness and a Higher way—whenever you choose to see it as such.

CHAPTER 13

Daily Practice

HERE IS YOUR SECOND CYCLE of Wholistic Fitness training. This is the chapter that pulls together the preceding five chapters and packages it for you in a day-by-day schedule that will deliver you your next level of amazing body/mind fitness!

All the following workouts have been cross-referenced to the appropriate chapters we've just covered in here and in Part One. I've put page numbers next to each movement and technique for easy cross-referencing.

Practice reminders:

Don't stress if unable to do all the workouts for that day. Do your priority disciplines if possible. Remember, you are still living a WF lifestyle if you can't do anything but eat consciously and in alignment with WF guidelines or even working your Breath and Posture. Don't think WF is just about doing gym or yoga or cardio workouts.

Don't try to make up missed workouts by cramming several workouts into the next day. Instead, just keep flowing through the week. You've got your whole life to become wholistically fit.

Consistency comes first, sequencing comes second. I've choreographed the fitness disciplines in the order that provides the optimal training effect. However, if you need to switch the order, you can.

Good luck, noble warrior! Train hard, choose softness, and most of all, be sincere in your effort.

THE COSMIC YANG DAILY PRACTICE

Wholistic fitness training precepts

1. Be prepared

2. Be on time

3. Give 110 percent

Monday. Recovery and Scheduling Weekly Workouts

Mondays are traditional WF recovery days, no physical workouts today.

Focus on your work while giving your body time to prepare for the upcoming training week.

Sometime today, go to your schedule book and block out the time needed to do your workouts each day. Mentally prepare for your training week, and learn from the prior week: Where could you have been more noble? How are you going to do better this week? Visualize yourself doing the upcoming workouts in a strong, elegant, and focused manner. Maybe this is the week you decide to incorporate a Cardio Commute or a Periodic Renunciation. If so, schedule it in and prepare for it. Energy follows thought.

Receiving bodywork (massage) on Mondays is wise.

Tuesday. Lower Body in the Gym

Meditation: Beeper Guru: Smiling (page 185).

Cardio: None or Cardio Commute (page 76).

Yoga: None or flow through a few rounds of one or more HP Yoga Sun Salutations as a warmup before your Strength Training workout.

Strength: Do the Cosmic Yang lower body workout. This is your main workout of today. Be brave.

Prescription Notes

- All sets to momentary failure, unless otherwise noted.

- Recovery phase: 45 to 60 seconds unless otherwise noted.

- Active warmup: Perform a few minutes of Cardio to raise your body temperature.

Gunther Hops (page 155)

Do 2 sets of 16 jumps.

Superset: Go from A to B without resting 5 times.

A. Back Squats (page 49)

Do 8 to 10 repetitions.

B. Jump Squats (page 50)

Jump like your life depended on it for 30 seconds.

Knee Tuck Jumps (page 156)

Do 3 sets of 20 seconds each.

Leg Curls (page 48)

Do 4 sets of 6 repetitions.

Seated Calf Raises (page 51)

Do 5 sets of 10 repetitions.

Triset: Go from A to B to C without resting 4 times.

A. Medicine Ball Crunches (page 53)

For 1 minute.

B. Suspended Leg Raises (page 54) for 1 minute.

C. Ab Wheel (page 157)

For 30 seconds.

Wednesday. Upper Body in the Gym

Meditation: Early Morning Cleaning Ritual (page 186).

Cardio: None or Cardio Commute (page 76).

Yoga: None or flow through a few rounds of one or more HP Yoga Sun Salutations as a warmup before your Strength Training workout.

Strength: Do the Cosmic Yang upper body workout. This is your main workout for today. Be brave.

Prescription Notes

- All sets to momentary failure, unless otherwise noted.

- Recovery phase: 45 to 60 seconds

- Active warmup: Perform a few minutes of Cardio to raise your body temperature.

Bent Arm Dumbbell Pullovers (page 159)

Do 3 sets of 6 to 8 repetitions.

Pull-Ups (page 57)

Do 2 sets of however many (or few) you can do.

Hang Cleans (page 163)

Do 4 sets of 6 to 8 repetitions.

Dips (page 59)

Do 2 sets of however many (or few) you can do.

Bench Press (page 61)

Do 1 set of 10 repetitions, then do 3 sets of 3 repetitions, and another 1 set of 10 repetitions.

Repetition Jerks (page 160)

Do 3 sets of 5 repetitions.

Barbell Curls (page 63)

Do 5 sets of 8 repetitions using Entre Nous recovery technique (see page 67). Maintain a physical touch with the barbell in between sets. Don't wander.

Concentration Curls (page 161)

Do 3 sets of 8 to 10 repetitions for each arm.

Lying Triceps Extension (page 161)

Do 3 sets of 6 to 8 repetitions using Entre Nous recovery technique.

Superset: Go from A to B without resting 3 times.

A. Dumbbell Arm Swings (page 158)

For 15 seconds.

B. Dumbbell Horizontal Swings (page 158)

For 15 seconds.

Recover for 15 seconds then repeat.

Thursday. Intervals!

Meditation: Early Morning Cleaning Ritual (page 186) and Beeper Guru: Smiling (page 185).

Yoga: None or flow through a few rounds of one or more HP Yoga Sun Salutations as a warmup before your Cardio workout or as a cooldown/stretch after it.

Cardio: Using any Cardio of Choice, do the "Minutes Are Forever" interval workout (page 166).

Friday. Yang Day in the Gym

Meditation: Early Morning Cleaning Ritual (page 186) and Beeper Guru: Smiling (page 185).

Cardio: None or Cardio Commute.

Yoga: None or flow through a few rounds of one or more HP Yoga Sun Salutations as a warmup before your gym workout or as a cooldown/stretch after it. If desired, you can do the entire Cosmic Yang HP Yoga routine.

Strength: Do the Yang Day workout.

Yang Day Workout

In the East, the balance of all that exists is represented by yin/yang. Yin is the female, the dark, the yielding. Yang is the masculine, the light, the forceful.

Yang Day workouts are special. They develop what is known as *ekagrata* in the yogic tradition: performance of physical effort with maximum mental concentration. During this workout, note how quickly your mind will want to wander. These sessions develop mental focus in life.

The recovery phase is 1 minute between all sets and movements.

Bench Press (see page 61)

Do 5 sets of 5 reps.

Back Squats (page 49)

Do 5 sets of 5 reps.

Power Cleans (page 162)

Do 5 sets of 5 reps.

Dips (page 59)

Do 2 sets of as many as you can perform at bodyweight.

Pull-ups (page 57)

Do 2 sets of as many as you can perform at bodyweight.

Saturday. Long, Steady Cardio

Meditation: Rasa Eating Exercise (see page 186).

Cardio: Using any Cardio of Choice, get out and enjoy 2 to 3 hours at a steady aerobic effort, staying within Zones 1 and 2 for 80 percent of the time. The remaining 20 percent can be at the lower end of Zone 3 (see Table 2.1, page 75).

Yoga: None or flow through a few rounds of one or more HP Yoga Sun Salutations as a warmup before your Cardio workout or as a cooldown/stretch after it.

Sunday HP Yoga Day

Meditation: Do the Rasa Eating Exercise (page 186).

Yoga: Do the HP Yoga Cosmic Yang Practice.

CHAPTER 14

Cycle Summation

UPON YOUR COMPLETION OF FOUR consistent weeks on my Cosmic Yang program, take seven days off from training. If desired, you can continue doing Yoga every other day. You may choose either the Green Tara or Cosmic Yang Yoga routines.

Limit Cardio to three 30- to 60-minute workouts done on nonconsecutive days and at an intensity level no higher than Zone 2.

You may practice Meditation as desired.

No Strength Training should be done during this week.

Use the extra time normally spent training to share with family, friends, or to be by yourself.

At some point, read the next chapter to prepare psychologically for your next program. The Frugal Realm is demanding. Get ready for it.

And if your arms are not too well trained to pick up a pencil, you may wish to answer the following questions regarding your performance during the Cosmic Yang program.

Cosmic Yang Cycle Summation

Date started:

Date finished:

Today's date:

Finish this sentence:
The main overall difference I felt between Cosmic Yang and Green Tara was:

Strength Training

1. Note your consistency during this discipline.
2. How did the upper and lower body workouts go? What did you notice most about them?
3. And the Yang Day Workout. Note the poundages you used for the following movements:

Bench Press

First Week:

Fourth Week:

Squat

First Week:

Fourth Week:

Power Cleans

First Week:

Fourth Week:

Pull-ups

First Week:

Fourth Week:

Dips

First Week:

Fourth Week:

4. Which gym movements seem harder than others? Why?
5. Which seemed easier? Why?
6. Any changes in physique?

Cardio

1. Any standout reactions in this discipline?
2. How did the Minutes Are Forever intervals go? Note any interesting physical or emotional resistance?
3. Were you able to do any Cardio Commutes? If not, why not?
4. What was your weekly average in terms of Cardio hours logged?

Yoga

1. What is your first reaction to the word "Yoga" these days? How has it changed from four weeks ago?
2. How did the Cosmic Yang Yoga routine go?
3. Were you able to maintain ujjayi breathing through the forms?
4. Name the three poses that you find most difficult. Note any commonality among them. (Coach's Note: These three poses hold your Highest teachings. Dive deep into them.)

Meditation

1. How did the Early Morning Cleaning Rituals go?
2. The primary lesson I learned from the Beeper Guru: Smiling was:
3. Note how you felt after doing the Rasa Eating assignment.

Nutrition

1. Did you notice any changes in your dietary attractions during this cycle?
2. Describe *exactly* what you ate and drank yesterday and the manner in which you consumed it. Include supplements, drugs, everything.
3. Did you order and use your Sunrider or other herbs? How do they feel to you?

Number the WF disciplines 1 through 5, starting with the ones you really need to focus on during the next program.

Strength

Cardio

Yoga

Meditation

Nutrition

Oh-oh . . . I sense something large coming. Could it possibly be the Frugal Realm?

PART THREE

THE ADVANCED PROGRAM: THE FRUGAL REALM

Make no mistake, the Frugal Realm is advanced training. Accomplishing this program might be the hardest thing you've ever done in your life. The spiritual, mental, and physical impact of this realm can be intense. Please remain alert to all five Fitness Disciplines here; the balance between them will be delicate during the next four weeks. Possible injury may occur if you are not consistent in each Fitness Discipline.

Whoever, wherever you are, I bow to you. If you've gotten this far in my program, you deserve high applause!

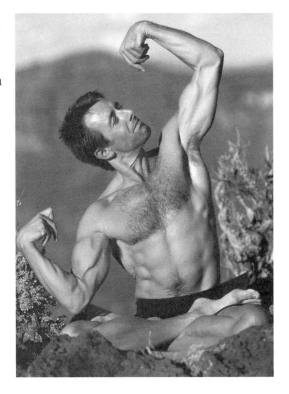

But the final pitch onto the summit of my basic training steepens. In fact, it gets downright extreme. My final program—the Frugal Realm—will blur your everyday life. The edges of your world will soften because this program is going to bend you, shake you, and test you until you have met and have become intimate with your higher self.

Albert Einstein said, "Imagination is more important than knowledge." Imagination is the seed essence to all life goals. I used to imagine competing in world championships in several different sports until my imagination and reality combined. Each night you fall asleep within the Realm program, you will need to imagine yourself flowing through the difficulty of the next day's training. I have faith that if you can complete the next four weeks of training, you too will have gained world-class capability. I am serious. You will see.

I have designed this cycle to basically "make you or break you." This cycle will rid you of useless emotional clutter, energy-wasting activity and desires, and outdated attachments. Your life will become spartan but focused.

| Frugal | = | The practice of providence; marked by sparsity |
| Realm | = | An area or spaciousness. Also, a kingdom |

Journey now into the Frugal Realm and live the kingdom of your dreams!

Pure logic is the ruin of the spirit.

—SAINT-EXUPÉRY

Strength Training

Most people's minds are anywhere but within the body part they are training.
—Coach Ilg

THE STRENGTH TRAINING WORKOUTS OF the Frugal Realm will push your physical limits and stretch your mental skills to the point of pandemonium. There are few recovery days and each workout is alternated with high-rep and low-rep versions. In other words, you will be in the gym six out of seven days. You will train each body part twice per week; once using heavier weights and low repetitions (your yang workout), and again using lighter weights and higher repetitions (your yin workout). Each workout will have its own special flow—listen for it. This prescription requires acute attention to its wholistic nature; forsake one part of it, and you violate its power. There is nothing to do but your best.

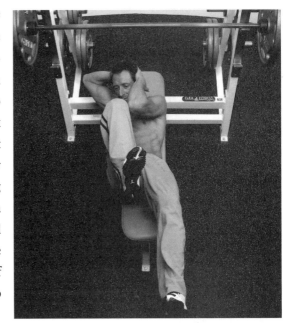

Because of the intense nature of the Frugal Realm, I've limited the number of new Strength Training movements to just a few. Let's take a look at the Strength Training workouts now and describe any new movements along the way.

Note: Take only 30-second recovery intervals except where noted.

CHEST AND BACK: YANG WORKOUT

Stiff Leg Deadlifts (page 47)

Do 1 set of 4 repetitions.

Dips (page 59)

Do 5 sets of 5 repetitions.

Note: Add weight by using a belt when needed.

Pull-ups (page 57)

Do 5 sets of 5 repetitions.

Note: Add weight by using a belt when needed.

Bench Press (page 61)

Do 10 sets of 5 repetitions.

Hang Cleans (page 58)

Do 10 sets of 6 repetitions.

Stiff Leg Deadlifts (page 47)

Do 1 set of 4 repetitions.

Dumbbell Flyes (page 60)

Use the Envelope Technique:

1 set of 1 minute

2 sets of 6 to 8 repetitions

1 set of 1 minute

Superset: Go from A to B without resting 5 times.

A. Bench Press (see page 61) for 12 repetitions.

B. Dips (see page 59) for however many you can do!

On left, I have reached the bottom transition at the end of my inhale. And on right, with an exhale, I push away from the ground, clap my hands in the top position, and prepare for the next repetition.

Plyo Push-Ups

Do 3 sets of however many you can do!

Assume the top of a traditional push-up position by supporting yourself on your toes and palms, parallel to the ground. Maintain a strong integrity throughout your body by firming your thighs and engaging your abdominals.

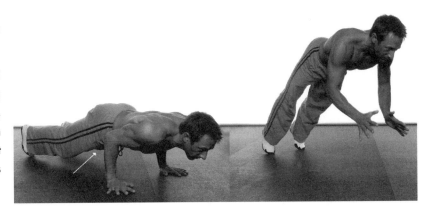

Inhale as you lower yourself toward the ground until your upper arm is parallel to the ground.

Exhale and dynamically push off from the ground with both hands. Your feet can stay connected to the ground (although master WF students should raise both feet off the ground as well). Use enough pushing-away force so that you can clap your hands at the zenith of your push away.

Upon landing, rocket back off again and repeat for as long as you are able. After reaching muscular failure (don't break your nose!), dissolve into standard push-ups until failure.

YANG PHASE: Pushing away from the ground

YIN PHASE: None . . . well, really it's the attenuation of the yang phase.

WHAT YOU ARE PRIMARILY WORKING: Explosive upper body strength, core stability, and chest, shoulders, and triceps.

WHOLISTIC NOTES: People generally have too many opinions and not enough convictions. As you blast away from the earth, dig down into that deep, powerful space within to find and develop your conviction. What some call genius is simply someone developing an infinite capacity to take life by the horns.

Superset: Go from A to B without resting 5 times.

A. Pull-ups (page 57)

Do as many (or as few) as you can.

B. Hang Cleans (page 58)

Do 8 to 10 impeccable and very fluid repetitions.

V-Handle Pulldowns (page 57)

Use the Envelope Technique:

1 set of 1 minute

2 sets of 6 to 8 repetitions

1 set of 1 minute

Sorry, but believe me, I am doing this for your own good.

SHOULDERS AND ARMS: YANG WORKOUT

Repetition Jerks (page 160)

Do 5 sets of 5 repetitions.

Seated Dumbbell Lateral Raises (page 62)

Do 3 sets of 8 repetitions.

Barbell Curls (page 63)

Do 6 sets of 5 repetitions. Get down, get ugly with it if you have to.

Concentration Curls (page 161)

Do 6 sets of 6 repetitions each arm; no recovery between arms.

Lying Triceps Extension (page 161)

Do 5 sets of 5 repetitions. Be there!

Superset: Go from A to B without resting 3 times.

1 minute each:

A. Medicine Ball Knee-ups

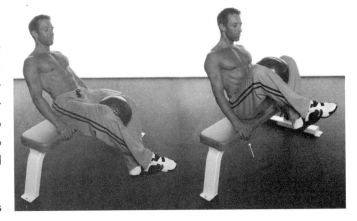

Begin this movement by sitting on the edge of a flat bench. Place a medicine ball between your knees. Squeeze and hold the medicine ball in place by adducting your thigh muscles and by raising your feet off the ground, crossing your ankles. Lightly grip the edges of the bench to stabilize your body. Invite elegant, pulled-up posture to your spine. Keep your eyes trained on the ball.

Exhale and flex your hips, drawing your knees (and thus the ball) toward your belly.

Inhale, and lower your knees (and thus the ball) toward the ground, but keep your feet from touching down. Repeat for the prescribed amount of time or repetitions, striving for fluidity of motion.

YANG PHASE: Bringing the medicine ball toward your belly.

YIN PHASE: Lowering the medicine ball toward the ground.

WHAT YOU ARE PRIMARILY WORKING: Core muscles (abdominals and obliques), hip flexors, inner thighs, torso stabilizer muscles.

WHOLISTIC NOTES: One of my all-time favorites, which teaches superb core-dination! Not to mention ripped abs.

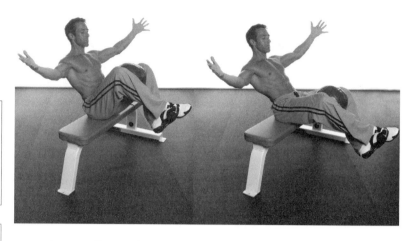

Note: Those of you who want a little more intensity, do this movement without holding on to the bench with your hands (see photo)!

Aspiring Warrior Students should do this Superset 5 times. Master Students? Tack on a 1-minute set of Ab Wheels (see page 157) after each set of Medicine Ball Crunches.

B. Medicine Ball Crunches (page 53)

SHOULDERS AND ARMS: YIN WORKOUT

Superset: Go from A to B without resting 3 times.

A. Seated Dumbbell Lateral Raises (page 62)

Enjoy yourself while doing a Staccato Technique: Hold the top position for 10 seconds, then do the exercise for 10 seconds, repeat that stick-and-go sequence until the 1-minute mark is reached.

B. Seated Dumbbell Press (page 62)

Melt your delts into butter during a 3-Stage Technique: Do the upper half of the movement for 20 seconds, then do the lower half of the movement for 20 seconds, then do a full range for 20 seconds—doing these three stages equals one set.

Superset: Go from A to B without resting 4 times.

A. Pulley Curls

Get enlightened during a Shivaya Technique: Do the full range of the movement for 3 repetitions then do repetitions 4 through 9 only through the upper half of the movement, then from repetition number 10 return to the full range movement until momentary failure.

Stand approximately 2 feet before a lower pulley apparatus holding a short bar attachment at arm's length with your palms facing outward (supinated, or an undergrip). Feet should be hip-width apart and your knees slightly flexed. Keep your head pulled up and draw your shoulders backward and away from your ears. Pin your elbows to the sides of your body.

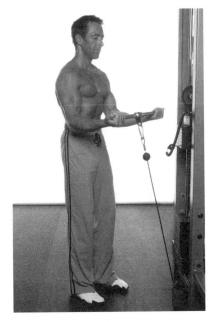

Exhale and curl the bar to your upper chest without letting your elbows wander away from the sides of your body.

Inhale as you lower the bar toward the starting position, feeling the exquisite stretch of your biceps controlling the speed of the descent. Once the arms extend fully, repeat for prescribed repetitions.

YANG PHASE: Curling the bar to your chest.

YIN PHASE: Lowering the bar.

WHAT YOU ARE PRIMARILY WORKING: Biceps, standing posture, kinesthesia (learning to listen to the feel of the muscles as they work).

WHOLISTIC NOTES: Be very disciplined about not letting your elbows travel . . . I press my elbows into my lower ribs to increase the purity of stress on my biceps.

B. Barbell Curls (page 63)

Do 15 repetitions. Using a "delayed yang style" 4 counts on the yang phase (as you curl the barbell toward your chin) and only 2 counts on the yin phase (as you lower the barbell to arm's length).

Two-Bench Triceps (page 64)

Do 3 sets of 1 minute with as much nobility as possible. Use the Escape Plans on page 64 if/when needed.

Superset: Go from A to B without resting 3 times.

Do 1 minute each.

A. Medicine Ball Knee-ups (page 211)

B. Medicine Ball Crunches (page 53)

Aspiring Warrior Students should do this Superset 5 times. Master Students? Tack on a 1-minute set of Ab Wheels (see page 157) after each set of Medicine Ball Crunches.

Stiff Leg Deadlifts (page 47)

One set of 6 repetitions. Get grooved with your breath and posture.

Overhead Squats

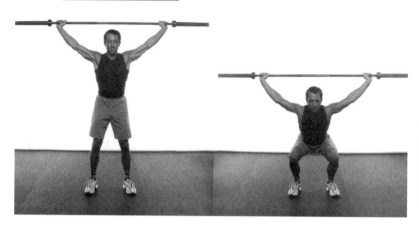

Open up your hips and get the chi flowing: Do 3 sets of 10 repetitions.

Stand upright with a light barbell held overhead. Grip the barbell with your palms facing out about 20 inches farther apart than your shoulders. Your stance is also wide, about 15 inches wider than your shoulders with your toes turned slightly out. Make sure the barbell is being held at complete arm extension and is behind your head (see photo).

Inhale and slowly lower your hips down by bending both knees evenly and in alignment with your toes. Keep your spine flat and look straight ahead as you perform this very "balancy" squat. Keep squatting down until the tops of your thighs are parallel to the ground. If your heels come up, adjust two things: (1) widen your stance, and (2) do more yoga.

Here I am in the start position of an Overhead Squat. The barbell must remain behind my head for the entire movement. Note also how wide my stance and grip is. In the bottom position of an Overhead Squat I reach a classic Strength Training position all but lost in our modern era of fitness training. Note the similarity between this position and the yoga postures of Utkatasana (page 91) and Malasana (page 103).

Upon reaching the bottom position (both thighs parallel; see photo), exhale and extend your knees but keep them in alignment with your toes. Do not let your knees collapse inward. Keep extending the knees until you attain the start position. Repeat for the prescribed repetitions.

YANG PHASE: Extending the knees.

YIN PHASE: Flexing the knees.

WHAT YOU ARE PRIMARILY WORKING: A lot of balance, significant hip and shoulder flexibility, grip strength, and ekagrata (one pointed concentration)!

WHOLISTIC NOTES: This relatively unknown movement captures the essence of what genuine Strength Training is all about: balance, fluidity, stability, perseverance. In this movement is a lot of yoga!

Leg Press (page 50)

Do 4 sets of 10 repetitions.

Back Squats (page 49)

Do 6 sets of 8 repetitions. Do your best to make each set heavier.

Leg Curls (page 48)

Do 3 sets of 4 repetitions.

Gunther Hops (page 155)

Crank off 2 sets of 30 seconds each. Beauty and the breath.

Jump Squats (page 50)

Jump into 2 sets of 45 seconds each. Beauty and the beast!

Calf Raises (standing or seated, page 51)

Do 10 sets of 10 repetitions. Champions only, please.

LOWER BODY: YIN WORKOUT

Stiff Leg Deadlifts (page 47)

Open your workout with 1 set of 4 repetitions for spinal satisfaction.

Leg Press (page 50)

Let's get it on with an Envelope Technique: 1 set of 1 minute, 2 sets of 6 to 8 repetitions, and 1 final set of 1 minute.

Touch 'n' Go Lunges

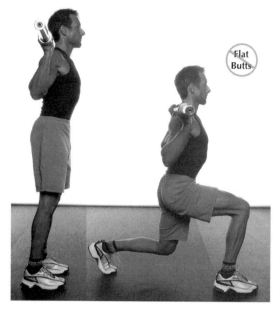

Flat Butts

Do 2 sets of 14 repetitions on each leg.

Stand upright with a barbell across the back of your neck, low on the trapezius (upper back) muscles. Assume a stance wider than your shoulders, toes pointed straight ahead. Your grip on the barbell should be with your palms facing out at a comfortable, steady position several inches wider than your shoulders. Look straight ahead.

As you inhale, lunge forward onto your right leg, landing softly, until the top of your thigh is parallel to the ground. Make sure your right knee does not travel in front of the right ankle.

Exhale and explode back toward your standing position by extending your knee. Keep your spine as perpendicular to the ground as possible throughout this lunging motion (see photo).

As your body comes upright again, just tap the toes of your right foot onto the ground beside your left foot then lunge back onto your right foot again as described above. In other words, I do not want you to step onto your right foot or release the tension in your supporting (left) leg. Repeat for the required number of repetitions on the same leg before switching to the other leg.

> An excellent athletic movement, though often overused, that develops and maintains beautiful posture and nicely sculpted buttocks.

YANG PHASE: Extending (pushing back off the lead leg) the knee from the lunge position.

YIN PHASE: Flexing the knee (bending the knee to lunge onto it).

WHAT YOU ARE PRIMARILY WORKING: Glutes (buttocks), frontal thigh, postural muscles, and fast-twitch neural development.

WHOLISTIC NOTES: An excellent athletic movement, though often overused, that develops and maintains beautiful posture and nicely sculpted buttocks. Maintain a sharp, crisp action to inspire power, agility, and balance. Advanced warriors: You guys don't even need to tap the right toes, but instead, just swing the right leg through the starting, upright position like a pendulum.

Jump Squats (page 50)

Do 2 lovely sets of my dastardly Staccato Technique: Hold the top position for 10 seconds, then do the exercise for 10 seconds, and repeat that stick-and-go sequence until the 1-minute mark is reached. Recover for 1 minute. That is one set. Welcome to the "Black Hold."

Leg Press (page 50)

Do 2 sets of 1 minute each. Did I say 2 sets of 1 minute? You are in the Frugal Realm now, baby!

Front Squats

Five sets of 20 repetitions. You sure you want to be a Wholistic Fitness warrior?

Stand upright with a barbell in front of your neck, high on the clavicular region of your chest muscles. With the barbell sandwiched between your throat and upper shoulders, crisscross your hands over the barbell and raise both of your elbows until they are parallel to the ground. Your hands do not even hold the barbell, but rather just float on top of it (palms rest on the upper surface of the bar-

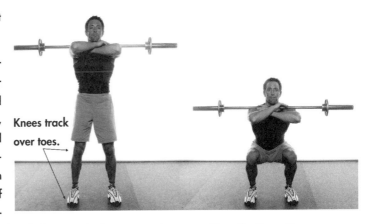

Knees track over toes.

bell, keeping it in place). *Note:* An alternative hand placement is the same as the top position of a Hang Clean (see page 58). Assume a stance wider than your shoulders, toes pointed straight ahead. Look straight ahead.

Inhale as you begin a controlled descent, bending and tracking your knees over your toes, until the top of your thigh is parallel to the earth.

Keep your spine elegant and pulled up (see photo).

Exhale and begin an explosive upward phase by extending your knees until you reach the standing position again. Repeat for prescribed repetitions.

YIN PHASE: Lowering the weight.

YANG PHASE: Rising from bottom position to top.

WHAT YOU ARE PRIMARILY TRAINING: Tremendous postural strength, frontal thighs, hips, midsection, erector muscles of the spine—and inner power, baby.

WHOLISTIC NOTES: Keep your knees slightly flexed in the standing position and never bounce in the low, bottom position. Besides building an endless reservoir of spinal strength, front squats are key for promoting dynamic balance. Metaphysical benefits include enhanced self-confidence. Many people fail to reach their dreams because they have a wishbone where their backbone ought to be.

Leg Curls (page 48)

Do 3 sets of 1 minute each.

Calf Raises (seated or standing, see page 51)

Bury this workout by doing 3 sets of a Staccato Technique: Hold the top position for 10 seconds, then do the exercise for 10 seconds, and repeat that stick-and-go sequence until the 1-minute mark is reached.

CHAPTER 16

Cardio

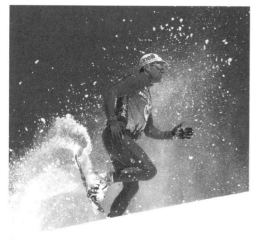

Coach Ilg snowshoe training at 10,500 feet in the Sangre de Cristo mountains above Santa Fe, New Mexico.

B Y THIS TIME IN YOUR WF training, you realize that to be true to Cardio is like studying your face in a mirror—the nature of who you are keeps staring right back at you. Every moment is a chance to look at yourself or to dissociate. It is my hope that you are using more and more of your Cardio moments as a form of self-reflection.

In the Frugal Realm training program, the Cardio discipline takes a lower priority as the Strength Training discipline shines front and center. But don't be fooled into thinking that I've let your Cardio fitness dwindle. There is method in my madness. As you will see, the intensity of the Strength Training workouts will tax your Cardio fitness more than you might think. Besides, the investment of your Strength Training during this cycle will make a lasting and positive imprint upon your long-term Cardio fitness.

In this new training cycle, I have reduced your mandatory Cardio volumes and you have no interval sessions. I've done this to create time for your Strength Training workouts and to save energy for recuperation. Knowing how to regulate amplitude—or the combined effects from week-to-week training—is a key factor in wise, effective training.

As I guide you deeper into WF, I lay more and more responsibility upon you to take command of your own spiritual warriorism. You will read on your Frugal Realm Daily Practice in Chapter 20, for instance, that I suggest doing Cardio Commute every day during the week. But, as always, Cardio Commuting is optional, not mandatory. You are free to not do any direct Cardio training during the weekdays of the Frugal Realm.

Or, you might rise higher and ride your bicycle or jog to the gym to do your workout. You might ride to work or just walk with your loved one to an afternoon cinema instead of driving. Such lifestyle Cardio choices are huge in WF. What if everybody did it? The difference between the two—electing not to do Cardio Commute through the week and doing it—is the difference between a novice student and a master student of WF.

Your weekends, however, are different. Weekends for you during the Frugal Realm will

IN THE GUTTER OF NOBILITY

After doing regular Cardio training for over twenty-five years and having much of my Cardio training come from Cardio Commuting, I know damn well how difficult it is to rearrange your life and make the sacrifices to ride your bike instead of drive once or twice a week. I've lost count of how many SUVs have run me off the road and into the rain gutter of my nobility. I am not interested in your excuses. I've heard enough of my own. What I am interested in is reading an e-mail from you like the one Martin Moore sent me:

Dear Coach Ilg—

I finally did it and had to tell you about it! *Why did it take me so long?!* Today, as you suggested eight months ago, I finally rode my bicycle to my yoga class! I cannot tell you how different it made me feel! As the cars whizzed by me, I felt so noble (your word, I know!) as I pedaled along trying to get to class on time. It was weird, it felt like the people in the cars really respected me with my yoga mat across my back, hunched over into the wind. When I arrived at class, I finally realized what you have written about in your website journal . . . the difference between a high-performance yogi and a "studio yogi"! My classmates looked at me as I rolled my bicycle into class . . . they *knew* I was being a brave and noble warrior, like Arjuna in the *Bhagavad Gita*! Oh man, Coach! My perspective of who you are and what you have tried to do through encouraging Wholistic Fitness has just jumped into clarity! But you are right, Wholistic Fitness must be lived to be understood . . . at least at its deeper, more profound levels! I want to ride my bike now to yoga class once a week! I want to be a Wholistic Fitness *warrior*! Easy on the earth and high within the spirit!

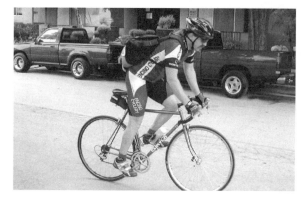

FITNESS COMMUTING IS HIGH NOBILITY

Steve Marlowe, age forty, during his daily 21-mile bicycle commute through L.A. traffic. Steve is a "zero tolerance" Cardio Commuter—he refuses to drive a car no matter what. Steve's extreme example of fitness warriorism is not for everyone, but spiritually helps produce a national shift in our society's laziness when it comes to commuting. Cardio Commuting is the spiritual and planetary solution for a healthier inner and outer world.

be consumed by Cardio and Yoga. Do not, however, attempt to do the higher range of the pre-scribed weekend volumes if you are doing less than two hours of Cardio during the weekdays. Your connective tissue is going to be prefatigued from all the Strength Training in the gym, so be wise and get in your Cardio in carefully measured amounts.

LOW-IMPACT LIVING EQUALS HIGH CARDIO FITNESS

One reason why so many Americans are overweight and have so little Cardio fitness is that we've engineered activity right out of our lives. A WF society would certainly embrace a return to the days when people would occasionally or regularly self-propel themselves to school, work, or on errands. It is important to live or relocate to an area where a fitness lifestyle—not shop-ping malls or hospitals—is the priority. Having quick access to parks, mountain areas, beaches, or open space is important. Find a gym or a yoga studio within a reasonable bicycle or inline skate distance from you. Living in an area conducive to fitness commuting is a WF version of engaged Yoga, which I will talk more about in the next training cycle: The Jeweled Lotus.

Most Americans die from diseases stemming from too many day-to-day choices for lux-ury and comfort instead of effort and exercise: Stray out of your comfort zone in at least one way, at least once each day. For some, this may mean smiling at a store clerk. As you progress in stretching your comfort zones, however, it is the integration of Cardio Commuting into your lifestyle that represents one of the highest and most transformative practices of this philosophy.

IT'S IN US

I was naturally attracted to Cardio training. So were you, whether you know it or not. Perhaps you've forgotten your initial love affair with Cardio, but it was there. As soon as you could crawl, what did you do? You tried to walk. Then, after walking, you tried to run. Then, remember your

DEPRESSION AND CARDIO

Eastern Masters such as Rinpoche Trungpa and the Dalai Lama concur with the Western psychology of Freud and Jung that depression comes from spending too much time in the mind. The mind dominates feelings and overrides the instinct to move and breathe. The body grows tense, circulation becomes inhibited, and all that remains is a robotic, automatic body/mind system that is stuck in depression and can't see a way out. Treating depression with drugs cannot work from a spiritual point, since pacification of symptoms misses entirely the karmic or energetic reasons for the depressed state.

Getting back into the body is vital for treating depression because you are not "treating" it any longer, you are using it as inspiration to grow. In my endurance races, the best way I grew more confident in my chances for winning came from passing other racers. In combating depression, the best way to rise out of it is to overcome an obstacle, no matter how small. In Wholistic Fitness therapy, this means moving the body and allowing breath (pran) to begin eroding the depression with life and light. Once movement and breath get going, the nervous system relaxes, blood and oxygen and nutrient delivery to the tissues increases, the mind eases its clutching, and life springs back into the spirit.

first tricycle? Can you recall the rush of joy when you rode your "two wheeler" for the first time? I am a state champion in bicycle racing. I've spent hundreds of hours training on bicycles, but my simple love of riding a bicycle has never left me. Riding bikes still exhilarates me!

If we sit for too long, we fidget. We need to run. We need to link breath with sustained, rhythmic movement. It's in us. People who don't move within the joy of their bodies become depressed and even suicidal. This has been proven in horrible experiments, but the point is principal. Our intuitive wisdom pleads and prods us to please move and breathe. Unfortunately the whirring of our overthinking mind too often drowns out the still, small voice of our inner wisdom. Too much thinking imbalances hormones and negatively affects blood chemistry.

Our body/mind system pivots upon frequent stints of heart elevating exercise for composure. My own records clearly show depressed and suicidal clients are those who also did not consistently do Cardio exercise in their lives. Hell, if I never moved and breathed in my body, I'd be depressed and suicidal too. You think I am kidding, but I am speaking of my family history. But we don't need to analyze it, we just need to feel the difference before and after just twenty minutes of Cardio activity like walking, running, cycling, or hiking. It is common sense to enjoy the rhythmic pulse of your heartbeat mixed with your breath. Those two things—heartbeat and breath—act like soothing metronymic balms for the body and soul once set in motion.

New guidelines from the National Academy's Institute of Medicine shows that getting thirty minutes of exercise per day is not enough for long-term health benefits. That figure needs to be doubled. Thus, the new standard for personal health is one hour of exercise per day.

Can you see where all these academics are leading us? Back to our natural state of lifestyle exercise. Chop wood, carry water! Ride your bike to work or to the gym. Hike with your family or friends instead of washing the damn car or watching football on the weekends. Move! Breathe!

By age twelve, I was running regularly from my elementary school in the mountain town of Durango, Colorado, to our home four miles out in the country. Instinct was making me run. It felt right to run. It felt wrong to cram myself onto a bus with screaming kids that weaved through country roads for an hour dropping other kids off before me. That wasted way too much precious after-school time. I'd rather take that hour and run home. Fresh air. Thumping heart. Roadside creatures. Sound of feet skimming across the earth. This, to me, felt right.

Though burdened by textbooks, school clothes, and a couple of terrifying St. Bernards (see sidebar), I favored the company of big, lazy sunflowers, flitting hummingbirds, and the rushing waters of Junction Creek over the school bus or a ride home with my parents. There seemed some essential, inner therapy being accomplished through my Cardio Commute. In sync with my growing body, the running was developing a spiritual dimension that offered a wider perspective to my adolescent challenges. Something about running strengthened my entire being. I could just feel it. I've never stopped.

Don't let the stress of modern society poison Cardio's innate healing joy. There is no need for fancy equipment or to know a whole bunch of fitness and medical data to enjoy Cardio exercise. In fact, too much input clutters the native Zen of Car-

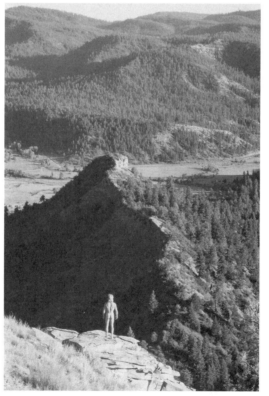

A young Coach Ilg on Southern Ute land near Pagosa Springs, Colorado.

IS YOGA CONSIDERED CARDIO ACTIVITY?

Since my definition of Cardio is any activity that elevates the heart rate and keeps it elevated for at least twenty minutes, the answer is yes. And no. If the yoga style is an ashtanga or power yoga style (like High Performance Yoga, the style unique to WF), then your heart rate will definitely be elevated for over twenty minutes. Count it as Cardio. Other styles such as Iyengar, restorative, and vinniyoga are slower and do not elevate the heart rate enough to be considered a Cardio activity. You should, however, count only the amount of time your heart rate was elevated during a power yoga class, say during the Sun Salutations. Most of my hour-and-a-half HP Yoga classes are good for about thirty minutes of strict Cardio training. An Iyengar-style yoga class, by comparison, never elevates my heart rate and thus provides no direct Cardio benefit.

COACH ILG ON HIS FIRST INTERVAL WORKOUTS

My childhood jogs home along (then) secluded Junction Creek Road from school were natural exchanges with the nature around me. But my Thoreau-like aerobic immersions were ceaselessly interrupted by an inevitable encounter with a pair of fearsome dogs. Dragons, they were, to me. Guarding the final quarter-mile stretch to my house were two territorial St. Bernard dogs. They protected a mobile home only slightly larger than they were. I never saw the owner of that mobile home, but I sure knew his dogs. Downwind days were better for me. I could slink past just opposite them, about thirty yards from their slobbery, snoring, horse-sized heads, then sprint away. But on upwind days, the beasts could smell me coming. On such days, I'd have to hunker in the tall wheatgrass just out of their range for long periods, waiting for them to lose interest or for the wind to change. For days after one terrifying skirmish left my left calf torn and bleeding, I hiked several miles up Logchute Mountain to avert another bloody encounter.

Sometimes I sought revenge on the monsters by traversing Superstition Mountain across the river from them and chucking fist-sized riverstones at their hulking hides. This maneuver, however, achieved all the noticeable effects of throwing popcorn at sea lions. But I never allowed those furry gargantuans to deter my enjoyment of running. In fact, dashing past those dogs was my first form of interval training. Later in my competitive life, if forced to a sprint finish in a race, I'd recall those St. Bernards chomping at my calves and use the resultant adrenaline spike to hammer ahead of my competitors. Moral: Even if you lose, learn not to lose the lesson.

dio. Get out of the machines and leave the monitors at home. Run as naked as possible along a beach or mountain trail. Let the pandemonium of your mind be pacified by the simplicity of breath linked with movement. By following my programs in this book, Wholistic Fitness restores the Zen to your Cardio workouts, and maybe even your life.

High Performance Yoga

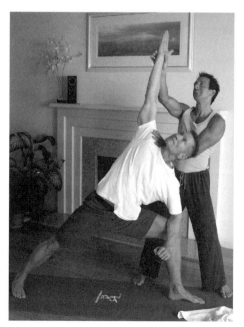

From Bulkiness to Buddhahood; Kurt Bruno is now a shining warrior of multidisciplined fitness.

K NOWN AMONG HIS FRIENDS AS "Captain America" for his superhero physique and chiseled jaw, Kurt Bruno always relied on bodybuilding as his main fitness training. But after spending twenty years in the gym, getting bigger and bigger but less and less flexible and more and more injured, Bruno, at age forty-one, came to one of my High Performance Yoga master classes in Santa Clarita, California. The Light of Yoga went on for Bruno. He realized that his muscles might have been big, but they were not very functional or fun to maintain. Bruno soon quit his gym membership, bought my yoga video, and with Marge, his lunch-hour stretching partner, used it every workday for two months.

The result was a new, leaner, more improved Captain America. Bruno lost over fifteen pounds of bulk, had much more defined muscularity, injury-free joints, greatly enhanced agility and flexibility, a happier state of well-being, and improved dietary patterns, such as less meat eating and coffee drinking, and more fruits and vegetables. Inspired by his upgrade in functional fitness, Bruno climbed Mount Whitney, the tallest peak in California, during the summer of 2002 with absolutely no problem. Next up for Bruno is an adventure race and my HP Yoga teacher training. Bruno's life has taken on whole new and exciting dimensions ever since he took up Yoga. Soon, other men will realize what Bruno and other Wholistic Fitness warriors know: Balanced fitness is best!

That is precisely what Yoga does best—it opens us.

During the Frugal Realm, you will just be attempting to maintain suppleness. The Frugal Realm is not a time to go for big flexibility gains, but rather to use Yoga to keep your joints healthy.

What I have done is made a small change in your Yoga routine. You will notice a strong similarity between your Frugal Realm Yoga routine and the Green Tara. I've intentionally kept most of the poses you have become familiar with so you can deepen your *asana* technique without learning a lot of new poses.

The new poses I have selected target hip openers. The amount and intensity of Strength Training that you will be doing requires attention to keep your hips open and your lower back strong. I think you will really enjoy this new Yoga routine and its effect upon you. In your next "maintenance program," the Jeweled Lotus, Yoga reestablishes itself as a high-priority discipline. For the next four weeks, however, I want you to focus on the preciseness of these familiar poses and releasing ever deeper into the new hip openers.

Have fun and enjoy the practice. Here is an overall look at your Frugal Realm Yoga routine.

HP YOGA: THE FRUGAL REALM PRACTICE

Begin by engaging ujjayi (see page 83) breathing and don't stop ujjayi until the final pose.

This is the same opening warmup as was used in your Green Tara HP Yoga practice (see page 85).

3 x Ardha Surya Namaskar (Half Sun Salutation)

2 x Series A Modified

1 x Series B (both legs = 1 set)

1 x Series C (both legs = 1 set)

5 x Series A

Then, do these movements, holding each for 30 to 60 seconds. Focus the mind with ujjayi breathing and the ego with honoring your edge.

Standing Vinyasa (Flow Sequence)

Start with right leg in lead position.

A. Utthita Parsvakonasana (Extended Side Angle Pose)

Exhale into:

B. Parsvottanasana (Side Extended Pose)

Into

C. Utthita Trikonasana (Extended Triangle Pose)

Into

D. Ardha Chandrasana (Half Moon Pose)

Swing your left leg through into

E. Garudasana (Eagle Pose)

F. Step back into Downward Facing Dog (Adho Mukha Svanasana)
Repeat A through F for left leg.

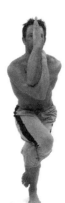

This is the same standing vinyasa sequence that appeared in your Green Tara HP Yoga routine except that I have substituted Garudasana (Eagle Pose) at the end of the sequence for Revolved Half Moon Pose. So, let's learn how to do the mighty Eagle Pose.

Garudasana (Eagle Pose)

Since you will be coming into Eagle Pose while balanced on your right leg, let's begin our description with you standing upright on your right leg with your arms held out to your sides for balance.

Exhale and slightly bend your supporting right knee. Cross your left leg over your right leg and pass the left shin behind the right calf muscle. Wrap your left foot around the inside of the right shin/upper ankle area.

Now that your left thigh is resting atop the right thigh, it is time to entwine your arms in a similar, but opposite, fashion. Stretch both arms out in front of you, parallel to the ground, palms facing the ground as well.

Exhale and cross the right arm over the top of the left arm, forming a scissor or X. Your right elbow should feel as if it is glued on top of the left elbow. Bend both elbows and draw your left hand toward your face enough to swivel your wrists so that your left fingers press into the palm of your right hand. Breathe evenly.

As your shoulders accommodate this stretch, slowly raise your elbows to shoulder level and deepen into the posture by bending your right knee a little more. Breathe and stay here for the prescribed time before releasing the arms and legs.

WHAT YOU ARE PRIMARILY WORKING: Sacroiliac flexibility; aligns the horizontality of the pelvis, improves circulation throughout the hip and pelvic musculature, strengthens the vascular and arterial walls by improving their elasticity, develops balance and mental concentration.

WHOLISTIC NOTES: A bewildering movement for those with tight hips and calves, but a splendid one. Do not worry if you are unable to get the nasty little ankle wrap move—with perseverance it will come. Work to synchronize the arm and leg movements. Try to bring your knees and elbows into alignment and extend the trunk up as you squat into the pose.

Dhanurasana (Bow Pose, page 101)

You may have done this pose as an option during your Cosmic Yang Yoga routine.

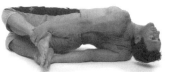

Option Pose: Parsva Dhanurasana (Sideways Bow Pose)

From Dhanurasana (Bow Pose), exhale and roll onto your right side while stretching your ankles against your hands (see photo). Stay here and breathe for the prescribed time.

Inhale and return to Dhanurasana (Bow Pose). Exhale and roll onto your left side for the prescribed time.

Inhale and return to Dhanurasana (Bow Pose). Exhale and release your legs.

WHAT YOU ARE PRIMARILY WORKING: All the benefits of Dhanurasana (Bow Pose), plus additional toning of the external and internal obliques, enhanced digestive and respiratory benefit, and frontal shoulder opening.

WHOLISTIC NOTES: This quaint posture is an elixir for gym people whose shoulders are overly tight from too many Bench Presses as well as for those who suffer from back pain.

Parivrtta Utkatasana (Twisting Chair Pose)

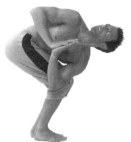

Stand upright with your ankles and knees together. Also press the knuckles of your big toes together.

Exhale and squat down by bending both knees and twist your torso to the right. Dig your left elbow and upper arm into the outside of your right thigh and bring your hands together into a Namasté (prayer) position. As you breathe and hold this position, keep trying to drape as much of your left upper arm across your outer (lateral) thigh of your right leg until your left armpit is pressed onto the outside edge of your right thigh. Stay here, breathe here.

Exhale, look down and place your left palm next to the outside edge of your right foot. Keep twisting your heart center toward the right as if you are trying to shine your chest up into the sky. Extend your right hand into the sky and gaze at your right thumb (see photo). Stay here, breathe here for the prescribed time before repeating for the other side.

WHAT YOU ARE PRIMARILY WORKING: Rotator trunk muscles, paraspinal muscles, shoulder flexibility, leg strength, and massage and strengthening of internal organs due to abdominal cavity compression, and detoxification of kidneys, liver, and spleen.

WHOLISTIC NOTES: This severe spinal twist produces exactly the deep kind of internal compression needed to counteract the detriment caused by years of sitting on toilets, sitting in furniture and cars, sitting in front of computers, etc. Use the leverage system of your arms to push your knees to the opposite side that your chest is facing. Hard work here will pay off handsomely in thousands of life-enriching ways.

Option Pose: Dwi Pada Koundinyasana (Two-Footed Sage Pose)

Perform Parivrtta Utkatasana (Twisting Chair Pose). Exhale and lower your right arm and place the right palm with fingers facing forward, approximately 18 inches across from the left hand, which is positioned the same way. Center yourself here for a few breaths.

Exhale and bend your left elbow deeply into the illiotibial band (outer edge) of your right thigh. Work your right thigh as close to your left armpit as possible (see photo). Center yourself here for a few breaths.

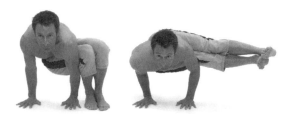

Inhale and extend your spine forward.

Exhale and raise your legs parallel to the ground as they rest upon your left upper arm. Ankles and knees should be stacked on top of each other (see photo). Gaze straight ahead and try to slow your breathing, which will probably be rapid due to the strenuous nature of this posture.

Exhale and bend your knees and return to Parivrtta Utkatasana (Twisting Chair Pose), before attempting the other side.

WHAT YOU ARE PRIMARILY WORKING: Core strength, baby! This five-star pose demands arm, leg, and abdominal strength plus balance while producing an incredible torque on the digestive organs, which leads to detoxification of the colon. Elasticity of the spine is improved.

WHOLISTIC NOTES: Let's see, it took me nearly five years just to bring both palms onto the ground, so take your time. Once your spinal twist deepens enough to allow both hands to be planted on the ground, raising your legs off the ground is easier than you might think, just keep finding the arm balance by shifting your weight forward as you learned to do in Bakasana (Crane Pose, page 104).

Floating Pigeon Pose

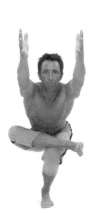

Stand upright with your hands on your hips. Raise your left foot off the ground and balance on your right leg. Bend your right knee slightly. Open your left hip by bending your left knee and lift (you can use your hands to help) your left ankle onto your right thigh just above your right kneecap. Make sure you have placed your left ankle bone, not your left foot, to this position. Stabilize here for a few breaths while gazing straight ahead.

Inhale and reach both arms overhead, palms facing each other with your fingers spread wide as in Utkatasana (Chair Pose, page 91).

Exhale and squat deeper into the pose by bending your right knee, but descend very slowly into this one-legged squat. Find where your edge is as you lower into this squat, then breathe there for the prescribed time (see photo).

Exhale and stand up slowly by extending your right knee. Release your arms down to your side and bring your left foot back to the ground. Repeat for the other leg.

WHAT YOU ARE PRIMARILY WORKING: Standing balance, leg strength, hip flexibility.

WHOLISTIC NOTES: Rely on conscious breathing as you squat deeper into the one-legged squat— millimeters can make a significant difference to opening your opposite hip, so go very slowly into this squat. I could not find this pose in the traditional Hatha Yoga texts, probably because Indians have such open hips from their lifestyle and culture that open hips are assumed. But this is not the case in our country.

Option Pose: Flying Pigeon Pose

Coming into Floating Pigeon Pose use your right leg as your supporting leg. Exhale and lower both of your arms and drape your armpits in front of your left shin. Place your right armpit directly in front of your left ankle. Flex your left ankle firmly to solidify the relationship between your right armpit and the front of your left ankle.

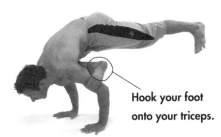

Hook your foot onto your triceps.

Exhale and lean forward as you reach both palms for the ground, fingers facing straight ahead of you.

Over the next few breaths, try to find the arm balance as you did with Bakasana (Crane Pose, page 104).

Once balanced on your arms, exhale and extend your right leg in back of you (see photo, previous page). Hold for as long as possible while breathing steadily before retracting your right leg, and reversing the moves above to regain Floating Pigeon Pose.

Exhale and stand up slowly by extending your right knee. Release your arms down to your side and bring your left foot back to the ground. Repeat for the other leg.

WHAT YOU ARE PRIMARILY WORKING: Intensification of all the benefits of Floating Pigeon Pose, plus far more core balance and arm strength.

WHOLISTIC NOTES: Just be glad pigeons aren't known for graceful flight. I know I am anything but graceful as I take awkward flight into this difficult pose. Trusting your arm balance will deliver confidence to your leg lift and extension.

Virasana (Hero Pose, page 102)

Option Pose: Supta Virasana (Supine Hero Pose, page 102)

Malasana (Garland Pose, page 103)

Option Pose: Bakasana (Crane Pose, page 104)

You remember these from your Green Tara Yoga practice.

Prasarita Padottanasana (Extended Foot Pose, page 173)

Option Pose: Sirsasana (Headstand, page 175) *from Prasarita Padottanasana*

You did these two postures in your Cosmic Yang Yoga practice.

Trianga Mukhaikapada Paschimottanasana

(Three-Limbed, Face, and One-Legged Western Extended Stretch Pose)

Sit upright in Virasana (Hero Pose, page 102) until your breathing is even and calm.

Do not disturb the left leg from its kneeling position, but carefully unfold your right leg and stretch it out in front of you. Press down through the entire back side of your right leg and strongly flex the right ankle as if you were trying to point all of your right toes toward your head.

Inhale and extend your spine out of your hips and reach both arms overhead. Make your spine as concave as possible. Look up between your arms.

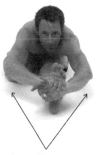

Inhales will lift and lengthen here.

Exhales will erase th[e] rounded spine here.

Float elbows away from the ground.

Exhale and fold forward, reaching your navel between your thighs first, then your heart center. Finally, capture your right foot by wrapping your right hand around the left wrist. Keep your elbows floating away from the ground and reach your chin down along your right shin (see photo). Stay here, breathe here for the prescribed time.

Exhale and slowly bring your torso back to perpendicular. *Note:* If you are attempting the option pose, Krounchasana (Heron Pose, below), practice it now before repeating Trianga for your left leg.

WHAT YOU ARE PRIMARILY WORKING: Toning of all the abdominal organs, muscles, and connective fabric. Repairs structural deviations within the pelvis.

WHOLISTIC NOTES: A fantastic, highly medicinal asana that is underenjoyed. This pose is a compound movement of Virasana (Hero Pose) and Paschimottanasana (Western Stretch, page 103) and thus opens both the front hip flexors as well as the hamstrings.

Option Pose: Krounchasana *(Heron Pose)*

Assume Trianga Mukhaikapada Paschimottanasana (Three-Limbed, Face, and One-Legged Western Extended Stretch Pose) with your right leg extended forward and your left leg folded back in Virasana (Hero Pose, page 102). Move your left hand to your left ankle, gripping it. Perform a yogic lock (page 103) with your right hand onto the right big toe.

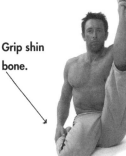

Grip shin bone.

Descend this thigh bone into the Earth.

Exhale and press the top of your left foot into the ground and raise your right leg off the ground and straighten it upward. (*Note:* If your right leg does not like this maneuver, set the right foot onto the ground with your right heel close to your groin.)

Inhale and make your spine as concave as possible.

Exhale, release your left hand from the left ankle, and capture the right heel with your left hand. Breathe here for a while.

Fine-tune the capture of the upraised foot by gripping the left wrist with the right hand around the sole of the right foot. Work the pose at this stage by bringing your heart center toward your right knee and gazing up at your right foot.

Exhale and slowly release the pose.

WHAT YOU ARE PRIMARILY WORKING: An intensification to all the benefits noted in Trianga Mukhaikapada Paschimottanasana (Three-Limbed, Face, and One-Legged Western Extended Stretch Pose).

WHOLISTIC NOTES: Pulling the extended foot off the ground should be done with a flat, not rounded, back. Once you have gotten the extended leg up into the air, you can repeatedly flex and extend the knee joint of the raised leg to create more lengthening to the leg. Imagine pulling the top of the raised thigh bone down into the ground.

Upavistha Konasana (Seated Angle Pose)

Lots of space between shoulders and ears

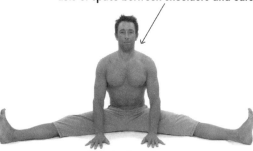

Breathe from here.

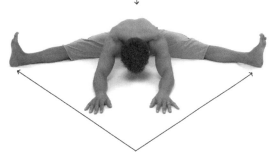

Keep feet flexed!

Sit elegantly upright on the ground with your legs spread wide at your comfortable edge. Your kneecaps should face toward the sky and your feet should be in line with your knees. Press down through the back of your thighs, spread your toes wide, and press out through the balls of your feet.

Inhale and elongate your core.

Exhale and carefully bend forward from your lower back (see photo). Your primary goals are twofold: (1) do not let your spine curve and, (2) imagine your belly button touching the ground before anything else. Get to your edge and breathe softness into the restrictions. Keep externally rotating your upper thigh bone, that is, keep rolling your inside thigh bone toward the back of you.

Inhale and draw the front of your body up.

Exhale and fold deeper into the pose by walking your hands in front of you (see photo). Stay here, breathe here for the prescribed time before pushing your hands against the ground and returning your torso to perpendicular.

WHAT YOU ARE PRIMARILY WORKING: Core strength. Creates space in the hip joints, lower back vertebrae, and pelvis. Brings circulation to all those areas while increasing flexibility of the hamstrings and adductors.

WHOLISTIC NOTES: Don't gobble up depth during this pose. Depth is not as important as keeping your spine flat. This is why I teach this pose with the hands behind the neck; it forces the core muscles to control the movement and the posture muscles to develop.

Option Pose: Parivrtta Upavistha Konasana (Revolved Seated Angle Pose)

Sit tall while assuming Upavistha Konasana (Seated Angle Pose). Turn your chest so that it is in alignment with your right leg. Place your right hand on the outside of the right thigh, and your left hand on the inside of your right thigh.

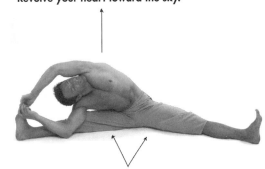

Revolve your heart toward the sky.

Exhale and walk both hands down toward your right foot while bending from your lower spine. As you reach your edge, breathe evenly for a while.

Listening for your breath to guide you toward softness, slowly start revolving your heart off your right thigh by twisting your torso toward the left. Move your left hand to your left hip and your right elbow to the inside of your right knee area. Use a yogic lock (page 103) to capture your right big toe with your right hand. Breathe here.

Externally rotate thigh bones.

Over the next few breaths, use your inhales to inch your spine longer and away from your hips and your exhales to keep your torso actively revolving.

As you reach your maximum edge of torso twist, remove your left hand from your left hip and reach it upward and then down and over to capture the right foot wherever you can (see photo). If this second foot capture is not happening just yet, simply hover the left elbow overhead at your edge. Stay here, breathe evenly for the prescribed time before releasing the pose on an exhale. Repeat process for the other leg.

WHAT YOU ARE PRIMARILY WORKING: All the benefits of Upavistha Konasana (Seated Angle Pose), but with a delicious opening of the upper ribs. This pose really frees a locked-up respiratory diaphragm and is great to do before and after Cardio workouts. By using this pose to soften the bracelet of the ribs, more oxygenation of the breathing tissues translates to more energy throughout the day. This pose is also great to do during difficult relationship times since it nourishes anahata chakra (heart center) like few poses do.

WHOLISTIC NOTES: Time keeps on turning—so should your torso. Keep the noninvolved leg active by extending it away from the more involved leg. Nudge the elbow that is on the ground against the inside of the involved leg to create a lever to help you revolve your torso.

Upavistha Dwi Pada Kapotasana (Seated Two-Legged Pigeon Pose)

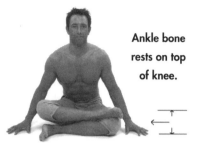

Ankle bone rests on top of knee.

Sit upright, near the top of a yoga mat. Using your hands to help, bend your right knee so you can place your right shinbone parallel to the top front edge of your yoga mat. Your right knee is near the right top corner of your yoga mat, and your right foot is nestled into the left top corner of your yoga mat.

Wriggle your hips around so that you can grab and place your left ankle bone on top of your right knee (which is bent). Make sure that it is your left ankle bone, not the left foot, that is on top of the right knee. Again, shift your hips around so that your left knee is directly on top of the right foot. Even though there might be a sizable gap between your left knee and right foot, just make sure that they are in alignment as described above. Rest your right hand on your left foot and your left hand on your left knee. You may even wish to press down with your hands if you need to deepen your edge. Breathe evenly here for a while. (*Note:* If either of your knees starts to squawk with pain, proceed very, very gingerly or just remain right where you are for the prescribed time.)

Inhale and make your spine concave.

Exhale and lean forward from your lower back. Walk your hands out in front of your shinbones, which remain horizontal (see photo). Rich sensations will start oozing from your buttock muscles as they are pulled and stretched. Relax into the intensity for the prescribed amount of time before releasing and repeating for the other leg.

WHAT YOU ARE PRIMARILY WORKING: Hips, hips, and . . . let me check here, hips!

WHOLISTIC NOTES: A real button pusher, especially for endurance athletes and others with tight hips. I want you to really respect this pose, which is a preparatory pose for Padmasana, or Full Lotus (see page 116). If you try to be too aggressive here, your knees will over-rotate and may get injured. You should never experience any pain in your knees during this pose. Focus your attention on releasing forward from your hips and lower back.

Salamba Sarvangasana (Supported All-Parts Pose, page 180)

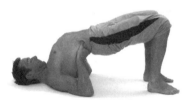

Do this pose, which you did during your Cosmic Yang Yoga practice, for 2 minutes.

Option Pose: Setu Banda Sarvangasana

Assume the pose, Salamba Sarvangasana (Supported All-Parts Pose, page 180), and bend your left knee so that your left heel drops behind your left buttock cheek. Breathe evenly and move your hands deeper into your rib cage.

Exhale and slowly lower, in a reaching way, your left foot to the ground behind your left buttock. You may touch down first with the toes, then lower the heel. Breathe here.

Exhale and lower your right leg in the same manner (see photo). Use the following breaths to open the chest and really plant all four corners of both feet into the ground. Knees and feet should remain at shoulder width and your toes should be pointed slightly in, as if pigeon toed. Breathe here for the prescribed time before raising the right leg again to its overhead position, then the left so you are back in Salamba Sarvangasana (Supported All-Parts Pose).

WHAT YOU ARE PRIMARILY WORKING: All the benefits of Salamba Sarvangasana (Supported All-Parts Pose), plus all the benefits of a backbend. This pose is particularly good for keeping the nervous and endocrine systems healthy and for restoring lost confidence, virility, and energy.

WHOLISTIC NOTES: If your lower back issues any radiating pain or strain, do not proceed deeper into the pose. Keep making micro adjustments with your hands pressed into your rib cage to amplify the opening effect of the chest. Once in the final position, press your shoulders and hands to lift your torso. If you want more? Extend your legs.

Navasana/Ardha Navasana (Boat/Half Boat Pose, page 107)

Savasana (Corpse Pose, page 108)

You did these two final poses to close your Green Tara Yoga practice.

HP YOGA: THE FRUGAL REALM PRACTICE

Begin by engaging ujjayi (see page 83) breathing and don't stop ujjayi until the final pose.

> 3 x Ardha Surya Namaskar (Half Sun Salutation)
>
> 2 x Series A Modified
>
> 1 x Series B (both legs = 1 set)
>
> 1 x Series C (both legs = 1 set)
>
> 5 x Series A

Then, do these movements, holding each for 30 to 60 seconds. Focus the mind with ujjayi breathing and the ego with honoring your edge.

1. Standing Vinyasa (flow sequence). Start with right leg in lead position.
   A. Utthita Parsvakonasana (Extended Side Angle Pose, page 96) exhale into
   B. Parsvottanasana (Side Extended Pose, page 97) into

C. Utthita Trikonasana (Extended Triangle Pose, page 97) into

D. Ardha Chandrasana (Half Moon Pose, page 98) swing your left leg through into

E. Garudasana (Eagle Pose, page 226)

F. step back into Downward Facing Dog (Adho Mukha Svanasana, page 99)
Repeat A through F for left leg.

2. Dhanurasana (Bow Pose, page 101)
Option Pose: Parsva Dhanurasana (Sideways Bow Pose, page 227)

3. Parivrtta Utkatasana (Twisting Chair Pose, page 228)
Option Pose: Dwi Pada Koundinyasana (Two-Footed Sage Pose, page 228)

4. Floating Pigeon Pose (page 229)
Option Pose: Flying Pigeon Pose (page 229)

5. Virasana (Hero Pose, page 102)
Option Pose: Supta Virasana (Supine Hero Pose, page 102)

6. Malasana (Garland Pose, page 103)
Option Pose: Bakasana (Crane Pose, page 104)

7. Prasarita Padottanasana (Extended Foot Pose, page 173)
Option Pose: Sirsasana (Headstand, page 175) from Prasarita Padottanasana

8. Trianga Mukhaikapada Paschimottanasana (Three-Limbed, Face, and One-Legged Western Extended Stretch Pose, page 231)
Option Pose: Krounchasana (Heron Pose, page 231)

9. Upavistha Konasana (Seated Angle Pose, page 232)
Option Pose: Parivrtta Upavistha Konasana (Revolved Seated Angle Pose, page 233)

10. Upavistha Dwi Pada Kapotasana (Seated Two-Legged Pigeon Pose, page 234)

11. Salamba Sarvangasana (Supported All-Parts Pose, page 180) for 2 minutes
Option Pose: Lower from #8 into Setu Banda Sarvangasana (page 234)

12. Navasana/Ardha Navasana (Boat/Half Boat Pose, page 107)

13. Savasana (Corpse Pose, page 108)

CHAPTER 18

Meditation

THERE ARE ONE OPTIONAL AND three mandatory Meditation assignments for you to practice during each of the four weeks of the Frugal Realm. Three of the four Meditation assignments are new. One of them is your old pal, Early Morning Zazen (page 119), from the Green Tara practice. Seems like you are a totally different person now, huh? You are! A leaner, fitter, and more focused one.

At this point, you are about to embark on the final training cycle of my

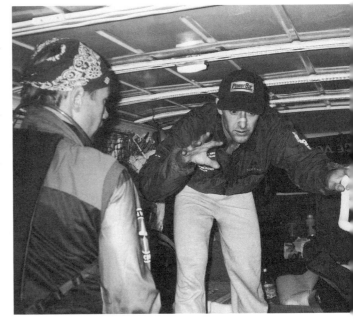

Coach Ilg, 3 A.M. after taking another 45 minute "pull" at the Furnace Creek 508 Ultra Distance bicycle race, Death Valley, CA.

program. You have learned by direct experience that WF is tough stuff. In fact, you may not have been able to complete all the prescribed workouts, no matter how noble was your effort.

That is fine. You can always return to the programs and do even better on them with your newfound fitness and disciplined mind.

What really matters is that you are learning more about your true self. You are learning that not running away from effort can often bring more joy and meaning into your life than the constant pursuit of happiness. Everybody has told you to chase happiness. The society that we live in teases you with the illusion of pleasure to be gained through material things and nonstop entertainment.

I am teaching you to create time for regular Meditation.

I am teaching you not to run away from effort, but to embrace it. Devote yourself to difficulty so you are freed from it. This may mean meditating in the wee hours or drinking one less alcoholic drink. It all depends on who you are and what your inner work requires from you to have you love yourself enough to be free. The mystic Rumi wrote:

Fall in love
With the agony of love
Not the ecstasy
Then the Beloved
Will fall in love with you.

> *I cannot imagine the darkness of my being if I did not have WF. This Path kicks into automatic whenever I need some light the most.*
> —DEAN KRAKEL, 1999

Rumi was amazing with words born from his meditative absorption. But my students are not Rumi. They are like you and me, and Sally and Jim. That's what makes their words, born from their meditations, that much more beautiful to me. If my students followed conventional personal training methods, not one of them would have meditated. But they did, because they studied WF. Listen to their words, fresh from their meditation sessions during the Frugal Realm.

Let's learn the three new Meditation tools for your Frugal Realm journey.

3 x 30 Assignment

In Chapter 20, you will see on your Frugal Realm Daily Practice sheet the following assignment:

Meditation: 3 x 30 Assignment

This Meditation is taken from a Theravada Buddhist mindfulness exercise. On this day, chew your first bite of food during your three main meals thirty times.

During this conscious chewing, feel the significance of the food being eaten. Draw from your previous Meditation training in this program, such as the Rasa Eating Exercise (page 186), to appreciate the fact that you are not different from the food you eat and one day, you too will be consumed by the Universe as well.

Use this "chew time" to honor, if not revere, your food. Tell the food that you will do your best to use its life-giving energy to refine yourself in order to help others.

Some common body/mind insights that arise for most students during this interesting assignment include how surprisingly effective is the act of chewing for easier digestion. Many times, the food has been long gone before the thirty chews have been completed. I've had many students remark that their "chronic heartburn" or other digestion or elimination difficulties disappeared once this assignment inspired them to chew more thoroughly.

Other insights include the decline of hurried, unappreciative eating habits and enhanced respect for the natural efficiency of more mindful chewing. As one student noted, "After practicing this assignment for four weeks, I am convinced that nearly all people who take heartburn and antacid medications don't need those medications. They just need to learn what you taught me: Chew your food."

> *I discovered the sanctity of Difficulty. I know more deeply than ever who I am.*
> —JEFF KILDAHL, 1996

> Steve—
> Before you left Durango for the Big City I never got a chance to thank you for all the materials and knowledge about meditation you have given me. They are gifts beyond price. They mean more to me than you will ever know. Thank you.
> YOUR MOUNTAIN BIKING BROTHER FROM COLORADO, RANDELL LABAUME, 1995

Gratitude Journal

On evenings when this meditation is assigned, take a few minutes before retiring to record ten things that you noticed during the day that inspired gratitude. Note also why you are grateful for it. This Gratitude Journal can be done with your children or spouse, or perhaps while lying in the softness of your bed, enveloped by your material world.

A sample entry might look something like: "I feel grateful for this bed, which will afford me a deep and refreshing sleep" or "I feel grateful for my car, which is so amazingly convenient . . . I couldn't imagine having to ride my bike to work every day or walk ten miles to get fresh drinking water."

Commit to keeping a simple journal for this assignment. Some students choose to keep the journal assignment going after this cycle, which is fine. Keeping this journal cultivates an attitude of gratitude: a child's smile, a flower growing in the middle of road construction, a stranger's polite eye contact—things that should be feeding your soul but you are not seeing until now.

Early Morning Zazen

You learned this during Green Tara (page 119). This practice now reemerges with higher volumes that build throughout your training week. Do your best not to miss one session. If you must reduce the prescribed time, that is fine. It is much better to sit fewer minutes more consistently than to pressure yourself into doing longer sessions. Remember to switch your leg position halfway into the prescribed sitting time.

Media Fasts

These are optional meditation practices that truly must be done for those wishing to reach master student levels of this path. Feel completely free to just do one Media Fast during the four weeks. Again, there is no need to pressure yourself into these practices.

MORE STUDENTS' INPUT ON MEDITATION WITHIN THE REALM

Dear Coach—

I have to tell you . . . I've really noticed a big-time difference in my attitude/outlook/philosophical approach on life, training, being . . . how I interact with others—both verbally and nonverbally . . . I know it because I'm losing my fears and trusting me, you, meditation, WF, and the universe . . . because each will provide if the effort and sincerity is there . . . I see what you mean . . . a dance . . . a flow . . . I sense the rhythm of the universe . . . and am more aware when I am in or out of tune with it. Like if I sit down on the floor . . . take a deep breath and really appreciate the smell and beauty of the food I am lucky to be able to have, prepare, and eat (and to be healthy . . . and have a nice apartment to sit in) . . . how much more nourishing both physically and spiritually . . . and emotionally the meal and life is . . . or before a yang day squat set in the gym . . . how being aware of where my mind/focus/spirit is . . . it's little things like this, Coach, that are meaning so much to me these days . . . I'm noticing the pauses in between the notes . . . and I'm hearing another facet to the music that enriches the whole song . . . I'm crying my eyes out now . . . I just really wanted you to know this . . . and how much I appreciate you . . . p.s. my wife says mega thanx too . . . she's noticed.

—STUDENT DANSAN SALIMONE

Choose between one of the two types of media fasts, Novice or Advanced. First, the definition of media:

> media. a. A means of mass communication, such as newspapers, magazines, radio, or television.

Novice Media Fast

When these days are prescribed, you may watch TV, radio, or cinematic forms of media, but you are not to watch or read any commercials or listen to any commercials. On this day do not read any newspapers or magazines. During daily life take care not to read billboards, ads on benches, beverages, sports arenas, etc. Note how bombarded you are by media. Personal CDs are allowed; music is not considered media at this level.

Advanced Media Fast

When these days are prescribed, you are not to watch, read, or listen to any form of media whatsoever. Personal CDs are not allowed; music is considered media at this level.

> Coach Ilg,
>
> I don't think I've ever said this directly but I want you to know how much this work means to me. It fills my need for spiritual work that I felt has been missing in my life over the last few years, as well as the awesome training. I really appreciate you being here and providing Wholistic Fitness for me and every one else who is led here. Sometimes, I never thought I could accomplish as many of your programs that I have! This work alone is worth doing. I consider it a bonus that I'm able to climb and play outside.
>
> —STUDENT JOHN CAMPBELL

CHAPTER 19

Nutrition

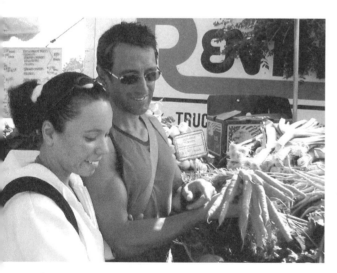

Kathy and I enjoy preparing nutritious mealtimes together but at least half the nutrition comes from the loving appreciation of having such easy access to so much beautiful food every day! Here we are visiting a farmers' market after taking a yoga class in Santa Monica. We just plain feel sorry for people who choose to eat fast food—they are missing so much!

YOUR BASIC EATING PATTERN SHOULD not differ from what I've already detailed in chapters 5 and 12. Adding an extra 300 to 600 calories per day might help you recover a bit more fully and faster from the high volume of Strength Training workouts inherent to the Realm. You may find yourself craving protein sources such as meat, fish, peanut butter, etc. Just do your best to maintain the 60-30-10 ratio of carbs, protein, and fat (respectively).

I've found that getting some help from herbs is a definite plus during this cycle. You might add some extra immune system herbs (if you are using the Sunrider herbs, which I suggest, this means additional Alpha 20C and Conco). There are also herbs that benefit quicker strength shifts and recovery, such as Wu Chia Pi. Adding a Protein Plus bar from PowerBar, Spiralina, or just increasing dietary protein a bit during the Realm are also wise options for the four weeks of the Realm (see Sources).

The Meditation assignments given during this phase are intended to work closely with your nutritional awareness. Ask yourself these questions when making your food choices during this cycle: Am I appreciating my foods? Am I eating slowly? Am I eating mindfully? Am I chewing thoroughly? Am I beginning to feel the energetics of my various food choices? Am I beginning to feel the energetics of my relationship nutrition? How does who I hang out with affect me? Is it conducive to my path? What is truly feeding me? And what is not?

> Remember, the students who make the most significant gains in Wholistic Fitness are those who *prioritize* the "softer" disciplines of meditation, yoga, and nutrition—not cardio or gym workouts!

Daily Practice

Although I have shown the means of liberation,
you must know that it depends upon you alone.
—THE BUDDHA

H ERE IS YOUR FINAL MAIN training cycle of Wholistic Fitness training before your maintenance program. This chapter pulls together the preceding five chapters and transforms it into a day-by-day schedule for your Frugal Realm experience.

All the following workouts have been cross-referenced to the appropriate chapters in Parts Two and Three. I've put page numbers next to each movement and technique for easy cross-referencing.

Practice reminders:

Don't stress if unable to do all the workouts for that day. Do your priority disciplines if possible. Remember, you are still living a WF lifestyle if you can't do anything but eat consciously and in alignment with WF guidelines or even working your Breath and Posture. Don't reduce WF to mere physical workouts. WF is much more about developing awareness than it is muscle.

Don't try to make up missed workouts by cramming several workouts into the next day. Instead, just keep flowing through the week. You've got your whole life to become wholistically fit.

> Consistency comes first, sequencing comes second. I've choreographed the fitness disciplines in the order that provides the optimal training effect. However, if you need to switch the order, you can.

Good luck, noble warrior! Train hard, choose softness, and most of all be sincere in your effort. I'll see your higher side on the other side of The Realm.

Wholistic Fitness Training Precepts

1. Be prepared

2. Be on time

3. Give 110 percent

Monday. Recovery and Scheduling Weekly Workouts

Mondays are traditional WF recovery days, no physical workouts today.

Focus on your work while giving your body time to prepare for the upcoming training week.

Sometime today, go to your schedule book and block out the time needed to do your workouts each day. Mentally prepare for your training week, and learn from the prior week: Where could you have been more noble? How are you going to do better this week? Visualize yourself doing the upcoming workouts in a strong, elegant, and focused manner. Maybe this is the week you decide to incorporate a Cardio Commute or a Periodic Renunciation or a Media Fast (new to this cycle). If so, schedule it in and prepare for it. Energy follows thought.

Receiving bodywork (massage) on Mondays is wise.

Tuesday. Lower Body Yang Workout

Strength: Do the Frugal Realm lower body yang workout (page 214).

Yoga: None or flow through a few rounds of one or more HP Yoga Sun Salutations series (page 86) before your gym workout or as a cooldown/stretch sometime after it. (*note:* If by week 3 you are adapting to the Realm okay, it would be fantastic to add the Frugal Realm HP Yoga practice (page 225) or you could do the HP Yoga video (see Sources) on this day to really deepen your fitness.

Meditation: Do the 3×30 Assignment (page 238).

Meditation 2: Passive Meditation: Gratitude Journal (page 239).

Cardio (optional): Cardio Commute.

Wednesday. Chest and Back Yin Workout

Meditation: Do an Early Morning Zazen session (see page 119) for 20 minutes (switch leg position halfway).

Yoga: None or flow through a few rounds of one or more HP Yoga Sun Salutations series (page 86) before your gym workout or as a cooldown/stretch sometime after it.

Strength: Do the Frugal Realm chest and back yin workout (page 209).

Meditation 2: Passive Meditation: Gratitude Journal (page 239).

Cardio (optional): Cardio Commute.

Thursday. Shoulders and Arms Yin Workout

Yoga: None or flow through a few rounds of one or more HP Yoga Sun Salutations series (page 86) before your gym workout or as a cooldown/stretch sometime after it.

Strength: Do the Frugal Realm shoulders and arms yin workout (page 212).

Meditation 2: Passive Meditation: Gratitude Journal (page 239).

Meditation 3 (optional): Media Fast. Choose either a Novice or Advanced version (page 241).

Cardio (optional): Cardio Commute.

Friday. Lower Body Yin Workout

Meditation: Do an Early Morning Zazen session (page 119) for 30 minutes (switch leg position halfway).

Yoga: None or flow through a few rounds of one or more HP Yoga Sun Salutations series (page 86) before your gym workout or as cooldown/stretch sometime after it.

Strength: Do the Frugal Realm lower body yin workout (page 215).

Meditation 2: Passive Meditation: Gratitude Journal (page 239).

Cardio (optional): Cardio Commute.

Saturday. Double Day: Chest and Back: Yang and Cardio

Strength: Do the Frugal Realm chest and back yang workout (page 208).

Cardio: After the gymwork, enjoy a Cardio of Choice (page 74) for 1.5 to 3 hours at Zones 1 and 2, some Zone 3 (see Table 2.1, page 75), but no more than 30 minutes total at Zone 3.

Meditation: Passive Meditation: Gratitude Journal (page 239).

Sunday. Double Day Shoulders and Arms: Yang and Yoga

Strength: Do the Frugal Realm shoulders and arms yang workout (page 210).

Yoga: Do the Frugal Realm HP Yoga practice.

Cardio (optional): If you are really becoming a WF animal, then enjoy an hour or so of Cardio of Choice done within Zones 1 and 2 (see Table 2.1, page 75). This is a low priority, however.

Meditation: Passive Meditation: Gratitude Journal (page 239).

Cycle Summation

T**HIS SHEET IS TO** be completed after four weeks of getting "Realmed." Pass out during your recovery week, get some IVs—and we'll see you in seven days to learn your maintenance program . . .

Frugal Realm Cycle Summation

Date started:

Date finished:

Today's date:

Strength Training

1. Since the Frugal Realm has only three words in it, describe in three words what you felt about the Strength Training.
2. Describe the effects from and your consistency in the Strength Training workouts.

Cardio

1. Note any observations during your efforts in this discipline. Record the average number of Cardio hours you performed during the Realm.
2. How do your joints feel?

Yoga

1. Were you able to stay somewhat supple even through the intense Strength Training of the Realm? Why?
2. Give me an indication of the insight you gained through your yoga during the Realm.

Meditation

1. Comment on your zazen sessions. Give me a depth of the insight gained through your practice. Do you have questions?
2. What did you learn about gratitude journaling?
3. If applicable, note insights from your Media Fast.

Nutrition

1. What angered you most during the Realm (a particular circumstance, an ongoing challenge, etc.)?
2. Why couldn't you breathe through it?
3. What can you learn from this anger?
4. Did the training in the Realm seem to trivialize other things that usually anger or get you away from center? Note them.
5. Describe exactly what you ate yesterday and the manner in which you ate it. Note any cravings.
6. Note any cravings that came up this cycle as opposed to during the Green Tara or Cosmic Yang.
7. Note physique/bodyweight changes experienced during the Realm.

Now that you have finished one of my most intense training programs, it is I who bow to you. You don't even need to think about training for the next few days. But when you do, you're gonna love y(our) final passage.

It's time to get free . . . It's time to do more yoga, enjoy a little less intensity and structure, and synthesize all of your great work of the past three months with the Jeweled Lotus Maintenance Program.

Enjoy your recovery week . . . you damn well deserve it! There ain't nothing like WF! And there sure ain't nothing like you, baby!

You should feel very go(o)d about yourself right now. Very few athletes (even elite ones) have traveled the inner and the outer, the hard and the soft, as you just have. Congratulations. I bow to your devoted practice.

PART FOUR

MAINTAINING AND MASTERING YOUR WHOLISTIC FITNESS: THE JEWELED LOTUS

The most fun of Wholistic Fitness starts right here. You, like the lotus flower, have survived the high difficulty of my three foundation phases. Green Tara was like your infancy . . . so much was new to you. Crazy new fitness training techniques, a new understanding of nutrition, formal meditation, and bizarre daily assignments planted the seed that would marry your physical workouts into your daily life.

Then, one week after you recovered from Green Tara, I slapped the power-packed

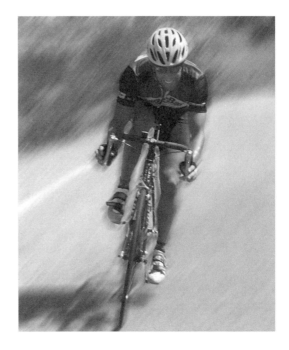

The lotus flower often symbolizes spiritual warriorism because it blooms into beauty from mud and floats on water yet remains dry. Similarly, fitness warriors should practice inner work while remaining immersed in the outer world. With lotuslike tenacity, a passionate yet nonattached devotion to life should be embraced, as the lotus pushes itself upward through dark, thick muck to embrace sunshine and blossoms into a most gorgeous flower. The lotus teaches a nonjudgmental acceptance of the muck we grew up in, a cleansing within the waters of our life, and an elegant strength from growth experience. Now you know why many Eastern deities are depicted sitting upon a throne of a lotus blossom (see page 39).

Cosmic Yang across your ego. These four weeks were like your adolescence in WF training. Like a teenager resistant to society's rules, you probably rebelled at the effort I required from you to step up to the authority of doing intervals and kinesthetically demanding strength and yoga movements. But somewhere within you, a shift occurred and brought with it a newly discovered sense of who you are. You fell in love again with notions of mastery and daily warriorism and random acts of kindness and compassion. Your workouts grew to more than mere appetizers or desserts to your "real life." They became the main nutriment for your spiritual and physical life.

Another recovery week later and all hell broke lose. The Frugal Realm entered your life and shattered any remaining fragment of your once proud sense of self. The Realm grounded you and metaphorically represented adulthood. There was no easy way out from the response-ability to the training within the Frugal Realm. The program functioned like a living Zen koan. The workouts were like a riddle impossible to solve by the intellect. Each day seemed to be a journey into your inner fire. How noble could you be? Would you do the Cardio Commute or blow it off? Would you do the Double Day workouts where one gut-busting gym workout preceded a two-hour Cardio session? How beautiful a fitness warrior could you be? Beautiful enough to recycle the newspaper instead of reading it and shut the television off for one day of Media Fasting?

The Frugal Realm was designed to make or break you. I designed the Frugal Realm so that you would become fatigued by the very brilliance of the cleverly constructed ego patterns of your past and your conditioned vision of your life. At the barrier of ego fatigue there was a mirror asking you to look at a much more pure version of yourself. Did you like what you saw? How clear was the reflection? Within the Realm of the

Frugal, if you were honest in your meditation sessions, all your hidden dragons were scraped front and center. I asked you to deal directly with whatever came up.

Notice how little I even talk about all the fantastic physical changes that have occurred in your body since you began work with me fourteen weeks ago. *This is because the essence of my work with you is that an improved body is a by-product of personal growth.*

HERE NOW

You have just enjoyed your recovery week from the Frugal Realm. You are probably quite curious about what I have cooked up for you in this maintenance program. How am I going to create for you a program that maintains the unprecedented level of body/mind fitness that you have achieved within the last three months? There is no way you can keep up the volume and the intensity of what you encountered during my first three programs, right?

Right.

I wouldn't want you to even try. The largest mistake most fitness athletes make is their attempt to maintain high-level, specific, year-round fitness. But what you have in this book are transpersonal fitness tools and techniques you can repeat, modify, and benefit from for the rest of your life.

My final program for you, the Jeweled Lotus, captures the core of everything you have been through with me. In the Lotus, you will take fitness out of your self and turn it inside out to the benefit of others. This program is a living connection with the yoga spirit. No longer just a physical fitness program with a cool spiritual spin, your foray into Wholistic Fitness, which began with three programs that kicked your physical butt, now matures and radiates with a lifestyle program designed to make a difference in the

Whether you fulfill 100 percent of the program's teachings or just 1 percent does not matter. Sincere effort does. Remember, in Wholistic Fitness, nothing matters but everything counts. For example, if every household in the United States replaced just one bottle of 28-ounce petroleum-based dish-washing liquid with a similar vegetable-based product, over 82,000 barrels of oil—enough to drive a car over 86 million miles—would be saved.

consciousness of society. The Jeweled Lotus program is the realization of what I see as America's highest and most practical form of Yoga.

It is said that all paths lead to Yoga, and Wholistic Fitness is not an exception. Yet, in America, Yoga has largely been reduced to asana practice. There are thousands of certified Yoga teachers who really are just asana teachers. Perhaps they don't teach yama or niyama (see page 79) or tie asana into meditation (dhyana) because they don't live it in their daily lives or have never been properly introduced to the larger sphere of Yoga.

While improving your body/mind fitness, this maintenance program allows you ample occasion to refine yourself as a human being. What I present with my Jeweled Lotus program is an ongoing opportunity for you to actually live classical Yoga precepts within the context of our modern fitness lifestyle. The Lotus program is designed to lift you out of indecorous ego patterns and elevate yogic ethical and moral inflow in fun ways. The Lotus maintenance program is my contribution toward a more fit and more conscious America.

PROGRAM NOTES

For optimal long-term physique and health effects, don't remain on the Lotus longer than eight weeks. By eight weeks, it is time to take a recovery week and restart the Green Tara program.

Once you have completed my full program—Green Tara into Cosmic Yang into Frugal Realm into the Jeweled Lotus—then you have the education and fitness base to sequence the various programs in a number of creative ways to fit your training year.

Here are some examples that have proven especially effective:

Month 1	=	Green Tara
Month 2	=	Jeweled Lotus
Month 3	=	Cosmic Yang
Month 4	=	Jeweled Lotus
Month 5	=	Frugal Realm
Month 6	=	Vacation!

or

Month 1	=	Green Tara
Months 2 and 3	=	Jeweled Lotus
Month 4	=	Cosmic Yang
Months 5 and 6	=	Jeweled Lotus
Month 7	=	Frugal Realm
Month 8	=	Vacation!

or

Autumn	=	Green Tara into Jeweled Lotus
Winter	=	Cosmic Yang into Jeweled Lotus
Spring	=	Frugal Realm into Jeweled Lotus
Summer	=	Jeweled Lotus

I even have students who enjoy doing Jeweled Lotus for a period of several weeks, then do Green Tara for four weeks, and go back to Lotus. They just repeat that simple sequence and express fantastic inner and physical rewards.

For this first time, however, the Jeweled Lotus capitalizes upon your high strength fitness gained during the Frugal Realm. Thus, the upcoming weeks utilize a unique and colorful blend of all your newfound fitness.

An emphasis on High Performance Yoga replaces the time spent in the gym (you don't even need a gym membership for the Jeweled Lotus).

SOMETHING SPECIAL

Since you are somebody special for even making it to this chapter, I wish to let you in on a special secret. I have not told you this secret earlier, because I teach in the same manner as did my Tibetan and Japanese teachers: The student must earn secret teachings from the master only through steadfast and intense practice. You earned this secret teaching.

The secret teaching is that I have secret teachings behind every one of my programs. There are secret teachings to the three previous programs, for example, but you were not ready to hear them. Now you are. For the Jeweled Lotus, I will share with you her secret teachings. Think of the following information as spiritual springboards. If you choose to go higher, research their meanings and whole new inner dimensions will arise from within you. Enjoy!

ASPECTS AND AIMS OF THE JEWELED LOTUS

TECHNICAL AIMS

To maintain prior body/mind fitness attained from the previous three main programs. To find your workout everywhere. To prioritize softness and acceptance over hardness and rebellion.

PRIORITY TRAINING DISCIPLINES

Yoga

Nutrition (physical and spiritual)

SPIRITUAL AIMS

Balance, Communication, Bliss, Awareness, Perception

PRINCIPAL CHAKRAS

Although svadhisthana receives particular emphasis, all seven chakras are stimulated by this program.

PRINCIPAL GEMSTONES

Lapis Lazuli, Rose Quartz

PROGRAM DEITY

Amitabha, the "Boundless Light." This ruler of an exquisite state of consciousness is extremely popular and important in both Chinese and Japanese Buddhism. He symbolizes mercy and wisdom. It is said that just calling on the name of Amitabha, especially during the death process, is enough to be reborn in paradise.

PROGRAM MANTRA

"Om mani padme om," which means, "Hail to the jewel in the lotus flower which blooms in my heart." There is complex meaning to the sound sequencing of this six-syllable and most popular Buddhist invocation. One who recites this mantra will be saved from all dangers. For Tibetan Buddhists, the syllables express an attitude of compassion and longing for liberation "for the sake of all sentient beings." This is the national chant of Tibet, arguably the most spiritually advanced—but nearly extinct—culture in our world.

Low but consistent practical and formal meditations dance throughout the week.

Weekends are highlighted with outdoor activity (it's important to let your feet connect with Mother Earth at least a little each week!).

Nutrition just flows along and the result is a lifestyle program unmatched for producing equanimity and blissful fitness.

May your in-joyment of the Jeweled Lotus sparkle with insight and radiate ever blossoming Joy for you!

Excellence in every workout performed.
—Coach Ilg

CHAPTER 22

Strength Training

*If you are true to your practice,
complexity will dissolve.*

—VENERABLE KHANDRO RINPOCHE

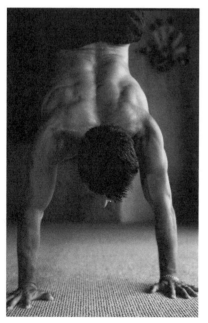

**Coach Ilg practicing
Adho Mukha Vrkasana
(Downward Facing Tree
Pose or Handstand) during
an HP Yoga session.**

ENOUGH OF THE GYM!
There is not one Strength
Training workout to do for the
next four to eight weeks! You
have just finished three training
programs that relied heavily upon
the "Iron Temple" to produce
incredibly deep strength fitness. Now, however, during the Lotus, I'm
going to turn your raw strength base into a more functional and more
multifaceted form of muscular fitness. How I am going to do this is by
jacking up the volume of your HP Yoga. So
basically, now is the time to say good-bye to
the barbells and hello to the Chaturgangas.

I purposely want you to remain out of
the gym so your joints and muscles and nerves

> *The Jeweled Lotus program forces the
> gym addict away from the Iron
> Temple to develop a more functional
> strength. Strength with flexibility is a
> truer form of warrior strength.*
> **—COACH ILG**

can properly recover and enjoy the benefits from Yoga. Instead of maxing out your strength in the gym, try testing your inner resolve in daily life. This is a truer form of strength. Use the time away from the gym to appreciate the role of strength in more transpersonal ways. I outline several key ways to apply such transpersonal strength in Chapter 25.

PRESCRIPTION NOTE

For those of you who choose to enjoy the Jeweled Lotus program for longer than four weeks, you will need to go to the gym once per week to maintain some of the deeper neural and chemical training effects for your muscle strength. So, if you do follow the Lotus for longer than four weeks, I want you to alternate an EEE-GAD workout (page 143) with a Yang Day workout (page 199) on each Tuesday. I've made a note of this in your Daily Practice in Chapter 27.

CHAPTER 23

Cardio

The real Porsche lies within.

—COACH ILG

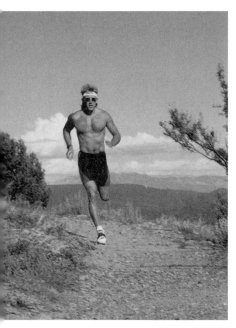

YOUR CARDIO TRAINING DURING THE Jeweled Lotus can be done in high, moderate, or low volumes. I've kept one Cardio session reserved for a playful form of high-intensity Cruise Intervals. I'll describe how to do those in a moment. For those of you who are still looking to drop bodyfat levels, you are really going to have to use the Lotus as a time to up your volume of Cardio training. There is no good reason not to. I do not have you in the gym at all, which will save you bucketloads of time and energy. Use this reservoir of time and energy to increase the number of your Cardio workouts. Sure, I would love it if you would integrate Cardio Commuting into your lifestyle, but if not that, then do some Cardio of Choice (page 74) that you enjoy. Remember, doing a fifteen-minute walk or jog is absolutely better for your body and fat-burning metabolism than nothing at all.

    If losing fat is not a priority for you by the time you enter the

Lotus, then use this cycle to do low volumes of the Cardio discipline to create more time in your week to concentrate on the Yoga component.

In the Daily Practice chapter coming up you will see listed the following options for your Cardio training: Cardio Commute (page 76), Cardio of Choice (page 74), and Cruise Intervals.

What are Cruise Intervals? Good question. Let's find out now.

> Cruise Intervals are an excellent form of free-flowing high-intensity Cardio training. They are more spontaneous and intuitive than structured interval training like Assigned Intervals.

CRUISE INTERVALS

When Cruise Intervals are prescribed, begin doing your Cardio of Choice (page 74) with an easy Zone 1–2 warm up for 20 minutes (see Table 2.1, page 75). You should have nice sweat triggered by the end of this warmup.

After 20 minutes, hit your inner turbojets and accelerate your pace up to high Zone 3—a difficult but sustainable pace. Hold this high Zone 3 "time trial" pace for 1.5 minutes. Then reach way down deep and push the booster jets, accelerating once again and reaching Zone 4, and hold Zone 4 for 30 seconds.

Immediately reduce your effort until your heart rate reaches Zone 1.

"Cruise" along at Zones 1–2 for several minutes before popping off another 2-minute interval.

Repeat that choreography until you have ticked off 5 of these 2-minute intervals. Then finish the rest of your workout coasting in Zones 1–2.

During the intervals, focus on smooth, powerful mechanics. Use the active intervals to focus on your technique—cycling, running, swimming, power walking, cross-country skiing, whatever. During the time spent between the active intervals, widen your focus to a more open perspective so you enjoy the nature or scene around you.

CHAPTER 24

High Performance Yoga

Why not apply your practice right now,
in the moment?
—COACH ILG

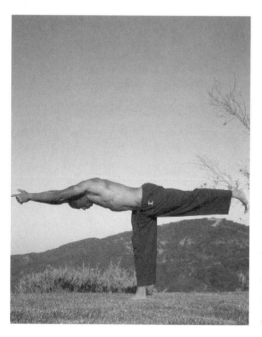

DURING THE JEWELED LOTUS, YOU have the opportunity to practice the three HP Yoga routines that you have learned in each of the three preceding programs. I have you scheduled for Yoga practice on Wednesdays, Fridays, and Sundays during this cycle. This doesn't mean that you have to do that much Yoga, but if you do you will be very healthy, fit, and glowing with inner power and energy.

More important, you will discover the answer to my question, "Why not apply your practice right now, in this moment?"

It works like this. On Wednesdays you do the Green Tara routine, Fridays are your Cosmic Yang routine, and Sundays are your Frugal Realm routine. Certainly, the more consistent your Yoga practice is during this cycle, the greater your chance of mastering certain poses, balancing out your body and mind, increasing your core strength, reducing bodyfat, and enhancing your flexibility and mental focus.

You can also use any day to take a Yoga class at your favorite Yoga studio, but don't do Yoga more than once a day. Some students do that, but inevitably the physical and mental quality of the practice suffers. If you just get bit big time by the Yoga bug and can't get enough, then do an extra "Pranayama Pump" session, which I will explain below. The point I want to make is to keep Jeweled Lotus vibrating at an easy level for you so your time is not strained by the structure of fitting in daily workouts. If you miss a workout, fine. No big deal. There is always tomorrow. Just return to your Breath and Posture and keep flowing with your moments as they unfold.

Since you already have all you need to do the various HP Yoga routines that will appear in your Daily Practice for this cycle, I want to explain a new, fun, and very effective Yoga session that functions as a Meditation but also an important way to increase your life force (pran). I call it the Pranayama Pump session. Here is how to do it.

PRANAYAMA PUMP

This amazing session combines three safe pranayama (breath control) techniques. The net result oxygenates all tissues and balances the body/mind energies by invigorating the body and calming the mind. I have relied on "the Pump" since the early eighties to get me centered and balanced before competitions and public speaking, or to help handle illness or other stressful challenges.

Your mind will achieve calm strength with this practice. Your life force (pran) will be stronger. Your neurohormonal chemistry will be more balanced. Your emotions will be more centered. Enjoy.

1. Go to your meditation space and make sure there is a clock with a second hand available and within sight. Light a stick of incense, a candle, and put on yoga or meditation music.

2. Assume your best zazen sitting posture. Engage Mula Bandha (Root Lock, page 169) and Jalandhara Bandha (Throat Lock, page 106).

3. Bring both hands into Jnana Mudra (Wisdom Seal) by stretching both hands onto the top of each knee, palms facing up. Bend the tip of your index finger into the base of your thumbnail. Extend the other three fingers. Make sure your bandhas and leg, spine, arm, and hand position are activated, strong, and stable.

4. Do 2 to 5 minutes of deep Ujjayi Pranayama (Victorious Breath, page 83). This is the same breath technique you use during your asana sessions, but now I want you to use it exclusively as a form of Meditation. Focus your full attention on matching the depth and lengths of your inhales and exhales. Seek a raspy, hollow sound to Ujjayi. Do not allow your mind to wander away from the breath awareness.

5. Do 2 to 5 minutes of Uddiyana Bandha Pranayama (Drawing Upward Lock breath control). This bandha cleanses chakras, intensifies pran, stimulates nadic (nerve) energy, and blocks apana (down breath, a principal life-force current that powers the body from its lower half).

    Make sure Jalandhara Bandha and Mula Bandha are activated.

    Finish an exhale completely.

    Inhale by drawing the navel toward the spine.

    Let your exhale "fly up" the spine toward *anahata chakra* (heart center).

    Repeat for prescribed time. Inhales should match exhales in duration. Do not hold breath. If you become dizzy, stop the practice. Try again later. Keep the mind focused only on the breath control. Here again is the choreography of the Uddiyana Bandha pranayama technique:

    a.   activate Jalandhara and Mula Bandha
    b.   inhale, draw navel toward spine
    c.   exhale, bring breath up the spine
    d.   repeat for prescribed or desired amount

6. Do 2 to 5 minutes of Nadi Sodhana Pranayama (Channel Purification breath control) technique. Maintain the correct pranayama posture and bandhas as above. This is vital.

    Stretch your left arm onto the top of the left knee, palm facing up. The left fingers were traditionally used for counting rounds but today are usually placed in Jhana Mudra (see photo and page 265).

    Bring your right hand toward your nose. Bend the right index and middle finger of the right hand into the right palm. Your right thumb opens and closes the right nostril, while the ring finger and pinky controls the opening and closing of the left nostril. This hand position is known as the "Deer Mudra" owing to the shape of the hand when this hand posture is viewed from the side.

    One cycle works like this: Close off the left nostril using two fingers. Exhale through the right nostril. Inhale completely but slowly through the right nostril while the left nostril remains blocked off. At the top of your inhalation, shut off the right nostril with your right thumb, release the left nostril, and exhale through it. Inhale through the left nostril, then shut it off and exhale through the right nostril. That is one cycle.

    Keep repeating this sequence. Start with 2 minutes, building up to 5 minutes. Inhales should match exhales in duration. Do not hold breath. If you become dizzy, stop the practice. Keep the mind focused only on the breath control. Here again is the choreography of the Nadi Sodhana pranayama technique:

    a.   exhale through right nostril to begin
    b.   inhale through right nostril

> When the five senses and the mind are still, and reason itself rests in silence, then begins the path supreme. This calm steadiness of the senses is called yoga.
>
> —FIRST WRITTEN REFERENCE TO YOGA AND MEDITATION; *UPANISHADS*, CIRCA 3000 B.C. AND 1200 B.C.

Here, WF student Lenore Fusano demonstrates correct pranayama posture. Note how her chin is resting in the notch between the collarbones. This contraction of the throat is Jalandhara Bandha. The left arm is stretched and the left fingers can be used for counting rounds (traditional) or placed in Jnana Mudra. The index and middle finger of the right hand are folded into the palm. The right thumb opens and closes the right nostril, while the ring and small finger control the opening and closing of the left nostril.

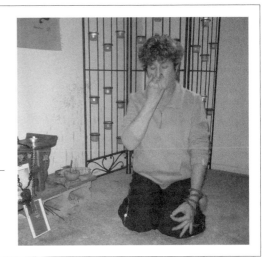

      c.   exhale through left nostril

      d.   inhale through left nostril

     Repeat as prescribed.

7.   Finish with 5 to 20 minutes of Savasana (page 108).

CHAPTER 25

Meditation

Practice and enlightenment are one.

—DOGEN

D EEP WITHIN THE LAYERED INTELLIGENCE of this cycle, the crux of the Jeweled Lotus program unveils itself. The Lotus is less about doing hard physical workouts and more about creatively integrating the nobility of fitness into daily life. To master the WF path, fitness must be clearly expressed in the way we choose to live our lives. The time to radiate your warriorism has arrived.

> The thrust of meditation during the Jeweled Lotus phase is best described as Engaged Meditation, bringing enhanced levels of awareness and insight into your daily life.

During this cycle, select and practice at least one of the following ten WF Mastery Pathways. Some are "big" and others are "little." Approach whichever one you choose with an even-minded will to rise higher in your life.

I have arranged these pathways to be in modern alignment with classical yoga's first and second limbs, *yama* (ethical guidelines) and *niyama* (personal guidelines).

1. Ahimsa (Nonharming): Prioritize Wholistic Shopping

Start prioritizing your food, household, and cosmetic shopping with the following qualities: perservative-free, natural, wholesome, organic, ecofriendly, no animal testing, cruelty-free. Begin with small things, such as lightbulbs, rechargeable batteries, or organic fruit. Choose to harm Mother Earth as little as reasonably possible when you make purchasing decisions. See Sources for a list of products that I and my Wholistic Fitness master students have used for years.

2. Satya (Truthfulness): Align Your Job with What Nourishes Your Soul

Recent statistics reveal over 85 percent of people don't like what they do for a living. If you are one of those unhappy people, then I want you to change your job to one more aligned with your soul. In the long run, nothing is more important than living your life from soul energy instead of the predictable path of fear-based ego and logic. It is wise to recall Rabindranath Tagore: "I have spent my life stringing and unstringing my instrument while the song I came to sing remains unsung." As your personal trainer and your Yoga teacher, I am telling you that the most important Yoga and the healthiest thing you can do for your long-term health and joyfulness is to lead a life of no regret. I am training you so that on your dying breath, you will know in your heart of hearts, "Wow, I did it! I lived in truth, for I lived my own life, not someone else's!" Your soul needs to live in satya, pursuing its own flight rather than following another's path. As you visualize your last few breaths, what is going to be the truth that you leave? Will it be a truth of noble adventure and bravery of heart, or will it be a sad song filled with regret at never really leaping into your own truthfulness?

3. Asteya (Nonstealing): Don't Steal from the Moment

Stay Here Now. Each moment is seen as perfect and beautiful in the eyes of God. Why should it be different for you? Why do you constantly pull yourself out of the moment? Leave the moment alone! Have no other agenda but to let the moment enrich you. Don't steal from the moment! You are only stealing from yourself if you do. Staying Here Now means you are connected to the totality of It All. Time and space become as unreal but as real as an unwritten number. Stealing begins when we think God has not provided enough for us in the moment.

He has. So don't steal from the moment and you will be less likely to feel a need to steal from others.

4. Brahmacharya (Modesty): Warrior Conduct

Enjoy, appreciate, respect, but don't abuse lower chakra energy. Sexual and sensual energy—be it in activity, thought, or words—is such a beautiful, mystic, and powerful spiritual privilege. Warriors do not addict themselves to the lower chakra energies but instead use them to grow consciously higher. Be careful about buying into modern status symbols such as fancy cars and houses. Often, these status symbols are clues to the spiritual impotence of their owner. Control over your lower chakras is difficult by design. Spiritual warriors must check the powerful animal, survival instinct and transform it higher. This takes a lifetime, so take your time, and by all means have fun. But keep it in balance and always be respectful of the sexual energies. Here are some ways to practice brahmacharya in today's society:

- Prioritize modesty and fuel efficiency when buying lower chakra things like cars, houses, and entertainment possessions.

- Be a gentleman or lady; place yourself in your partner's shoes. Treat your partner as if he or she were of royalty.

- Give plenty of occasion and make it easy and fun for your partner to treat you well. For instance, step to the side for a moment when approaching a door so that your partner has a better chance to open the door for you.

- Alternate lower chakra with higher chakra activity.

- Volunteer/Renunciate/Tithe. Think of this option as a triset: Week One, volunteer to speak to kids at a school or visit an elderly home. Week Two, gather nonfunctional clutter from around your house and donate it to a charity. Week Three, tithe to any cause that feels close to your heart.

- Alternate watching sports on TV (lower chakra) with watching PBS.

- Alternate day spa visits with museum visits.

- Alternate nightclub weekends with family or volunteer work the next weekend.

WF is not about being prudish, it's about balance.

5. Aparigraha (Greedlessness): Be Easy on the Earth

Traditionally, this means not accepting gifts, for doing so generates attachment. But another and perhaps more relevant aspect to aparigraha is not to hoard things that everybody needs: water, fuel, smiles, hugs, cheerfulness, and inspiration. So maybe work toward driving a fuel-efficient car or riding a bicycle, but also linger less in the shower. Conserve electricity but also be cheerful at work. Stay near home and do fitness things instead of taking a needless trip, but also hug someone who doesn't expect it. Be creative with your loving kindness. Here are some other less greedy ways to live upon this earth and save tremendous amounts of suffering and natural resources:

- Don't overeat and eat less meat.

- Switch to e-billing instead of using paper checks and billing.

- Get weekend-only newspaper subscriptions.

- Cancel subscriptions to magazines that do not serve your practice.

- Get rid of junk mail by contacting the sender ASAP.

1. Shauca: Use Yogic Personal Health Products

Purification is absolutely essential, for without it, you will have only distorted vision, not clarity. Yes, keeping yourself "clean" is important. But shauca also relates to a pure mind that can con-

> ### NIYAMAS—PERSONAL GUIDELINES (FIVE STEPS TO INNER HARMONY)
>
> There are five niyamas according to Patanjali's classical yoga:
>
> 1. Shauca (purity)
>
> 2. Santosha (contentment)
>
> 3. Tapas (inner fire)
>
> 4. Svadhyaya (study)
>
> 5. Ishvara-pranidhana (devotion to the Lord)

centrate like a laser at your decision or expand in perspective like a floodlight. When I am inline skiing down a steep asphalt road, my mind must be completely focused to analyze and react to the incoming data at high speed: gradient changes, sounds of oncoming cars, debris and dirt on the road surface. Pavement and skin do not mix well; ask any bicycle racer or inline skater. I need a pure mind to process the data. But when I am with Kathy, I need to expand my mind, take in the gestures of her body language, absorb the look in her beautiful eyes, think back and consider what type of day, week, month, year she has been through, and respond to her with sensitivity. This, too, requires shauca.

The body needs to be clean so that the mind can be clean. It does no good to keep the rest of your house clean if the kitchen stinks to high hell with trash. Meditation will take care of the kitchen, but begin using one or more of the following products regularly or periodically so that the cleanliness and openness of your body supports the purity of your mind:

- ayurvedic tongue cleaner (see Sources)

- toe spreader (see Sources)

- neti pot (see Sources)

2. Santosha (Contentment): Have Not a Vacuum Within

Not wanting more than what is at hand may not be an American ideal, but it should be. To be satisfied with what is and not with what we think "should be" provides a base for equanimity. It is said that to a yogi, there is not much difference at all between a clump of dirt and a brick of gold. Such even-mindedness allows a spiritual warrior to traverse the ups and downs, successes and failures, pleasures and sorrows of life without ever losing his or her natural state of joy.

On a less philosophical level, you must bring some degree of santosha into physical training or you will damage yourself. For instance, if I am not "content" with the decades-deep restriction in my left hip and hamstring, I will overstretch it during Yoga in an attempt to achieve space in my body that is not realistic for where I am. With santosha as a guiding principle, however, I accept that my left hip and hamstring need a more careful and sensitive approach. This allows me to breathe and relax more into the intensity of a stretch, and my pay-off is self-advancement instead of ego reiteration and possible injury. Be content with where you are and surprisingly enough the speed of the universe rushes in and you will progress higher than ever imagined. Paramahansa Yogananda taught: "Whether you are suffering in this life, or smiling with opulence and power, your consciousness should remain unchanged. If you can accomplish even-mindedness, nothing can ever hurt you."

3. Tapas (Inner Fire): Dare to Do

In the second chapter of the *Yoga-Bashya,* the oldest commentary on the *Yoga Sutra,* tapas is described as the "endurance of extremes." The word "tapas" is most often translated as "austerity" and refers to such heat-building practices as prolonged standing, sitting, and fasting. What we are really talking about is what WF is best known for: intensity. When we do a fitness workout, we create tapas. The fruit of tapas is heat. Yogic scholar Georg Feuerstein, Ph.D., wrote in his book *The Yoga Tradition,* that "yogins use this energy to heat the cauldron of their body mind until it yields the elixir of higher awareness." Feuerstein goes on to remind us that in the third chapter of the *Yoga Sutra* (3.45), Patanjali says that "the fruit of such asceticism is the perfection of the body, which becomes robust like a diamond." This certainly makes sense to us fitness warriors. We know all too well how fat and flabby our bodies become when we lose our inner fire and become lazy, and our spirit cools off. But there is no need for us to climb into caves and sit motionless for hours on end. We are not Hindu ascetics—we are fitness warriors! Therein lies the yogic connection. Workouts create tapas, but tapas is also created within the very essence of your day-to-day life. To generate tapas means not just realizing your workout is everywhere, but acting on it. Of all the niyamas, I feel that tapas is surely the fastest way toward igniting any latent spiritual energy within you. The following are some very practical ways to enkindle your spiritual fire, your tapas, in your life.

Be brave enough to follow through on at least a few of them and self-transformation is assured.

Get Out of the Furniture

Replace your most used mealtime table and chairs with a low table and zafus, sitting cushions (page 115).

Poop Naturally, Not "Normally"!

Outfit at least one toilet with a Nature's Platform squatting device (see Sources). The modern toilet is a leading cause of low back pain, disease, illness, and digestive/elimination problems. For being such a "smart" society, we are really stupid about the way we poop, and it causes so much pain and illness.

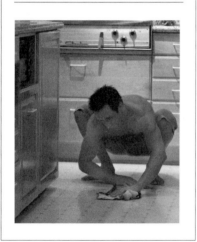

Find every excuse to do the yogi squat—this squatting position was literally my "wheelchair" in the years following my spine injury.

Yogi Squat!

Find every excuse to do the yogi squat, a.k.a. the Asian squat (see photo), instead of sitting in chairs or standing. The yogi squat is performed by most people in the world. Americans are an exception and we have the obesity, the constipation, and the low back pain to prove it. The more time you spend in a yogi squat, the more flexible your spine and hips and knees and ankles become. Your nervous system relaxes, digestive organs get rejuvenated, and all your internal organs get massaged. The yogi squat was (and remains) my "wheelchair" during the first several years following my spine injury. You can find me yogi squatting whenever there is a line to wait in or any prolonged standing: at airports, markets, concerts, when shopping. Of course, the ideal situations for doing the yogi squat include morning cleaning rituals (see page 186) such as cleaning, dusting, gardening. Any modern household device that limits your range of motion, like mopping, should be countered with doing just the opposite: squat, scrub, and stay close to the earth.

Get a PhysioBall and Sit on It!

This pathway is for anyone who spends more than an hour per day at a desk. Replace your office chair with a large PhysioBall (see Sources) and use it instead of your office chair. I don't care if you work in a huge fancy corporation or at home. This is a matter of life and death for your life energy and long-term health. I have used one as my main office chair for about ten years and recommend them regularly for students who work long hours at a desk. Your sacrum and hips are constantly "floating" when you sit on a PhysioBall so the craniosacral and spinal fluids are kept just that, fluid! Your core muscles are constantly kept in motion to stabilize and support your posture and movement so spinal alignment is always present. Best of all? You can enjoy all sorts of mini-yoga moments like backbends, lateral flexions, hip openers, and abdominal work, while you work.

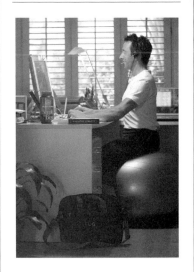

Forget those "ergonomic" office chairs that cost several hundred dollars! All you need is a simple, inexpensive PhysioBall!

4. Svadhyaya (Study): The Science of You

The Sanskrit translation of "Svadhyaya" breaks down like this: "sva" means "own," and "adhyaya" means "going into." The yogic masters relied on this niyama to have their students study spiritual literature, but continuously reminded them to feel the truth of any spiritual text by direct, personal intuition and wisdom. In other words, this niyama reminds you that you are an experiment and an experience of one. Intellectual knowledge about spiritual scriptures is great but is devoid of spiritual power. Spiritual study of books is the first step to access ancient wisdom. But that wisdom only comes alive when you animate your own path of self-discovery. Here are three tried-and-true WF practices that lie in accord with the intent of svadhyaya:

Assigned Reading

Following are five books suggested for most beginning Wholistic Fitness online students. Each book develops a degree of spiritual awareness that I build upon in other areas of Wholistic Fitness. Assigned reading is my version of getting Westerners into the practice of svadhyaya. Now that you know that, make reading the following books a ritual. Prepare a cup of calming tea. Snuggle up in bed before retiring. Do not rush to get through the book. Instead, linger within the pages. Let each book's teachings go deep so their potency has a better chance to come alive in your daily life. Highlight passages that touch you. Make personal notes in the margins. Talk about the book with your loved one(s). Quality sleep, not to mention an enviable state of mind, is impossible if you chronically fall asleep while watching television, or reading a murder mystery or gossip material, or bickering with your partner. Nourish your conscious mind into the sleeping state with the higher vibrations emanating from the following books. I've selected these five because they are all quick reads with simplicity as their common thread.

Peace Is Every Step, by Thich Nhat Hanh. Written by a Vietnamese Zen monk, this beautiful quick read articulates perfectly a yogi's everyday mentality and emotional equanimity.

Jonathan Livingston Seagull, by Richard Bach. Fun, vintage metaphysics. Jonathan Seagull would have loved WF! He was (is) a total fitness warrior bird! Extra credit: Read *Illusions,* also by Richard Bach. Shimoda lives!

Zen Mind, Beginner's Mind, by Shunryu Suzuki. An enduring classic that has not been bettered in my opinion.

Way of the Peaceful Warrior, by Dan Millman. I know you've read it because Dan is a member of our spiritual tribe. Worth at least a half-dozen rereads. Honorable Mention: *The Alchemist,* by Paul Coelho.

Beyond Words, by Sri Swami Satchidananda. "If you want to see a world free of greed, hatred, and jealousy, you must first see that your own mind is free of those qualities. As long as there are disturbances in your own mind, you will see disturbances in the world outside. So first put the man together and automatically you will be helping to put the world together." S.S.S.'s ability to articulate massive transcendent philosophies of the East into simple parables and metaphors makes this simple, joyful book a favorite of mine.

Extra-credit books:

The Tibetan Book of Living and Dying, by Sogyal Rinpoche. A teacher of mine at Naropa University, Sogyal Rinpoche penned this exquisite version of *The Tibetan Book of the Dead* and made it quite palatable to understand that if you are not preparing for death, what are you preparing for?

How to Know God: Yoga Aphorisms of Patanjali, by Prabhavananda and Isherwood. I have no idea why these two titled their book this way, since the yoga sutras are completely nondenominational and Patanjali made certain that there was no sutra with the "G" word in it. But, aside from that, this is one of my favorite translations, written by a devotional (bhakti) yogi and his guru on the practice of yoga and meditation.

The Bhagavad Gita. Pick any translation that appeals to you. Devour this stunning, historical yogic love poem that is the most famous of all Yoga scriptures. The central teaching of the *Gita* is counsel toward balancing conventional religious ideals with personal ethics and well-intended action. Still pretty timely advice for today.

Think on These Things, by J. Krishnamurti. As much of a must-read for the spiritual warrior as is Ram Dass's *Be Here Now.*

Tomboy Bride, by Harriet Fish Backus. Nonfiction. Takes place in my childhood home, a long time ago. Harriet could outsurvive any of those punks on those damned "reality TV" shows. Deepens appreciation in a most riveting, real-life way.

The Enlightened Heart: An Anthology of Sacred Poetry, edited by Stephen Mitchell. Spiritual/ecstatic poetry. Go for it. Crack open your anahata chakra (Heart Center) with poetry from any of these mystics, sages, poets, and ancient ones: Rumi, Tagore, Lao-tzu, Kabir, Issa, the Upanishads, Bassho, William Blake, Robert Frost, et al.

Fridge Quotes

Get a small magnetic dry-erase board. Put it up on your refrigerator. Right there, next to your clutter of magnets and shopping lists, write on your dry-erase board a spiritual or inspirational quote. Leave each quote on the board for at least three days. Memorize it. Extra credit for making up your own quotes! Here is the one I had up last week:

> *We dance round in a ring and suppose,*
> *But the Secret sits in the middle and knows.*
> —ROBERT FROST

The week before, our dear and powerful friend Kurt Bruno earned honor on the Ilgs' quote board for three days when he came up with this one, remarking on his lack of focus during a yoga class after a long day at work:

> *My mind was everywhere but on the mat.*

Spiritual quotes keep our hectic minds channeled on higher things. They function to re-mind us of our practice.

Music as Meditation

This assignment requires you to find a piece of music that you can just "go within." My father-in-law, Dave Faulstich, a self-described "recovering hippie" and former professional radio DJ, is a devout practitioner of this particular Meditation style. Dave used to "discipline" Kathy and her brother, Michael, when they got into trouble as kids by (1) kindly lecturing them for hours on end, elaborating at length on various reasons why it is important not to do bad things, and

(2) having them listen to songs. I mean, "real songs" by "real songwriters" that had lyrics that could shudder your soul in a given moment. Dave would have Kathy and Michael come into the living room, lie down, put their feet up, kill the lights, and then say, "Kids, close your eyes and listen!" With that, Dad would play one song from an artist like Bob Dylan, Carole King, Cat Stevens, Paul Simon, or Joan Baez over and over again.

I want you to take Dad's advice. Do the same thing some night. Just merge with the lyrics in the way a bhakti yogi might merge into a kirtan chant. Keep disappearing into the music until nobody remains and the song sings itself through your cells.

5. Ishvara-pranidhana (Devotion to the Lord)

This niyama gets narrow-minded folk all in a tizzy because of the "L" word. Essentially, this niyama is just trying to draw us closer to our inner guidance. It's trying to get you to connect your actions to their sacred source. It's really hard to do "bad things" or get off track if you learn to connect what you do with the source of its sacredness.

Ishvara-pranidhana might best be translated in English as "heartfulness." Practicing this niyama means that whether you are going to go to work or to do a workout or to pull weeds out of your garden, you do it from your heart.

Another aspect of this niyama involves surrendering your effort to whatever you feel is your Highest Source. Do your noble best, but let God handle the controls. Or, as the Christians might say, "Let go and let God!"

Playing around with Ishvara-pranidhana does not involve changing anything you already do. It does mean changing the way you do it. Do what you will, but do it all as an offering to that which created you and that which (one day) will also destroy you. Do your workouts not to become more physically fit, but to fill your heart with the Divine. Can you do that? If you can, you are living this niyama.

The absence of Ishvara-pranidhana is precisely why so many professionals feel lost and empty after they retire. All their years of training, sweat, focus, and sacrifice were never done as an offering to their Higher Source. They missed the link between their physical training and their spiritual connection. Most people, in my experience, suffer from the same malaise.

No one teaches us that there is a spiritual dimension to what we do. I mean, who taught you how to listen to your voice within? Anyone? Who taught you that it is not only helpful, but vital to have a trusting relationship with your inner guidance as opposed to your logical/egoic thought? Anyone?

That, to me, is a shame. But I understand. No one taught me either. I had to learn it for myself. In the *Yoga Sutra*, Patanjali distinctly refers to this inner voice as "Ishvara," our fore-

DEVOTIONAL ATHLETICS

Athletes as Holy Ones; Competition as Ishta-Devata

I devote my training and competition efforts as my personal offering to my own intimate connection with the Universe. Yogis know devotional energy as Ishta-Devata, which means "chosen deity." Because I've benefited so much from my devotional athletics, I imagine what our nation would be like if all us fitness warriors would unite in a simple, single, nondiscriminating and nondenominational spiritual purpose: to make our workouts our Ishta-Devata! As a nation, we would offer our collective efforts to our own particular sense of the Lord. Each workout would be done to better us as human beings first, and as more physically fit human beings second. Chakra-based workouts would replace ego-centered ones. Spiritual physiologists would be equal in number to exercise physiologists. Although I do feel that athletes are naturally more suited for spiritual work than sedentary, unfit people, I do not feel that this makes us any more "holy" than others. I do feel, however, that the hours a person invests in fitness training forms a unique spiritual devotion that helps us become more "whole."

most teacher (I.26). These days, even when I vacuum my carpet, I offer my action to the Divine, to Ishvara. Before I teach a yoga class or work privately with a fitness student, I offer my service and effort to Ishvara. In the middle of my ku top form bench presses, I offer my muscular failure to Ishvara.

I have had, throughout the years, people ask me how I stay so calm and peaceful all the time. Well, for one thing, I am not calm and peaceful "all the time"! That would be boring. But whenever I catch myself getting stressed or tight, I invoke WF Lifestyle Principle 1: Breath and Posture.

Upon my next conscious exhale, I release all my stress to the Universe.

I figure the Universe is large enough to adequately handle my comparatively feeble drama and stress. I then center myself by devoting my next few minutes to the Universe (Ishvara). I give it to God.

Of course, I soon forget that I am supposed to be offering my actions to the Divine (Ishvara). Instead of vacuuming my stairs for God, I am lost once again in my usual whirlwind of mental drama. I've let myself become disconnected not only from the vacuuming but from God. But that is the way the game is played. I don't worry about it, in fact, I smile at my spiritual failings. I pretty much trust that God is used to us humans forgetting Him so much of the time. Sometimes we remember (with) the Divine. Then we forget and buy into the illusion (maya) of the world. But that's okay, because even our lame and endless forgetting is part of the game. I say that it is okay, because God (Ishvara) knows intent. Just be pure in your intent and all will be okay.

Here is one approach I've found helpful in cultivating Ishvara-pranidhana in my own life and in the lives of my students of Wholistic Fitness.

Plants take substances out of the air through the tiny openings in their leaves. Some research has determined that plant leaves, roots, and soil bacteria are all important in removing trace levels of toxic vapors. Philodendron, spider plant, and the golden pothos seemed to be the most effective in removing formaldehyde molecules, while flowering plants such as gerbera daisy and chrysanthemums appeared superior in removing benzene from the atmosphere. Other good plants for detoxifying your home are dracaena, massangeana, and spathiphyllum.

Name Your Possessions with Spiritual Names

The more often we feel gratitude for stuff we normally take for granted, the happier we become. The reason is that when we feel gratitude, we feel more connected. That is why we like to name things that we identify as "our own." Didn't you name your bike or doll when you were a kid? Heck, yeah, because it was yours! You loved your bike and your dolls. But then you grew up and you stopped naming things because it was too silly, right? Well, as John Cage once said, "When they tell you to grow up, they mean stop growing." So I want you, as a clever practice of Ishvara-pranidhana, to start naming things again. Consider it another passage for spiritual growth and don't argue with me.

You name your dog and cat, don't you? Why not your car? Or that plant that has lived with you so long. I can't believe you haven't named it yet! It is important for your long-term health to begin to deepen your connection with all the stuff you have. To facilitate this, begin by giving your significant possessions names that bring you a sense of peace, happiness, inspiration, or sacredness.

Many people visiting my home think I am kidding when I introduce them to my plants. Of course I am going to introduce you! The plant is living and is my friend. Why wouldn't I introduce you? All of Kathy's and my houseplants have names. So do our bicycles and cars. Many are named in honor of spiritual gurus, deities, saints, and qualities, or for inspirational athletes. This naming stuff is both fun and effective as a spiritual growth tool. The plant that sits near the top of the stairs is Ramana Maharshi, named for the great Indian Jnana Yoga Master. I've got a pothos plant called Dalai, for the Dalai Lama. Kathy's stunningly beautiful split leaf philodendron (which I once left on a busy sidewalk and which was miraculously returned to us) is called Grace for good reason. We rescued another strange plant that grew into amazing health after nearly dying. We call it Lance in honor of Lance Armstrong. We also have a wiry, very determined spider plant named Bruce (for Bruce Lee) and a golden pothos called Marley (for Bob). My mountain bike's name is a decidedly unspiritual name—Grunt—because he often makes me do just that on tricky and steep uphills. My road bike's name is Andrew, in honor of my former student and Tour of Italy and Tour of Switzerland bicycle racing champion, Andy Hampsten.

My naming of things has become a bit too well known. Now people want me to come over to their house and name their stuff. I explain to these people that I actually don't "name" anything in a verb sense of the word. I just listen. The thing names itself. For example, after we first met, Kathy asked me to name her car. She thought it was "cute" that I named everything with such odd names (she was not a yogini back then). So, to please her, I agreed. Closing my eyes and laying my hands on her car, I went within. In a flash came the word, "Meru," which in Hindi means the center of the earth. In yogic literature, it is a term for the central axis of the human body and is also the designation for the center bead of a Buddhist rosary, or mala. But I felt a strong female presence about the car, so I turned "Meru" into "Miranda." She loved it. And, as the speed and the humor of the Universe would have it, when Kathy and I moved to a new apartment, guess what the name of the street was leading to our house?

Miranda Street.

You gotta love synchronicity. That's just the thing. The more fun we have with life, the more fun life has with us. Don't stop growing just because you are grown up.

BLUE LIGHT HEALING MEDITATION

The only new Meditation you have during the Jeweled Lotus is a fantastic one. It is my most commonly prescribed healing meditation. It is very utilitarian, durable, and effective. It is wonderful to use if you are injured, stressed out, or lacking in energy. May you enjoy it and benefit from it for years to come. I call it my Blue Light Healing Meditation.

Assume zazen posture.

Take several deep ujjayi breaths while inhaling a calming, golden light (pran) through the crown of the head (sahasrara) and exhaling a cleansing white light through the navel area (manipura).

In several deep ujjayi breaths inhale calming, blue light through sahasrara, and exhale cleansing white light through manipura.

Bring your awareness into manipura. Invoke a roaring fire in this energy center. Into this inner fire throw that which is troubling you: destructive habits, undigested feelings, injuries, fears, worries, etc.

Burn them completely. See them turn to ash, then vapor.

Stay with this burning for a while, then allow the fire to die. Replace it with a healing sphere of cool, blue energy. Stay with this blue, healing energy for a while. Let the blue permeate your physical body, especially at injury or trauma sites. Allow the blue to escape the confines of skin and bone.

Immerse yourself into an ocean of blue, healing energy.

Open your heart area (anahata) with the color green. Be aware of love, safety, and terrific power here. Allow images to come. Allow love to come. Stay here for as long as desired.

Bring the green back into your physical heart. Reduce the green into the size of a pea. As the green reduces in size, it turns brilliant white and full of concentrated love and acceptance.

Hands into prayer posture (namaskar). Head bows toward earth.

Chant "OM" three times.

Open your eyes.

Feel better?

CHAPTER 26

Nutrition

The most nourishing meal you can share is the one within yourself.

—COACH ILG

THERE ARE NO SPECIFIC DIETARY or philosophical changes to your nutrition discipline while on the Jeweled Lotus.

It would be wise to revisit the Nutrition section of the Green Tara program and reabsorb the principles of WF Nutrition.

If bodyfat loss is still a priority for you at this time, then I suspect you might be cheating on the program or have deeper, perhaps karmic, issues with your food intake. For those of you who still need to drop fat, follow the Lotus Fat Loss Diet below for the four to eight weeks of this program.

THE WHOLISTIC FITNESS LOTUS FAT LOSS DIET

Acclaimed worldwide for dropping the fat fast.

Read carefully through each mealtime to get a feel for the diet. Before beginning your first day of the Lotus diet, go shopping for the first few days of your diet.

USING SUNRIDER HERBS FOR OPTIMAL FAT LOSS AND RESULTS

For those of you who are using Sunrider herbal foods, the official Nutrition program of WF, losing bodyfat is no problem at all. It merely depends on how aggressively you are willing to work with the herbs to lose the weight. Here is how to do it.

SUNRIDER HERBAL FORMULAS NEEDED

1 bottle of Slim Caps

1 bottle of Action Caps

Fortune Delight (any flavor)

Sunny Dew

Large Sunrider shaker bottle

METHOD

Slim Caps—take 1 or 2 caps at night for 2 days.

Action Caps—take 3 to 6 caps 3x daily, when not taking Slim Caps, for 3 days.

Drink Fortune Delight w/Sunny Dew in your large Sunrider shaker bottle continuously throughout the day, every day.

Repeat the steps above until you lose the amount of weight desired.

Slim Caps, Action Caps, Fortune Delight, and Sunny Dew are available through Sunrider International (see Sources)

Snacks While on the Lotus Diet

One serving of any one of the following snacks is allowed per day, if needed:

- PowerBars, Harvest, or Pria bars from PowerBar (see Sources)
- Sunbars or NuPuffs from Sunrider (see Sources)
- flavored rice cakes or "healthy" popcorn
- fresh fruit or sorbet
- "healthy" vegan cookies

Note: For coffee addicts, you may have 1 cup of coffee (small) every day except Day 4.

Every Day

1 "Ilg Supreme" Sunrider herbal drink. Drink this before noon whenever possible. If you want more energy, drink one Ilg Supreme in the morning, and another in the afternoon. This recipe is found in the Sources section.

Option: If you are not using Sunrider herbs, a high-quality multivitamin/mineral "Nutrition" product (preferably one recommended to you by a doctor or nutritionist) for an alternative to the Ilg Supreme.

> To facilitate this diet plan, I've included some of my favorite recipes, from Part Seven.

Fortune Delight with Sunny Dew throughout the day.

Option: If you are not using Sunrider herbs, make sure you choose high-quality water and some "cleansing" teas throughout the day for an alternative to Fortune Delight.

Day 1

Breakfast: Oatmeal (slow cook if possible), yogurt, fresh fruit, herbal tea.

Lunch: Vegetable or bean soup and whole grain bread or tuna salad sandwich. Side salad.

Dinner: Grilled fish, rice, steamed or stir-fried veggies. Side salad.

Day 2

Breakfast: Fresh fruit, toast, herbal tea.

Lunch: Baked potato with salsa. Side salad.

Dinner: Stir-fried veggies with tofu. Side salad.

Day 3

Breakfast: Breakfast quesadilla, Huevos Rancheros, or egg whites on top of a bagel with fresh fruit.

Lunch: Tofu and rice.

Dinner: Pasta and tomato-based sauce. Side salad with tuna.

Day 4

Breakfast: Waffles, fruit, soy sausage, herbal tea.

Lunch: Tuna and rice.

Dinner: Garden burger and veggies or veggie burrito.

Day 5

Unstructured Day! Eat intuitively and like a Noble Warrior.

Option: Use mealtime choices in Part Seven.

Day 6

Students who are prioritizing bodyfat loss should return to Day 1.

Other students can have two more unstructured dietary days before returning to Day 1 (that is, weekdays = structured, weekends = nonstructured).

Water

If our bodies are mostly (about 70 percent) water, then it should be the best water possible. Fitness variables such as recovery from workouts, regeneration of muscle and connective tissue, and toxin flush are compromised unless you drink a lot of high-quality water every day. Basic cellular health is in question if heavy metals, pesticides, nitrates, overchlorination, fluoride, and harmful bacteria are finding their way to your drinking water. In America, there are several factors contributing to diminished water quality and pollution, which is why Kathy and I use bottled water to mix our herbs, drink, and cook.

One primary adversary to healthy water quality is industrial animal farming. The Environmental Protection Agency regards non–point source pollution, such as agricultural runoff, as one of the greatest threats to water quality. Agricultural runoff from industrial and conventional farming includes pesticides, chemical fertilizers, high amounts of nitrates, and sometimes dangerous levels of bacteria from animal feces.

I spoke to WF student Bradley Saul, who authors a wonderful newsletter, *The Organic Athlete* (www.organicathlete.com), and who also happens to be a professional road bicyclist. Besides being a very tapped-in and wholistic athlete, Bradley is married to a hydrologist. He knows a little something about healthy eating and quality water. Bradley told me that in the state I live in, California, 85 percent of water used goes to farming. He said that much of that goes to produce meat. Most meat in supermarkets comes from animal feeding operations, or AFOs. According to the EPA website, "AFOs generally congregate animals, feed, manure, dead animals, and production operations on a small land area. Feed is brought to the animals rather than the animals grazing or otherwise seeking feed in pastures. Animal waste and wastewater can enter water bodies from spills or breaks of waste storage structures (due to accidents or excessive rain), and non-agricultural application of manure to crop land."

Bradley kept the statistics coming at me like he was attacking me up the 7,700-foot vertical up Mount Lemmon in Tucson, Arizona, where he lives and trains. He says that the EPA estimates that hog, chicken, and cattle waste has polluted 35,000 miles of rivers in twenty-two states and contaminated groundwater in seventeen states. A two-year study of government reports and records on animal feeding operations by the Sierra Club revealed "massive water pollution resulting from millions of gallons of animal feces and urine flowing into waterways, workplace deaths, injuries and worker safety violations, 134 million pounds of contaminated and potentially contaminated meat, and repeated, gruesome violations of the federal Humane Slaughter Act."

Almost imitating the philosophies of WF, Bradley urges that those who eat meat (he does not) should consider purchasing organically raised and grass-fed meats. These are usually available at your local natural foods store, or search the Internet for suppliers. Bradley finished with this, "You're not only doing the world a good, you're saving your health by not consuming the harmful pesticides and chemicals stored in the animal fat."

Following the Nutrition principles of WF provides an easy way to help ensure quality drinking water for generations to come. Practicing WF is a practical way toward low-impact living. Be brave in your Nutrition choices and awareness. Dare to do that which is higher, not "normal."

Daily Practice

Listen to the language of your body, so you can learn to love the language of your life.
—COACH ILG

H ERE IS YOUR DAILY SCHEDULE for the Jeweled Lotus maintenance cycle. Remember, your training on the Jeweled Lotus is more of an exploration into living a high-fitness, low-impact lifestyle. Much of the Lotus is designed to have your intuitive fitness become elevated. There is much more flexibility in your Daily Practice during this cycle, so enjoy the more laid-back approach. The Jeweled Lotus comes into full bloom after four weeks and will remain at optimal bloom for up to eight weeks. After that time, you can feel free to create your own WF program using my suggestions on page 254.

All of the following workouts have been cross-referenced to the appropriate chapters. I've put page numbers next to each movement and technique for easy cross-referencing.

Practice reminders:

Don't stress if you're unable to do all the workouts for that day. Do your priority disciplines if possible. Remember, you are still living a WF lifestyle if you can't do anything but eat consciously and in alignment with WF guidelines or even working your Breath and Posture! Don't reduce WF to mere physical workouts. WF is much more about developing awareness than it is about muscle.

Don't try to make up missed workouts by cramming several workouts into the next day. Instead, just keep flowing through the week. You've got your whole life to become wholistically fit.

Consistency comes first, sequencing comes second. I've choreographed the fitness disciplines in the order that provides the optimal training effect. However, if you need to switch the order, you can.

Enjoy your Wholistic Fitness with focus and fun!

Wholistic Fitness Training Precepts

1. Be prepared

2. Be on time

3. Give 110 percent

Monday. Recovery and Scheduling Weekly Workouts

Mondays are traditional WF recovery days, no physical workouts today.

Focus on your work while giving your body time to prepare for the upcoming training week.

Sometime today, go to your schedule book and block out the time needed to do your workouts each day. Mentally prepare for your training week, and learn from the prior week: Where could you have been more noble? How are you going to do better this week? Visualize yourself doing the upcoming workouts in a strong, elegant, and focused manner. Maybe this is the week you decide to incorporate a cardio commute or a periodic renunciation or a media fast. If so, schedule it in and prepare for it. Energy follows thought.

Receiving bodywork (massage) on Mondays is wise.

Tuesday. Take Your Pick

Pick one of the following and do it. Those seeking Warrior level should do at least two, and Master Student level all four of the following:

Meditation: Do Early Morning Zazen for 30 minutes (page 119).

Yoga: Do a slow flow through at least two HP Yoga Sun Salutations (page 86).

Cardio: Do Cardio of Choice (page 74) for 1 to 2 hours at Zones 1–3 (see Table 2.1, page 75).

Meditation: Beeper Guru: Breath and Posture (page 112).

Wednesday. Green Tara Yoga

Yoga is your only mandatory discipline today. Do the Green Tara Yoga routine sometime today.

Those seeking Warrior level should add at least one and Master Student level should add all three of the following:

> **Meditation: Do the Early Morning Cleaning Ritual (page 186).**
>
> **Evening Meditation: Sit a 10-minute zazen and then do Blue Light Healing Meditation (page 279).**
>
> **Cardio: Do a Cardio Commute or 1 hour of Cardio of Choice at Zones 1–2.**

Thursday. Cruise Intervals

Cardio is your only mandatory discipline today. Do 1 to 1.5 hours of Cardio of Choice with 5 Cruise Intervals (page 261) sometime today.

Those seeking Warrior level should add at least one and Master Student level should add all three of the following:

> **Meditation: Do an Early Morning Zazen for 30 minutes (see page 119).**
>
> **Yoga: Do a slow flow through at least two HP Yoga Sun Salutations (page 86).**
>
> **Meditation 2: Choose a Media Fast option (page 240) and do it all day today.**

Friday. Cosmic Yang Yoga

Yoga is your only mandatory discipline today. Do the Cosmic Yang Yoga routine sometime today.

Those seeking Warrior level should add at least one and Master Student level should add all three of the following:

> **Meditation: Do the Early Morning Cleaning Ritual (page 186).**
>
> **Evening Meditation: Sit a 10-minute zazen and then do Blue Light Healing Meditation (page 279).**
>
> **Cardio: Do a Cardio Commute or 1 hour of Cardio of Choice at Zones 1–2.**

Saturday. Cardio, Slow and Steady

Cardio is your only mandatory discipline today. Do 2 to 4 hours of Cardio of Choice today.

Those working toward Warrior and Master Student level should make it a "Double Day" and add one of the following:

- Do a slow flow through at least two HP Yoga Sun Salutations (page 86).

- Take a Yoga class.

- Do the Pranayama Pump (page 263).

Sunday. Frugal Realm Yoga

Yoga is your only mandatory discipline today. Do the Frugal Realm Yoga routine sometime today.

Those seeking Warrior level should add at least one and Master Student level should add both of the following:

Meditation: Do the Pranayama Pump (page 263).

Cardio: Do 1.5 to 2 hours of Cardio of Choice at Zones 1–2.

Cycle Summation

T HIS SHEET IS TO be completed after four to eight weeks of becoming "bejeweled." Enjoy a recovery week phase before resuming your Wholistic Fitness journey with a return to the Green Tara program.

Jeweled Lotus Cycle Summation

Date started:

Date completed:

Today's date:

Strength Training

1. Sometimes Strength means overall energy. How do you feel now, in terms of overall energy levels, at the conclusion of the Jeweled Lotus as compared to when you started it?
2. How did your ego handle not being in the gym at all?

3. Your body?

4. Were you attached to the gym? If something happened to you that made it impossible to return to a gym, could you still be happy? Why?

Cardio

1. Note your consistency to doing Cruise Intervals and what you learned about yourself through doing them.

2. Note allegiance to or attempts at Cardio Commuting.

3. Record the number of Cardio hours performed during the 4 to 8 weeks of this cycle.

Week 1:	**Week 2:**	**Week 3:**	**Week 4:**
Week 5:	**Week 6:**	**Week 7:**	**Week 8:**

Yoga

1. Fun cycle, eh? What felt most improved when you revisited the Yoga routines from the previous training programs?

2. What part of your Yoga practice needs more work, mind or body? Elaborate.

Meditation

1. You had a lot of flexibility to either do or not do Meditation during this cycle. Consider why you embraced or stayed away from Meditation.

2. Wholistic Fitness is the only personal training program that incorporates classical Yoga ethics (the yamas and niyamas) into the actual fitness method. Note your progress on the Ten Wholistic Fitness Mastery Pathways that were available to you during this cycle.

Yamas—Ethical Guidelines: Five Steps to Social Harmony

- Ahimsa (Nonharming)—Prioritize wholistic shopping. For example, purchase preservative-free, natural, wholesome, organic foods and eco-friendly, no animal testing, cruelty-free products, as well as low-impact household items such as extended life lightbulbs, rechargeable batteries, low-flow plumbing.

  Note Progress:

- Satya (Truthfulness)—Align your job with what nourishes your soul. For example, make minor or major lifestyle changes to enable you to enjoy your work more.

  Note Progress:

- Asteya (Nonstealing)—Don't steal from the moment. For example, stay present, focus on purity instead of drama.

  Note Progress:

- Brahmacharya (Modesty)—Warrior conduct. For example, prioritize modesty and environmental consciousness when buying lower chakra things like cars, houses, and entertainment possessions. Practice politeness; alternate lower chakra with higher chakra activity; volunteer/renunciate/tithe.

  Note Progress:

- Aparigraha (Greedlessness)—Be easy on the earth. For example, don't overeat and eat less meat, switch to electronic banking, get weekend-only newspaper subscriptions, cancel magazine subscriptions that do not serve your practice, reduce or get rid of junk mail.

  Note Progress:

Niyamas—Personal Guidelines; Five Steps to Inner Harmony

- Shauca—Use yogic personal health products. For example, have a pure mind that can shift from sharp focus to wide perspective; use an Ayurvedic tongue cleaner, a toe spreader, a Neti Pot.

  Note Progress:

- Santosha (Contentment)—Have not a vacuum within. For example, don't want more than what is at hand, be content with where your body is and don't over-stretch or overdo it.

  Note Progress:

- Tapas (Inner Fire)—Dare to do. For example, get out of the furniture; poop naturally, not "Normally"; yogi squat as often as possible; get a PhysioBall and sit on it!

  Note Progress:

- Svadhyaya (Study)—The science of you. For example, do some assigned reading, make fridge quotes, try music as meditation.

  Note Progress:

- Ishvara-pranidhana (Devotion to the Lord). For example, offer your actions to your higher source, name your possessions with spiritual names.

  Note Progress:

Nutrition

1. In 2001, Americans spent nearly $300 billion at restaurants yet complained about being confused about what and how much to eat. WF guidelines are easy to live by. Rate yourself on how well you did on my ten WF Nutritional Guidelines, introduced in Chapter 5 (1 = I need to do much better; 5 = excellent):

   take a sacred pause

   eat mainly raw, whole foods

   eat several servings of fruit and vegetables per day

   limit fat intake, eat moderate volumes of protein and carbohydrates

   consider nutrition in both physical and spiritual ways

   half of effective nutrition is about cleansing and elimination

   reduce dairy and meat to nominal levels

   eat high-fiber foods

   generally maintain a one-third food, one-third fluid, one-third air ratio of stomach contents

   your "diet keyword" is Moderation!

2. Note changes in bodyweight and physique during the Jeweled Lotus:
3. Yesterday, what and how did you eat, exactly? Include all supplements and fluids.
4. How did you eat each of those meals: Elegantly and consciously or hurried and unconsciously?
5. If the latter, why were you in such a hurry?
6. Number the WF disciplines 1 through 5, starting with the ones you really improved in.

   Strength

   Cardio

   Yoga

   Meditation

   Nutrition

7. Compare your answers here to your answers in the Green Tara Cycle Summation. Consider how your entire body/mind has been changed in the process of becoming more balanced in your personal training.

Well, good and faithful WF student, I want you to feel very, very good about yourself. You have completed my course in Wholistic Fitness personal training. May you use your new insights and energies for the benefit of all beings.

I bow to you. Well done, Noble Warrior!

OPTIONAL STUDY

Retake the WF Quiz at the beginning of this book (page 34) and enter your score here:

Note area of most progress:

Note area of least progress:

Comment on your self-transformation through Wholistic Fitness:

PART FIVE

THE WHOLISTIC FITNESS SUTRAS

CHAPTER 29

Thirty-five Aphorisms to Help Guide You

Don't just do fitness; be it. Fitness is the most natural expression of wholeness.
—WF SUTRA 35

AT ITS SIMPLEST, THE SANSKRIT word "sutra" can be translated as meaning "threadlike." The poignancy of a sutra is usually only decoded through years of practice, although some function like insight spark plugs, igniting you toward higher awareness with the velocity of a rocket. On the surface, these cute little threads may at first seem almost trite. Go deeper into them, however, and you will find thirty-five kernels of body/mind fitness wisdom. These sutras are the literary essence of my life's work. Take them with you into your workouts—into your daily life—and watch their seed essences spring into your own creative wisdom!

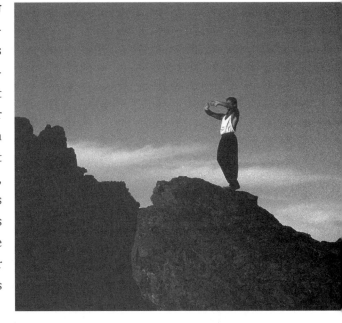

Sutras 1 through 15 describe the principles and qualities of Wholistic Fitness.

Sutras 16 through 24 describe primary emotions and the specific fitness disciplines that balance them.

Sutras 25 through 35 describe the ethics of Wholistic Fitness, the characteristics that are the hallmark of a WF Master Student.

PRINCIPLES

Wholistic Fitness Sutra 1

Your body/mind is a masterpiece, intricate in function, unique in her mix of attributes
and abilities. Give praise—you are wonderfully, singularly made!
The necessity of wholesome foods and lifetime exercise is
a Divine technique for giving praise.
Being able to work out is a Divine gift.
Give praise.

Wholistic Fitness Sutra 2

The cells of your body/mind are composed of matter
recycled since the birth of the UniVerse.
Uni = One. Verse = Poem.
The message of your life is a contribution to the One Poem of All Time.
You are made from the stuff of stars, let your Light shine!
You are made from the stuff of dirt, let Humility usher your Awakening.

Wholistic Fitness Sutra 3

Your body is so beautiful just the Way it Is.
It is a living, breathing Truth of God.
Cosmetic surgery cuts more than skin. It cuts Soul. Be careful.
The world has long imposed shifting and false standards for human beauty.
You need not measure up to outer ideals.
So doing causes suffering, dis-ease, and spiritual retardation.
Humans only grasp at relative truth and thus snatch at relative beauty.

Genuine beauty shines with the truth of God.

Focus therefore on inner Truth.

Tides of fashion quickly change, but Truth always remains beautiful.

To become more beautiful? Become more Truth-ful.

Wholistic Fitness Sutra 4

If you are unhappy with some part of your physical self,

dialogue with it.

Listen to the wisdom of your body,

your mind needs the rest!

Don't pursue what you don't have, pursue what already lies within. No champion

has ever lifted a trophy that was not already being held inside.

Pay little mind to "genetic limits," for you can always rise Higher than where you are.

Our perceived flaws are there by Divine design. They form the spiritual architecture

within which our Souls can play and learn.

Spiritual elevation is woven inexorably into our hearts and brains.

Wholistic Fitness Sutra 5

To even exist within a body is a magnificent gift from God.

Keeping fit honors the sacredness of that Divine gift.

Your body is a Temple.

Efforts in fitness creates the Scripture of Self.

What makes your brief life so sacred is the omnipotent flow of Truth through your

Temple and expressed through your Scripture.

The purest and most beautiful Prayer is sung

from perspiration, not pews.

Get Real.

Stay Real.

Your Higher Source

is divined through sweat,

not through stars, stones, cards, or the reading of palms.

Wholistic Fitness Sutra 6

*A fitness program is not punishment for an imperfect body, but a Vehicle for
Awakening. Consistency in fitness is a sign of care and understanding of a Higher Way.
Love your body as it Is.
Train to keep it well suited for the life tasks and natural Joy to which you are called.
Your Soul will benefit and pay you back, later, in a Way only seen through steadfast
Practice.
Human motivation comes in three Levels: external, internal, and Divine. Awareness is
the first and remains the common denominator of all three.
Appreciation is the catalyst for the second.
The third arrives from practicing spiritual surrender.*

Wholistic Fitness Sutra 7

*You have many spiritual guides during life.
Teachers and Teachings of various degree are encountered continuously. They arrive at
the speed appropriate to the pace you set for Awakening.
You live with many, yet do not recognize them as such.
Skillful Awareness determines the worth of each.
True Teachers embody your mind's yearning through the Light in their eyes and the
strength of their posture. These grace-full beings walk their talk through their actions,
which define their character and charisma. Study potential Teachers over a period of
time. True Teachings, similarly, will attract your heart; that is their first token. Omens
will arise to validate your Finding during seeking.*

*Once a Teacher or Teaching is accepted, trust them. Do not challenge them, otherwise,
sensing ego, they will offer lower level teachings and the ex-change will be shallow.
True Teachers teach by
subtle spiritual Seed Planting. Some Seeds will lie dormant for years. Guides must
therefore be carefully chosen. Then, commit entirely without flaw or doubt.*

Wholistic Fitness Sutra 8

Personal fitness is a journey; establish your own unique route.
With overtraining, or "too much, too soon," you will lose interest and
Higher learning will become difficult.
Begin slowly.
Progress at your own pace.
Accomplished endurance on a Spiritual Path is easily found in true Guides;
their life messages have weathered the barrier of fatigue and represent potentiation.
These qualities distill True Teachers from false ones.

Wholistic Fitness Sutra 9

Just breathing is enough.
Take Cleansing Breaths as often as possible during your day; long nasal inhale
followed by a mouth exhale. A Cleansing Breath lets the world breathe with you.
Conscious breathing lets you perform more smoothly.
Just breathing is always enough.

Breath awareness equals concentration of mind. Mind steers body toward out pictured
goals. Hurtfulness is stoked by the power of breath and provides all the spiritual fuel
you will ever require.
If this is your lifetime to succeed in worldly matters, outward manifestation occurs.
Regardless of manifestation, we all keep moving Higher by breathing.
It is the Way of the Higher Dance.

Wholistic Fitness Sutra 10

Present a graceful posture to the world, this awakens your spine.
Pretend your head is suspended from above.
An awakened spine sends joy and energy throughout your body.
And to other beings, as well.

Elegant posture is like peacefulness insurance. You are quick to buy life insurance or
car insurance or even stereo insurance, yet peacefulness insurance is freely purchased

by postural awareness. An elegant posture fulfills and provides the four foundations for
sustaining excellence and genuine happiness in all that you do:

Truth

Beauty

Goodness

Unity

Your mother told you to "Sit up straight," for they Knew.
Moms all-ways Know.
This is why they are called (m)oms, after-All.

Wholistic Fitness Sutra 11

Include Strength Training in your fitness plan, particularly during the formative years
of practice. This keeps your joints strong and develops inner power.
You achieve unity of breath, posture, and mental focus.
Strength Training is Structure.

To strengthen your sinewy Connection to the Divine, your structure must first be
secure. Of the Five Fitness Disciplines, Strength Training is foremost, for without deep
fiber Structure no tree bears fruit nor can any river flow. Strength, procured through
resistance, is the preeminent fitness tool. From the gym one gains powerful mental
concentration for spiritual advancement while increasing symmetrical muscle mass . . .
this produces body/mind balance. Those who ignore the Unlikely Temple of the gym,
self-create all other obstacles to genuine Wholistic Fitness. Beginning Students must
practice Strength Training deeply. The Master Student requires but occasional sips
from Strength Training for their well-grounded Connection is easily maintained.

Wholistic Fitness Sutra 12

Include Cardio Training in your fitness plan so that your inner breath learns to dance
with the Cosmic breath.
Every Cardio workout prepares the individual soul to become omnidirectional with
Universal soul . . . this is the very definition of yoga.
Cardio is Flow.

You must develop, regardless of affinity, year-round Cardio activity. This dedication alone is spiritual victory and will deliver many High teachings. Cardio teaches you to dwell not upon pleasure or pain. That delayment of gratification leads to even-mindedness. Cardio grounds ego and cleanses undigested emotions. This second of the Five Fitness Disciplines empowers our heart and lungs and maintains appropriate body composition. Introspection, rhythm, and perseverance is gained.

Wholistic Fitness Sutra 13

Practice Hatha Yoga year long, at least every third day.
This brings suppleness, patience, acceptance, and inner grace. You breathe more efficiently and more consciously and therefore live more efficiently and more consciously. You walk intuitively with the earth, instead of on top of Her. Trust the UniVerse arrives, so you no longer worry. In such daily union, there comes indescribable Joy.
Yoga is Wholeness.

The rapture of surrendering into your restrictions, feeling decades of tightness give way to openness will soon taste as sweet as sugar to your soul. Your true happiness rests in union. This third Fitness Discipline of Yoga reflects your Middle Way . . . When you are at h(om)e with your body, you are fearless and in love with It All. All sickness is h(om)esickness. Do not leave your Yoga on the mat; your Highest Yoga is done off the mat.

Wholistic Fitness Sutra 14

Have quiet times in your fitness program.
Meditation fuses inner and outer selves allowing receipt and experience of the Divine.
Meditation is Equanimity.

In the stillness of the fourth Fitness Discipline you attain true knowledge of self. Pain is caused by attachment. Meditation is the breaking of pain by a return to inner spaciousness. You exist in consciousness so you may play in the One Poem through bodily experiences. Practice of meditation melts the brain into mind so your True Nature re-members (with) eternal Joy.
Meditation is the glue that bonds the Five Fitness Disciplines into Wholistic Fitness.

Wholistic Fitness Sutra 15

Be attentive to Nutrition, both physical and spiritual.
Our body is fashioned from earth, and from the earth's harvest it draws well being.
Listen to your body; it will tell you what it needs.
Nutrition is Harmony.

Do not limit your Nutrition—the fifth and final Fitness Discipline—to physical food,
for it is the least efficient source. Higher Nutrition lies within the spiritual realm such
as occupation, conversation, relation, self-talk, pranayama, and meditation. Physical
foods are categorized as either Cleansing or Empowering. Balance the two. Do not
worry about food combining; just eat the foods that are easiest for you to digest. Take
as many meals as possible seated on the earth. When the hips are open, the stomach
fills appropriately. Approach meals with appreciation, leave them while still hungry.
Feed the physiologic body, not the ego body.

EMOTIONS

Wholistic Fitness Sutra 16

Lack of Confidence, low Self-Esteem, and depleted Mojo
are symptoms of inadequate Strength Training.

In the grip of a Pull-Up bar, inner power is magnified.
When Mind is immersed within a 10 repetition × 20 set back squat session,
your Warrior Self arises like the Phoenix from the ashes of self-doubt.
When thighs, screaming from lactic acid burn, are forced by your Willpower to crank
off 1-minute jump squat sets, your ego will vaporize into the mist of the Divine.
Practice in the Gym Temple will empower realization that nothing is
separate from your-self . . .
all Things are different forms of you looking at yourself in order to learn.
Especially barbells.

Wholistic Fitness Sutra 17

Anger, Restlessness, Frustration
are callings for Cardio.

Go for a run, a bike ride, or a walk.
Feel the tempo of your breathing within the rhythm of nature.
Your entire life can be lived as a flowing meditation.
See all things courageously and energetically as all things fall with Joy into
the present moment.
Cardio teaches us not to run-away but to run-into.
The long run is accomplished by staying present with what is.
That is not just a technique for Cardio training,
it is a metaphor for the rest of your life.

Wholistic Fitness Sutra 18

Stress, Anxiety, Depression
are re-Minders that you are in need of Yoga.

Noticeable tightness—physical or mental—is the body shouting for release.
Do yoga. Dance. Ski. Climb some rocks. Throw the frisbee on the beach.
Just move and breathe!
Feel the dance. Feel the flow.
Soon, you will regain breath, posture,
and your natural elegance.

Wholistic Fitness Sutra 19

Confusion, Impatience, Meaninglessness
are nothing but Zen gongs signaling you to sit in Meditation.

To Spiritually Awake, practice two essentials:
1. be where you are going and,

2. be what you are doing.
Your aim is not to be a great meditator.
Or a great yogi or businessperson or athlete or homemaker or religious devotee.
Your aim is to be impeccable in whatever you do.
This will get you Free.
To Awaken, we must open our eyes to See.
Meditation brings a Higher Vision
so you can open to what you are,
not what you "think" you are.

Wholistic Fitness Sutra 20

Tiredness, Agitation, Lack of Motivation
are Divine hands, tugging at your consideration of Nutrition.

What you eat directly affects how you feel and perform.
Eat gently when you feel anxious;
eat strongly when you feel weak.
Life is many things at once, so don't gulp at all the food around you,
especially likes and dislikes. Doing so causes lethargy of body and spirit.
When tired, rest.
When agitated, step back.
When unmotivated, change.
You need no more books. No more miracle diets. No more expensive "engineered foods."
The true soup for the soul is that which you eat all the time
when you are quiet enough to realize it.

Wholistic Fitness Sutra 21

Self-congratulation
is a necessary form of communication with your body. Reward yourself for your fitness
efforts. Positive transformations need encouragement.

Self-congratulation differs from pride.
Pride is ego-born and is useless baggage tarnishing your natural luminosity.

The spiritual warrior does not celebrate in the end zone, he merely hands the ball to
the referee. He knows that the Game is not yet over.
Practice elegance, not pride.
Be kind to yourself. Treat yourself well.
This is the Wholistic Fitness Way.

Wholistic Fitness Sutra 22

Rejection
is a testing tool from the Divine. It cannot harm genuine Practice and is needed to
filter counterfeit warriors from the Real ones. Nothing has power over your fitness
training unless you give it power.

Approach difficulties with a quiver of spiritual swords; use small ones with crafty skill
for small difficulties and large ones with unforgiving force for big difficulties. Become a
master swordsperson in the Art of Difficulty.
You are freed from difficulty by devoting yourself to it.
Look excuses in the eye, and gently toss them from your Path.
This is known by some as willpower and is trainable component in every human.
Willpower is fueled by rejection and difficulty.

Wholistic Fitness Sutra 23

Change and Impermanence
are essential for Higher growth in all things and all beings.
Seek small changes, not big end points.
Enjoy the process of change or you will leave the best part behind; yourself.
A drunk should remain a drunk until change becomes a better high than alcohol.
A yogi should not do the splits if he can't touch his toes, he should reach his edge,
breathe and wait for change to arise from within.
Change and Impermanence are only difficult for those with preferences;
prefer nothing and all things Dance before you.
Expect nothing, and you shall never be disappointed.

Wholistic Fitness Sutra 24

Greed
is distrust of the UniVerse.

Trust this: The UniVerse will always provide.
Ego specializes in "scarcity complexes."
Using too much water in the shower is as greedy as inside trading on Wall Street. Such
actions produce no inner elegance and ruin spiritual progress.
Hoarding your workouts also leads to stagnation of spirit.
Welcome family and friends to share your workouts.
They help unfold your enjoyment and progress.
God has a religion, it's you.
What exactly is the "glory of God" if it's not you?
So share yourself, honor yourself.
Don't be greedy, you are not yours.
We must give everything back, so why try hoarding the unhoardable?

ETHICS

Wholistic Fitness Sutra 25

Do workouts with animals and children.

Study how they move.
They are True fitness masters and love to teach.
Their teachings never stop.
Observe and imitate them.

Wholistic Fitness Sutra 26

Have a friend photograph you doing something physical that you enjoy.

Notice how energetic and freeflowing you look.
Photographs can make the Tao freeze in time.

So can art,

if done from the spirit.

Make sure you know the difference between yourself

"within"

and

"without."

Take your Practice within.

Wholistic Fitness Sutra 27

Occasionally, do these things:

Work out with a fitness expert in a private session.

Take classes from other Teachers.

Attend the Performing and Fine Arts.

Do an outdoor adventure sport.

Go to a retreat.

Road trip.

If you drive a fancy car, drive an inexpensive one for a while.

If you drive an inexpensive car, rent a fancy one for a while.

These things shift Perspective and bring out Potential.

Afterward, practice by yourself what you learned

to foster individual creativity and understanding.

Think of your fitness work as artwork.

It is.

Wholistic Fitness Sutra 28

Smile often

so you enjoy the path to unity and wholeness.

Smiling is an underused form of prayer

and perhaps the best way for you

to discover you.

Smiling is not an aftereffect of merely experiencing happiness,

it is a catalyst for becoming genuinely Joyful.

Wholistic Fitness Sutra 29

Drop your guises.

Staying physically fit means actively merging with the UniVerse
which constantly plays inside and all around you.
Participate fully in this game, as
nakedly as you dare.
You were born in Original Skin—not Sin.
That is why things are always more meaningful
—and way more fun—
the more naked (True) you are.

Wholistic Fitness Sutra 30

Your physical condition can be a letter from your unconscious.

When your body shows signs of stress, strain, or dis-ease, pay attention.
Your unconscious is warning you that your life is out of balance.

Wholistic Fitness Sutra 31

Give your body the best, and it will give you its best.
When your body is failing you in some way,
consider if you have failed to honor its needs for healthful

rest,

nutrition,

and exercise.
What the lazy do not understand: Action always rewards you with more energy.

Wholistic Fitness Sutra 32

Just as a plant thrives on water and the caress of sunlight,
so your body thrives on touch and warming up to other beings.

Get and give hugs each day.
Get and give massages.

Wholistic Fitness Sutra 33

Positive thinking is a health tonic.
Think well enough of yourself to treat yourself well.
Body follows mind; think yourself well.

Wholistic Fitness Sutra 34

Play out your fitness everywhere.
This moment is your chance to empower and transform your body. Your workout is
everywhere.
Do these things as much as possible:
walk barefoot,
yoga squat,
clean,
sit cross-legged,
smile,
see with soft eyes,
move with spine straight and the breath low.

Most of all, prioritize self-propelled movement and fitness-enhancing action. Every
time you linger in the shower, complain, manipulate, are mean, unconsciously drive a
car, or gossip . . .
You contribute to greed, ingratitude, insensitivity.
Are those the verses you wish to contribute to the One Poem?

Wholistic Fitness Sutra 35

Don't just do fitness; be it.
Fitness is the most natural expression of wholeness.

Don't try to love fitness.
True Loves are never found, they are within us all along.

PART SIX

QUESTIONS AND ANSWERS

CHAPTER 30

A WF Dharma Talk with Coach Ilg

It's nice to be important, but it's more important to be nice.

T HE FOLLOWING QUESTIONS REFLECT A wide spectrum of transpersonal fitness top-
ics and hopefully will provide some of the wit and wisdom that arises from my exchange
with students, friends, and fans of Wholistic Fitness. Much of the following has been gleaned
from my columns in various magazines, some has come from seminars and workshops. Most,
however, come from my online coaching archives, particularly my daily online web journal,
Direct Lines, at www.wholisticfitness.com.

I chose a few that are sport performance related, but most are questions from real people dealing with common challenges associated with trying to live a fitness life. Names may
have been changed, but content has not.

Subj: Drunk Student
From: F.S.

Coach Ilg,

I think I am a drunk. I only feel good when I am buzzed. I also smoke pot and gamble. I want to be like you and the cool, fit "warriors." That's all.

Dear F.S.,

There are no rights or wrongs in the spiritual journey, there are only consequences from our choices. Besides having lost your common sense, you've lost your "Cosmic sense." Attractions toward alcohol or drugs are not uncommon because they reduce tension of the mind. With a release of mental tension, your heart energy is more easily accessed. That is why you said you feel "good" when you are buzzed. That's a way of saying that you feel God when buzzed. In India, very high gurus are said to be God-intoxicated. But instead of drinking alcohol or doing drugs, they have learned how to get high on Divinity. There is nothing spiritually wrong with getting drunk or buzzed, it is the attachment to the altered state that kills the warrior spirit and weakens the body. The trick is to remain drunk (or high) when sober. That requires spiritual warriorism. Besides extracting an unrecoverable toll on the body/mind/spirit, the high from drugs is a far lower and shorter one than a Divine High.

One day—this lifetime or another—being a brave and noble spiritual warrior will make more Sense to you than alcohol. The lazy way to enlightenment is not the true Way. Intoxication may be seductive and give glimpses of spiritual consciousness, but one must be sober and grounded to follow the true, the spiritual warrior Way.

When it becomes more painful to suffer than change, we will change.

Subj: Broken Bones
From: Cris

Coach Ilg,

Help! Today I broke my shoulder and a couple of ribs, managing to get both sides of my body. I will have surgery on Friday. I am a Cat. 3, 38-year-old woman road bike racer and I have been training seriously since October. I was working toward a peak in June for Master's Nationals. I have between 10–15 hours a week for cycling. Any suggestions for time best spent during these next weeks of bone knitting? Nutritional advice? Thank you so much for your help.

Dear Cris,

Currently, you are out of my field of expertise. After surgery, it's best to work with a sports-knowledgeable physical therapist. I usually begin my work after students are released from medically prescribed treatment. However, a couple of things might help you in your healing.

Use the injury to learn. The only thing that hurts worse and is more expensive than an injury is repeating it in the future! Contemplate the "accident" to discover clues about factors that led to the "accident." Honestly assess your training. Was it lacking any component that could have prevented or minimized the injury? Strength training? Flexibility? Bike handling? Cornering? Descending? Cat. 3's have a lot of accidents. Fitness levels are high, but bike handling skills may not be up to balance with the aggressive nature of the peleton [the main group of racers in a bicycle race].

Bones are not "hard" by nature. They represent the most concentrated energetic structure in the body. Broken bones can represent a conflict in our spiritual energy. If meditation is not part of your training program, this injury might indeed be a beacon alerting you to more than just a surgeon and a fix-the-broken-part attitude. Use this time to cultivate a wholistic perspective to your training.

Healing visualizations are of utmost importance right now. Give your mind an accurate image of how you want the body/mind/spirit to heal, feel, and perform as you take responsibility to regenerate. Although this forum is not the appropriate vehicle for me to prescribe a series of healing meditations for you, contact me privately or another expert in this field to assist you in this area.

Good luck in your Journey. This situation will make you a stronger racer and a more whole person in the long term.

To work out gracefully is to live gracefully.

Subj: Not Quite Sore Knee
From: Sanda

Dear Coach Ilg,

I'm a triathlete. For the last few weeks I've had a tender right knee after training runs. It started after 6 miles (on a 7-mile run) four weeks ago, pain on the outside of my right knee (more toward the lower leg than the upper). It responded to ice and a couple days later actually got better after a 70-mile bike ride. I've gone easy on it. But it gets a little tender when I run on it—especially downhill.

And it isn't swollen, it isn't enough to cause a limp or for me to favor it, but it keeps wanting to get tender. Any advice? I am a 26-year-old female.

Dear Sanda,

Patellar tendon distress is common among all kinds of endurance athletes, regardless of sport. This time of the year—the end of the summer season—the connective tissue of the athletic body is often worn and vulnerable to aches, inflammations, or worse. Factors that compound this affliction appear to relate to two main avenues: inadequate nutrition and poor periodizational structure.

1. Inadequate nutrition. According to Wholistic Fitness tenets, nutrition is one discipline that must be maintained "full throttle" all year long, seven days per week. Many cases like yours stem from a negative nitrogen balance, which results from poor quality and/or quantity of amino acids.

2. Poor periodizational structure. Make sure your year-long training plan is one that provides a balance of intense training stimulus with properly timed restoration/deep regeneration phases. Examine your training structure to make certain your connective tissue is thoroughly strength trained in the off-season phases. Joint inflammations can be traced to inadequate strength training and kinesthetic (yoga and postural alignment) training. Connective tissue cannot withstand long months of endurance-specific work necessary for peak performances without rest and expansion.

Finally, do not disregard the energetic lesson behind the physical manifestation. When the knees begin to act up or weaken, it sometimes reflects an inner fear of moving forward in some important area of our personal life. In other cases it means a certain type of inner arrogance or stubbornness. An image of a "locked-out knee" stance conveys rigidity and lack of being open. Take time to consider in depth why this injury has come into your experience. Learn from it. Awareness is your biggest issue here, not sport performance.

Worry and fear come from the belief that we are powerless.

Subj: Back Pain
From: Jim

Dear Coach/Guru:

Last summer you gave me some excellent advice about a back injury. One thing you advised was to ditch a back support belt, and I must confess, that was absolutely the correct thing to do. Almost immediately, some secondary symptoms disappeared. You also advised me to pay attention to my personal relationships, as the injury was in the pelvic region and related to a chakra that was closed. Again, excellent advice, as I was able to heal both.

Subj: Lower Back Pain
From: Tim

I was recently diagnosed by orthopedics with an inflammation or, possibly a degradation, of the SI5 (Sacroiliac) joint near my right hip. I've had back problems for 11 years and cycling has never seemed to bring them on. Now my doc wants me to give up my road bike for something more upright like a mountain bike or hybrid to prevent long periods of time spent down in the drops. I live in Hawaii where wind is constantly 15 mph or higher, so riding low is common. Any recommendations on a pre-bike stretch routine or something else that might help? Have been riding a Lifecycle recumbent for the past 4 weeks to try and stay in some semblance of shape and my back still hurts.

Dear Tim,

Conventional medical training insists that doctors treat the symptom, so it comes as no surprise to me that your doctor wants you off the bike. That might be the cure, but it's not the healing. Neither is switching to a recumbent, a hybrid, or a MTB. That's just shuffling. Your true healing lies within, not in something external.

Lower back musculature and skeletal tissue are prone to injury in all fitness enthusiasts, but even more so among sport-specific athletes. Even sports like golf and darts commonly produce back injuries. It's possible that a lack of structural balance has predisposed this area to your current injury. A couple of immediate notes: Make certain your training year includes at least three months of noncycling specific strength training. Those three months should also include yoga to help realign structural, spiritual, and biochemical imbalances.

The more cycling specific we become, the more the psoas [hip flexor] musculature and associated connective tissue tends to harden, causing rotation of the pelvis actuating physical conflict. I suggest getting some structural bodywork such as rolfing [a type of deep massage and skeletal alignment] to "open" and "soften" this stockpiled rigidity. Look at your training: Do your training volumes reflect significant imbalance between contractive training like cycling and expansive training like yoga, regenerative nutrition, bodywork, and meditation? If so, this injury is a signal to get you onto a higher level of awareness. Giving up your road bike is not the way to learn from this injury!

Communication is a giving of light and vibration. Nutrition is an absorption of It. Fitness is choosing wisely.

>Subj: Cancer Concerns
>From: Lori

LORI: I want to focus on releasing into the beauty of this moment, as you said in yoga class. In my application to you, I expressed that I was motivated to study Wholistic Fitness to help me live with mindfulness, love, acceptance, and compassion for myself and others, and to live in the "now," in the presence of my true self. This has always been my motivation, even before I heard of Wholistic Fitness. I really do want to live this way.

COACH ILG: You already are, at some level.

LORI: I understand that fear, worry, and stress can cause things to happen that wouldn't have otherwise.

COACH ILG: Fear, worry, and stress are not causes, Lori. They are manifestations of not receiving the true presence of the moment.

LORI: I am scared about getting breast cancer. The fact is that my mom had it at age 42, and again at 64 years old; her sister had it at age 33, and again at 62 years old; their mom died of it and their aunt died of it at age 42 years old. There are genes called the BRCA1 and BRCA2 genes. The oncologist said that if I inherited an alteration in the genes, I have an 80 percent lifetime chance of getting breast cancer, a 50 percent chance of getting it by age 50 years old, and a 50 percent chance of getting ovarian cancer. How do you feel that genetics play a role in things, in terms of the development of our body/mind/spirit?

COACH ILG: What we call "genetics" are what yogis know as *samskara* or impressions, tendencies, and possibilities present in consciousness that arise and have arisen through one's actions and thoughts, including those of possible previous lifetimes. Let's pretend that your vehicle for this lifetime of learning is to learn how to deal with being a rich and famous athlete. If so, then your soul will experience a Michael Jordan type of lifetime. If your soul needs to go through dealing with breast cancer to learn, it will invite a body with breast cancer. From a soul perspective, one is not higher than the other. It's just what is needed for spiritual learning.

LORI: I have always wanted to develop my spirit.

COACH ILG: You are. You cannot help it.

LORI: Now, to me, it just makes sense to empower myself with the knowledge of research.

COACH ILG: The only true research is you . . . the only scientific evidence that matters is when you live it and become the evidence!

LORI: I am sure that my fear of getting cancer is partly responsible.

COACH ILG: Your true fear may be that you have not lived enough yet. We all must die. Is leaving the Stage by way of cancer worse than some other way? What if your soul needs to learn breast cancer? What then? Are you going to quit the Spiritual Journey? That would be like quitting your first marathon just a stone's throw from the finish line! All your prior effort would have been wasted. Do not waste one moment more, Lori! The Divine is here now! Lance Armstrong used his cancer to win the Tour de France. There are many ways of experiencing anything. Even cancer. It's about which perspective you choose.

Getting real is the only choice we have.

Subj: Body Fat and Exercise
From: Jill

Dear Coach,

I am a 25-year-old female, 5'3" and 132 pounds. In the summer I ride my mountain bike recreationally and also jog and hike and weight train. Since moving to Breckenridge three years ago, my fitness level has increased tremendously and my diet has improved. But I have always carried extra body fat in my upper thighs and particularly my butt. I have become more firm, but have not had the significant muscle building and fat loss I expected.

My question is: What activities and in what amounts would you recommend to eliminate some of the extra fat? I work a desk job forty hours a week and have to contend with the chilly mornings and rainy afternoons of Summit County. I have a trainer (rollers), which I used this spring, but even while watching TV, two hours is the most I can take of that. Any advice you have would be appreciated. Thanks in advance.

Jill,

If you are 25 and have only been training for three years, then practice some patience! If you grew up with those fatty areas, three years is a pretty short time to reverse over a decade of accumulating fat, don't you think? Appreciate your body for doing as well as it is without injury.

You are an efficient cyclist. Too efficient. Begin doing other Cardio activities at which you are not as efficient. Start cross training.

Additionally, get into the gym and do some high-intensity movements targeting the glutes and thighs: squats, lunges, and leg presses. Incorporate plyometric movements [exercises that develop fast-twitch or speed-strength type of fitness] to stimulate fresh neural service, which increases metabolic fire to the area. Use your off-season to compete in snowshoe races; that's major glute/thigh work, as is running up ski slopes during dryland training. In-line skating is okay, but still too much glide most of the time. Classic Nordic skiing should be prioritized this winter for you as well. Enough to go on? As with any Cardio training, volumes and intensities need to undulate throughout the seasons. Proper choreography includes sessions of high intensity plus low intensity.

Not deciding is choosing. What we choose to do is what we love. Love what you choose.

Subj: Motivation and Meditation
From: Leftside

Dear Coach,

Having a little bit of a motivational problem with the training. I have kept up with all the volumes and items but am still filling stuck in the mud. Have done some extra zazen to try and calm my racing mind. Have had many questions with the book by Sogyan, The Tibetan Book of Living and Dying. *The whole idea of every thing we say, do will have repercussions on future "lives." Thus leading to a global responsibility for all beings . . . man that is big! The idea of getting free from our minds and realizing our own trap . . . to really see what is important, to not be a slave to our thoughts. I just have not been capable to do these things as of yet. I have done a pathetic job in the Tapasaya day (saying "no" to desired, but unneeded actions), really not that great. I am just falling back into similar patterns of wants and desires . . .*

Student Leftside,

Be patient in your spiritual seeking to Big Questions. Just keep practicing—through boring weeks and through exciting weeks—just keep as even-minded and as steadfast as you can with your prescribed daily practices. Suzuki taught, "If you lose the spirit of repetition, your practice will become quite difficult." Work on forgetting yourself more. Merge into your awareness and leave the self behind. Your letter had several errors. Worry less about the Big Questions and more about mindful spelling.

Don't overthink. The spiritual journey is a long trek filled with many high mountains and low valleys. Be careful not to be too greedy for results in this journey. If you reach for the highest of Highs, be prepared to deal with the lowest of lows. For that is precisely what the UniVerse will produce to condition you. The Master Student of WF learns to cultivate the tranquil spiritual self that lies beyond the highs and lows of worldly living.

Yes, the idea that every thought, word choice, and action influences our next life and has global and even universal implications is a tremendous responsibility. Does it all count? Yes, every little bit counts. As we say in Wholistic Fitness: "Nothing matters, but everything counts." Just practice.

Finding my Inner Child? Hell, when I first started to meditate, I could not even find my inner family! When I did, they were all dysfunctional. We are all full of strangers.

Subj: This isn't fun
From: CG

Hi Coach,

I have a few questions about my "reactions" to Wholistic Fitness training. They have not all been joyous times of bliss, in fact, I am starting to feel a little down. It seems to be getting more difficult to maintain any kind of mindfulness for each day. I feel myself becoming detached during my recovery weeks. A feeling of almost floating in space.

My new awareness is telling many things about myself that I do not like, in fact, might perhaps even be afraid to admit. The real truth still is something I do not understand in myself and about myself. Have I spent so long on this earth without noticing? Why? Is this grogginess I feel normal? Am I finally noticing my dragons? Why am I confused about these reactions?

Dear Student CG,

Wholistic Fitness is about waking up. It's designed for self-understanding and greater spiritual wisdom. Magical solutions do not exist in spiritual training. What matters is finding inner tools such as mindfulness, meditation, and self-discipline, and using them wisely to chart your own Journey.

Depression, confusion, lethargy are commonplace dragons on the arduous trek up the path of self-cultivation. Every now and then, we may stumble upon moments of outright beauty, oneness, and joy. Along our trek, we see some people enduring very difficult, joyless lives while others seem to take their outlandish prosperity for granted. Doesn't matter. Everyone has their own unique karma.

Wholistic Fitness teaches mindful living and will eventually impart an inner peace and a sacred happiness far more profound than the typical Western model of linear success and material wealth. Your immediate work is to be as even-minded as possible through the highs and lows of everyday life.

Work on equanimity. Work within the present moment.

Waking up is something each of us must do for ourselves. No one but you can choose to move out of ignorance and awaken. That is why the Buddha taught his disciples to "be a light unto yourself."

Trying to "have it all come together" is like trying to eat once and for all. Wholeness is a dance, not a place.

Subj: Reincarnation
From: Sheryl

Dear Steve,

First, thank you for all your wonderful energy during yoga. I am so different now! Much happier! However, a lot of the things you say in class and some of your "dharma talks" have really thrown me into a confusion about dying consciously. I never even thought about how I was going to handle my last few moments until I starting taking your classes and reading your newsletters. Do I have to believe in reincarnation to do better in yoga? Oh gosh, I am feeling silly writing this to you. You don't have to reply. I am going to "practice being brave" as you say and just hit my send button instead of my delete button! . . .

Namasté.

Beautiful and Brave Student Sheryl,
You are so brave! Honor your confusion. Too much stillness equals stagnation. The UniVerse is change. Chaos is the preferred playground for spiritual shifting. That is why shamans use rattles and sufis whirl in their dancing! Do not lean too far in any direction; balance is what is important.

Reincarnation? It matters little if reincarnation is "true" or not. We do not know the exact whereabouts of heaven or hell, although my teacher, Sensei Kishiyama said that heaven and hell are in our mind.

What happens after our last gasp? I have no idea. I've studied the sacred literature on the dying process in several traditions, but "the map is not the territory." I won't know until I travel that astral terrain. Neither will you. Even the Buddha called such ruminations "imponderable" and advised that we not waste time on the matter. In Buddhism there are no comments on after-death, just the "bardo states," which are the transition zones between life and death. Himalayan yogi masters have evidently overcome the state of what we call death, but I certainly cannot provide comment on such mastery.

Modern physiology confirms that brain cells remain active for days after physical death, so there is plenty of consciousness still left in play after physical death. This much we know, all else are metaphysical and religious issues that really have no concern for me as a fitness instructor. My work with you is about cultivating here and now.

Dogen said, "The firewood cannot see its ashes." He meant that the firewood was life, and ashes were death. As when you hold a yoga posture, focus on the Now moment and let the more complex matters shift (like your bones will with continued yoga practice) on their own accord. It's not so necessary to believe in reincarnation or tarot cards. Any belief is a limitation and creates boundaries to your freedom. Don't make too many categories. Just live. Firewood cannot be rebuilt from ashes. Don't die too soon. Live fully. Burn cleanly. Do your practice and live here now.

The best athletes are like spiritual masters; they really don't compete, they create.

Subj: Fantasy or Visualization
From: SS

Dear Teacher,
I have a question that has arisen from my practice. What's the difference between visualizing something and fantasizing or wishful thinking? I suspect that attachment has something to do with it, but I'm having trouble discerning the subtleties.

Dear SS,
To visualize something involves a distinct step-by-step process having an origin, a middle, and a conclusion. Fantasies or wishful thinking lack the detailed, structured process. Visualization normally requires formal meditation whereas fantasies (at least the best ones!) are more spontaneous.

Things are not what they appear. They are what they are.

Subj: Q-angle and Lactate Threshold
From: Laura

Dear Steve,

I have two questions. I keep telling my indoor cycling class about how you always say to keep bringing the knees toward the midline of the body because of the Q-angle. Could you clarify what exactly the Q-angle is and how it influences indoor cycling? And also, clarify the lactate threshold and how to train it. Thanks!

Dear Laura,

The Q-Angle (aka, the femoral angle) is the natural angle between the upper leg and lower leg. Females generally have a less than 125-degree angle between the neck of the femur and the shaft of the bone. The smaller this angle, the more knockkneed the physique. Contrary to common belief, this knockkneed stance results in less injury than more due to a wider articulating surface between the femur and the tibia. Cyclists benefit from a knockkneed position because it is more stable for the knee. Where there is more stability, there is also more power. Trying to pedal with the knees out or even straight forward—like headlights—results in soft tissue transmission stress at the knee joint, especially in females due to their wider pelvis. The more knockkneed the better in terms of injury prevention and power development for cyclists.

About the lactate threshold. A cyclist can perform to a certain intensity without building up too much lactic acid in the blood. When this intensity is exceeded, the acid in the muscle rises and the muscle fatigues. The point at which the muscle's contractile mechanism begins to shut down due to acidosis is called the lactate threshold (LT).

Training the LT is important because, all other things being equal, the higher one's LT, the faster the speed over long distances or steep climbs. LT training takes on two basic forms: long intervals and tempo training. Recovery is vital in LT training and should be done no more than twice per week by anyone! You can increase the intensity and length of LT sessions, but not the frequency.

Long Intervals: 5 to 12 minutes each interval. Gradually build the heart rate to your LT level and maintain it to the end of the interval. Recovery between the intervals should range from 2 to 5 minutes.

Tempo Training: Gradually build your heart rate to your LT level with a group of riders and maintain a steady LT pace for 5 to 10 miles. Emphasis is on "pace."

Holy water is just another name for sweat.

Subj: Training First Aid
From: Samuel

Dear Coach Ilg,

My achilles tendon in my right legs hurts—my right ankle even swole last wk to the point that I couldn't even stand up on itt for about 3 hrs after waking up. Since then I have been off my bike but would like to resume ASAP. Now it's just the achilees. I was given Ibuprofen, which I have been taking, I haven't iced it though. HELP, Please.

Dear Samuel,

Help yourself by following through on that icing! Any swollen joint should be given a cold pack. Your degree of inflammation (not even being able to stand on it for several hours) may indicate a medical situation. Do not take this injury lightly. You did not inform me on the nature of the injury, but your first aid remains the same: RICE as in

Rest

Ice

Compression

Elevation

I suggest consulting a physician. A bursa (fluid-filled sac located beneath the tendon) may be inflamed. If this is the case, you've got several weeks of R&R ahead of you. I'm not intentionally pessimistic here, I want you to take care of this thing immediately.

If it is the bursa, consider yourself lucky. It's better than a ruptured Achilles tendon. You don't want this to escalate into a chronic condition, because then chances for a rupture increase. One thing: Test your uric acid level. If it is high, you are predisposed to Achilles ailments. If that is the case, warm up and cool down very seriously and rethink participating in explosive lateral sports like basketball and tennis.

WF excels at injury prevention. In the gym, WF students develop ligaments and tendons with the strength of aircraft cable. Then, we do yoga to make sure that that strong connective tissue is also supple. Strength without flexibility is dangerous. This injury is a blessing in disguise. Take care of this injury, get in the gym to work on your joint health, and eat well.

Pay more attention to your spelling. Lack of awareness in writing a letter invites lack of awareness in sport performance. Lack of awareness is not a quality to be cultivated by a fitness warrior!

It's weird that we hire indifferent and expensive friends and call them "therapists." The best therapist is a fit and comfortable body. The best therapy couch is a meditation cushion.

Subj: Too New Agey
From: John

Dear Steve,

Well, your approach certainly has caught my attention . . . is it just me or do lots of people think your approach is a bit "soft" or too "New Agey"? Does the physical side of your training take the same soft focus?

Dear John,

I can tell you are trying to understand Wholistic Fitness without doing the workouts. That won't work at all. WF workouts are the most intense, gut-busting, ego-withering, puke-inducing, godforsaken painful workouts a person can experience. Just follow for one week any one of my workout programs. You'll realize that this stuff is the most grounded, non–New Agey spiritual experience one can practice. WF is best approached by the Zen state of mushin or "mind without thought." Don't think about it, just do it. This requires much training because mushin is an effect, not a technique. No-mind comes from a highly concentrated mind, not a lazy one.

Mastery of WF takes a lifetime. Some appreciation for this notion can be found in a Sanskrit saying: "All skillfulness, all strain, all intention is contrary to ease. Practice 1000 times and It becomes difficult. Practice 1000, 1000 times and It becomes easy. Practice 1000 times TIMES a 1000, 1000 times and It is no longer Thou that doeth It but It that Doeth Itself through Thee! Not until that is that which is done well done."

People want everything very fast. But, genuine body/mind fitness is a yogic art. It's not about getting things fast. It's about Awakening to that which has already arrived.

If we can't find happiness in our efforts along the way, we will never find it at the end of the journey.

Subj: @#$#%#@!!
From: RJ

Ilgbro,

My mom-in-law just had breast surgery. They did a radical on one side and cut out some of the muscle tissue. No further evidence, so no chemo—that's all good news and we are relieved. I immediately was concerned about her normal function with her left side. She is petite and frail already and has poor strength. You know what they gave her to get her arm back to a normal level of function? Physical therapy? Some personal training? A membership at the gym? Hell no! They gave her a pamphlet with three exercises to do at home!

I told her a few generic exercises that she had to do on her own without instruction were not sufficient. I told her to go to her doctor and get a prescription for a physical therapist to restore function on her left side. All pretty basic, standard stuff or so I thought. The doctor told her there "was not a protocol for breast cancer rehab." So, I had my poor mom-in-law, still traumatized from the operation, call a PT (physical therapy) firm. The PT firm said they didn't honor referrals from doctors for breast cancer rehab because there is no protocol.

My God, Ilg . . . who needs a &%$% protocol to recognize and treat loss of function on her left side? How ridiculous! It defies all logic to me, man. Her arm does not work with normal function. Other regions of her body are hurting already because she's compensating and the doctors are scratching their heads waiting for a protocol to drop out of their asses!

This system we have is fucked-up man! Because there is no "protocol," a senior woman has to figure it out at home and lose functional movement, then when she's totally disabled she can then get a freakin' Rx for Physical Therapy! Ahhh! Save us, Ilg, from the Western idiocy, man! Write that book and open some eyes!

How can three generic exercises fit every single woman in the U.S. who is recovering from a mastectomy? And how can a woman with absolutely no background in physical fitness, training, and rehab know how to train back to normal function with three bullshit "work out by the numbers" exercises? Ahhh! —RJ

My Tribal Brother RJ,

I'm sorry for your mom-in-law. That sucks. Man, if I had a dime for every story like that one. One would think that over twenty years, even our medical system would have brightened up in terms of a more whole-person perspective. All you and I can do is do what we can and not take the fear-based doctors out of our heart. Most are too scared to take a piss these days without it being AMA-approved and insured for a bijillion dollars! It's a sad scene, which makes your Light all the more important. One day, fitness instructors like you will be paid like doctors, but until then, let us continue to be Warriors of the Heart.

You and Now are the best Teachers you'll ever have. Learn from the Now and treat Yourself well.

Subj: A New Student and Yoga
From: McConnaughey to WF Teacher Sheader

Dear Teacher Sheader,
I have really neglected the yoga side of things this cycle. A) I am really inflexible and have never historically liked it. B) I don't know what I'm doing and had not gotten the program, which gave me a convenient excuse to neglect it. C) When pushed for time, tried to get in the strength and cardio to exclusion of yoga.

Teacher Sheader,
Yoga is not so much about the tightness of the muscles and rigidity of the joints . . . those are simply manifestations of the deeper realities. As one moves deeper with the breath and mindful awareness a letting go occurs that facilitates increased flexibility of joints, ligaments, and muscles. When one gets frustrated or even hurt doing yoga it is not because they were doing yoga but because they were doing the ego.

Therefore, just be with the pose. Avoid "shoulding" on yourself—"I should be more flexible," "I should have more balance"—just be with the pose, right then right there no matter how tight or how loose you are. To illustrate: One yoga teacher I know studied in India with the master Iyengar. She had a gymnastics background and was very flexible. Iyengar told her it would be most difficult for her to truly learn yoga because her extraordinary flexibility limited her ability to grasp the essence of poses and their teachings.

Wasting energy is wasting life.

Finally, here is an excerpt from an interview I did with Hakado Ru. Kuhlman for *Santa Fe Live* magazine:

HAKADO RU: My impression is that Steve Ilg is fed up with fitting into the starving artist/athlete mold that says you have to run your business solely out of the kindness of your heart.

ILG: Sometimes, yes. Most of the time, no. I began Wholistic Fitness from my efforts in karma yoga; a Path of selfless service. I would train athletes for free because I knew they did not have money. Neither did I. I guess I was influenced by the whole Zen monk practice of mendicancy and renunciation. Also, I heard that in India, the best teachers never charged for their services but would receive huge donations from those they helped. I reckoned that if I did my Work well, the UniVerse would take care of me.

HAKADO RU: If you had the Catholic Church to take care of you, you could pull a Mother Teresa and teach Wholistic Fitness to everyone for free. Last time I checked, you were not a Catholic priest. But now you have only yourself to put a roof over your head, cycling tires on your bike, pay the rent, put food in your belly, and provide for a future family. Thus, you have to combine a passion with the ability to make a living.

ILG: Oh, I have all the money I'll ever need for the rest of my life. As long as I die by next week [laughing]!

HAKADO RU: Now, you can continue on what I assume is a relatively unstable and modest income. The thought-provoking question is: What do you see Wholistic Fitness, as a business, doing twenty years from now?

ILG: Along the Way, I've lost interest in that. To me, it's like discussing where the world will be one hundred years from now. My focus is on individual transformation, since the World is but a reflection of individuals. No matter what happens in the future, the best I can do is stay present to the moment, open to it, soften to it, embrace it. My business success (or lack of it) is a reflection of that philosophy, for better or for worse.

All I know is that I have been Blessed to have the courage to live what I have felt to be a very successful life, inwardly and outwardly. I have always been able to do what makes me feel good, which to me, means feeling God. I continue to live a full and adventuresome life. I still ride my bike or ski or climb whenever I want. I wear play clothes to my "job" and over the course of my life, I've had a pretty low impact on Mother Earth. I have quality time to nourish my soul and my relationships, my "job" is both my passion and my Path Higher. Most of all, I have been able to help and sometimes even inspire others.

HAKADO RU: You know, it's funny, this whole thing about allowing your passions to be your source of income . . . like my business as a website designer and manager, as far as me getting wealthy off this, it's not in the plans. I enjoy doing the work for someone who lets me out of my conventional business cage to do something fun and creative. Yes, I won't turn any money down when it comes in. I've always thought I could pull this self-made millionaire plan off.

> **People just want to be understood and loved. Wholistic Fitness gets us to understand, and eventually, love who we really are. That's truly personal fitness.**

This is America, dude. Although having a million shekels in my bank account wouldn't be a bad thing to have, I would be more satisfied in knowing that I created that wealth. If I inherited it or won the lottery, I would feel like a failure or a cheat. Bizarre, but true.

ILG: Henry David Thoreau said, "No man can be happy in wealth he has not earned." I know what you mean, there is more and more money being made off of image instead of substance and/or integrity. There are definitely vaporous spiritual areas to what "wealth" really means. There are many people who make an awful lot of money, but truly wealthy people, who radiate a higher light and put forth light-giving principles, are still quite rare. Technology is really pushing us toward ethical and moral edges unfelt before now. We have producers making a ton of money off of popular "Reality TV," whereupon we reward people for letting us inflict pain, starvation, and mockery on them. The way we choose to make our money is one of the highest spiritual thresholds we cross.

If you are not feeling wealthy, maybe you are making yourself poor.

PART SEVEN

RECIPES

CHAPTER 31

Realistic Daily Meals for WF Warriors

There is not another, more potent spiritual workshop than that of our nutritional discipline.

—COACH ILG

KNOW YOU ARE BUSY.

To practice our inner work in a society as chaotic as ours means we've got our work cut out for us. Big time. Why do you think Masters and monks retreat to caves and forlorn jungle huts to accomplish their spiritual work? They do so because when faced with the ever-accelerating pace of modern society, the busy-ness takes too great a toll on their austerities.

Because you and I are "householders" and not cave-dwelling sadhus or monks, we must learn to forgive—again and again—our inconsistent spiritual endeavor. We must learn and relearn how not to get down on ourselves, especially for not eating as slowly or consciously as we'd probably like. It's damned hard creating enough decompressed time during the day to mindfully prepare one, let alone three, meals. So be easy with yourself when it comes to dietary challenges, but stay firm with your inner desire to constantly improve as a fitness warrior.

Yet, having acknowledged the need to forgive ourselves often in terms of choosing wise and mindful mealtimes, I also need you to realize there is truly not another, more potent spiritual workshop than nutritional discipline. The senseless war of aggression and domination is too easily embraced by the typical American diet, particularly by supporting fast-food joints and large, chain grocers. Though there is no way around each of our unique personal and karmic predicaments, we certainly can choose to lead clearer, more focused, and more globally conscious lives through our nutritional patterns. Eating herbs helps significantly, but even WF warriors cannot live on herbs alone. To help you navigate the ever-changing seas of personal nutrition, I've enclosed some WF recipes that provide quality nutrition without requiring you to step into a time warp to prepare them. I merely ask that you do your best to treat each meal, regardless of preparation time, as a blessing from the UniVerse. Many, many beings and energies contribute to the abundance of food we eat during our lives upon Mother Earth. Respect, even revere, this fact.

May these staple recipes from my humble Path contribute toward a more sensitive nutritional awareness within and without.

MORNING MEALTIMES

Not Very Tidy Tofu and Eggs

Fun and messy to prepare. It's also quick and nutritious. High in protein so your muscles will be stronger and your day more powerful.

PREPARATION TIME 10 minutes   SERVES 2

1 teaspoon safflower oil

1 clove garlic, crushed

$1/4$ cup chopped onion

1 pound (1 package) firm tofu, drained

4 beaten egg whites (or $3/4$ cup liquid egg substitute like Egg Beaters)

$1/4$ teaspoon raw sesame seeds

2 teaspoons tamari

toppings: salsa or green chile sauce

Sauté oil, garlic, and onion in a large skillet using medium-high heat. When onions grow translucent, reduce heat to low-medium. Add tofu by squeezing it through your fingers over and over until the tofu has been squished into small pieces. Let tofu brown for a minute or two, stirring occasionally. Pour the eggs into the simmering tofu, and cook for 1 to 3 minutes, or until eggs are tinged brown. Add sesame seeds and tamari to taste. Top and serve.

Ilg McMuffin

My easier-on-the-earth, cruelty-free, and more nutritious alternative to that weird fast-food breakfast stuff.

PREPARATION TIME less than 10 minutes   SERVES 1

1 English muffin (fork-split, both sides)

1 soy breakfast patty (such as Morningstar Farms)

2 beaten egg whites (or ½ cup liquid egg substitute like Egg Beaters)

Salt and pepper

Jam of choice

1 slice of soy cheese (American or Cheddar style, such as Yves)

Place a medium-sized skillet on medium heat. As the skillet warms, toast the English muffin to desired level of crispness and microwave the breakfast patty. If you don't wish to microwave, cook the frozen breakfast patty in the skillet as directed on the package label. (This no-microwave option will add about 8 minutes to the preparation time.)

After the breakfast patty and muffin are ready, pour eggs into skillet and cook to desired consistency. As the egg cooks, add salt and pepper as desired and apply jam to the inner surface(s) of the toasted muffin.

Place the cooked eggs on the bottom muffin. Add breakfast patty, slice of soy cheese, and finally the top muffin. Press into a sandwich-style muffin and enjoy.

MEALTIMES FOR MIDDAY

Tofu Sandwich

PREPARATION TIME 10 minutes   SERVES 1

½ tsp. safflower oil (or any light oil)

¼ block extra-firm tofu (cut into 2 slices), drained

½ teaspoon tamari

2 slices of your favorite bread

Garnishes: mustard, lettuce, sprouts, tomato, onions, pickles, chilies, soy cheese, catsup, avocado, pepper, or create your own

Coat a large skillet with oil. Using medium-high heat, brown both sides of tofu. Braise the tofu with tamari. (If using soy cheese you can melt it on the tofu after the first side is browned.) On plain or toasted bread, add your favorite garnishes. When tofu has been browned, add it to the bread. Serve!

Electra Lentil Soup

Named for Electra Lake, located north of Durango, Colorado, a beautiful playground of my childhood.

PREPARATION TIME **60 minutes**   SERVES **6**

1 cup dried lentils

6 cups water

3 tablespoons olive oil

1 medium potato, peeled and cut into $^1/_2$-inch cubes

$^1/_2$ teaspoon black pepper

1 cup chopped celery

1 cup chopped swiss chard

1 teaspoon ground coriander

$^1/_2$ teaspoon cumin

2 tablespoons lemon juice

$^1/_4$ cup chopped parsley

$^1/_4$ cup chopped coriander leaves

Sea salt, to taste

In a large soup pot over medium heat, cook water and lentils. Simmer 35 minutes. In a small frying pan, sauté potatoes and pepper in oil for 2 minutes. Add celery, continue to sauté for another minute. Add sauté mixture to lentil broth. Boil for 10 minutes. Add chard, ground coriander, cumin, and lemon juice, cook for another 10 minutes. Add parsley, fresh coriander, and salt to taste. Serve.

Bok Choy with Rice

A great dish: subtle, cleansing, and invigorating on all planes.

PREPARATION TIME: **20 minutes**   SERVES **2 to 3**

$\frac{1}{2}$ **pound firm tofu, drained and cubed**

1 tablespoon safflower oil

$\frac{1}{2}$ **small onion, chopped**

1 clove garlic, minced

1 medium stalk bok choy, chopped

$\frac{1}{4}$ **cup water**

2 tablespoons lite soy sauce

2 tablespoons mustard

2–3 teaspoons curry powder

2 cups cooked basmati rice

Add tofu cubes and oil to large skillet. Brown slightly using medium high heat. Put in the onion and garlic. Cook for a minute then add bok choy and water. (Add more water if bok choy gets too dry.) Cook for 5 minutes or till bok choy has softened. Add soy sauce, mustard, and curry powder, and simmer for 3 more minutes. Serve over a bed of rice.

Spinach Staple

Kathy and I never tire of this meal, though we have it frequently. This is an especially valuable meal for vegetarians. The simplicity is astounding. The dark green, leafy nutrition is an important energetic choice. Feel free to experiment with the seasonings.

PREPARATION TIME: 20 minutes   SERVES 2 to 3

$1/2$ **pound firm tofu, drained and sliced or cubed**

1 tablespoon safflower oil

1 clove garlic, chopped

$1/2$ **small onion, chopped**

2 bunches fresh spinach

$1/4$ **cup water**

$1/4$ **cup yellow mustard**

2 tablespoons lite soy sauce

1 tablespoon Bragg Liquid Aminos

$1/4$ **teaspoon ground ginger**

2 cups cooked basmati rice

Garnish: soy sauce, mustard, or Bragg

In a large skillet, sauté tofu in oil on moderate high heat until browned. Add garlic and onion. Let it cook for a couple minutes before adding spinach and water. Cover. Once the spinach softens, top with mustard and add soy sauce, Bragg, and ginger. Add more water if spinach is drying out. Cover and cook for 1 to 2 minutes. Garnish and serve over rice.

Ab Wheel

Pay what you want for any number of fancy abdominal machines, devices, and outright ripoffs. But if you are serious about ripping up your abs and not your wallet, you can pick up an Abdominal (or "Ab") Wheel at most major sporting goods stores. They are also known as Abdominal Rollers. Cost usually hovers between $12 and $15.

Ayurvedic Personal Care Therapies/Items

Ayurveda is the oldest traditional healing system practiced in India and the most comprehensive wholistic healing system in the world. This ancient knowledge is more than five thousand years old and was initiated by sages and seers for the well-being of humans. It has been called the mother of all healing systems. It is the original source of many allopathic and naturopathic therapies. The Sanskrit term "ayurveda" is composed of two words, "ayus" and "veda." "Ayus" means life and "Veda" means knowledge. So the literal meaning of ayurveda is science of life.

In this book, I have mentioned only three ayurvedic health products that I have found most helpful and least "weird" for Westerners to incorporate into their personal care routines:

Tongue cleaner (or tongue scraper) These are becoming more and more common. Shaped like the letter "U" and made from metal or plastic, this item is dragged across your tongue upon awakening in the morning to clear accumulated mucus and God knows what else that gathers on your tongue during sleep. Try it once, and you'll never know how you lived without it!

Neti pot A bit more "weird" for most Americans, neti is done by pouring a small but steady stream of water into one nostril and allowing it to flow out the other (technically, this use of water instead of other materials such as thread, is called *jala neti*). This action flushes out all sorts of rather interesting particulates that are otherwise trapped in the phlegm and mucus of the nasal and sinus passages. I've had great success at erasing conditions like allergies, headaches, and respiratory ailments from my students brave enough to do and keep doing neti. I also did neti before endurance competitions because it greatly improved the efficiency of my breathing. I do neti nearly every day and always after air travel.

Toe spreader If you were to have seen me write this book in my office, you'd laugh as hard as my wife does. I sit on a PhysioBall (see below), hips wide open, with my knees plastered against the sides of filing cabinets. I shift my pelvis back and forth, to and fro, do little side flexions and backbends—anything to keep my sacrum and spine fluid and mobile. Upon my feet? Rainbow-colored toe spreaders! Thick ones! Why? Just ask a reflexologist how important supple, wide toe spread is! Each toe and its connective tissue is associated with a major nerve and organ system. If the toes are kept tightly squeezed together and suffocated in shoes, the toes lose gross amounts of neural activity, which compromises organic health. So go ahead and laugh. But after an entire life of squeezing my feet into rock-climbing shoes, ski racing boots, running shoes, etc., I had zero toe spread by age thirty. My toes were very stiff, which meant my organs were getting less neural service. Today, ten years later, although I still have limited toe spread, the softness and spread of my toes has greatly improved. Interestingly, I find that my entire foot strike upon the ground has changed, as has my gait. My standing one-leg balance poses in yoga have gotten firmer, and emotionally I find myself more cheerful and relaxed as my toes continue to spread and soften! Try it, you'll like it. But your spouse will laugh!

These ayurvedic products can be found at many New Age bookstores or online catalogs, such as www.ayurveda.com.au.

Bicycle Advocacy
League of American Bicyclists, www.bikeleague.org. See also Ron Jones, below.

Eco-Friendly/Low-Impact Living
Here are some of my most commonly used sources for efforts in living a little more lightly and consciously upon this beautiful planet:

www.GreenMarketplace.com To start reducing toxins, pollution, waste, and cruelty, begin by shopping smarter and greener. This source makes it easy to find truly healthy, earth-friendly alternatives that make a difference.

www.seventhgen.com One of the original eco-friendly companies that has survived and thrived. Their mission is to provide "high-quality, environmentally conscious quality products that are safer for your home, your neighborhood, and the earth's environment."

www.naturalhighlifestyle.com Produces casual and active wear using all-natural hemp, which is particularly suited—stylistically and philosophically—to the yogi and fitness warrior lifestyle.

High Performance Yoga Video

Available through the online catalog at www.wholisticfitness.com.

Meditation Cushions

Some online sources are www.tshirtplanet.com, www.huggermugger.com, www.yogaprop.com.

Sai Baba's Nag Champa Incense

"Got Nag?" The "official incense" of Wholistic Fitness warriors! Made in India. A small box (40 g) costs around $4 while a larger supply (250 g) of Nag sells in most New Age bookstores for around $20. I usually order online, specifically through www.tshirtplanet.com.

Nature's Platform Squatting Device

Every WF warrior's household should have a toilet outfitted with one! www.naturesplatform.com.

PhysioBalls

Once seen only in the domain of gymnasiums and physical therapy offices with those little udders sticking out of them, a whole new generation of PhysioBalls has emerged in all sorts of sizes for all sorts of activities. In this book, however, I wrote about using a PhysioBall to replace your office chair in order to save the health of your pelvis and spine. It works. For this purpose, a 65 cm ball seems a good choice for most people, although a 75 cm ball might be better for people over six feet. Make sure you order the little hand pump that usually comes with the ball. Keep the ball inflated so there is less than 12 inches of "squish" when you sit on it. Have fun. Try www.huggermugger.com, where they have, I think somewhat arrogantly, renamed these "Yoga Balls."

Tithes

Tithing has long been a practice of self-cultivation in many traditions. Some religions (I won't point a finger) and spiritual cults have tarnished the indigenous spiritual intent of tithing. I think of tithing as volunteerism made manifest. I always feel better when I tithe and so do many of my students.

Some longtime Wholistic Fitness tithes include Campaign for Tibet (www.savetibet.org), People for the Ethical Treatment of Animals (PETA, www.PETA.com), and Greenpeace (www.Greepeace.org). But you should really follow your own heart on this one. There are so many beautiful ways to help.

PowerBar

I've been with PowerBar since long before they became the world's best-selling energy food. I sample tasted some of the first "goo" that came off Brian Maxwell's oven pans back in 1982. To this day, if I eat a "processed" food, usually it is a PowerBar. As a member of PowerBar Team Elite, I often gauge the duration of my training by the number of PowerBars needed to complete it. For example, a three-hour backcountry run would be a "1 PowerBar" excursion. Riding my bike thirty miles to and back from the start of the three-hour backcountry run would elevate the training session to "PB Status 2." It got to the point where if I called my training partners to see if they wanted to join me for a training session, they'd ask, "Ilg, how many PowerBars are we talking here?"

I stay with PowerBar because their products work. Although they have expanded their product line well beyond Malt Nut and Chocolate PowerBars (which, by the way, remain my favorites!), they have never compromised the nutritional integrity of their bars. Their ingredients are very intelligently profiled to give short-, medium-, and long-term energy, and they use very high quality sources to get their amino acids and other nutrients.

In fact, I use their PowerGels for yoga practice. These carbohydrate gels also have branched-chain amino acids, which help foster muscle strength. And, since having an empty stomach is vital for a quality yoga session, consuming a PowerGel twenty minutes before class provides great energy without filling your stomach. Most grocery stores now carry PowerBars, but the PowerGel is harder to find. Check out www.powerbar.com, where you can order online as well. Their new line, Protein Plus, is an excellent after-training bar to help regenerate muscle strength.

Ron Jones

www.RonJones.org

This website was created by my ultra-bike racing teammate and a true mind/body tribal elder, Ron Jones. This dude has got the chi baby! Anything you want to know about what Ron calls "High Performance Health" can be found here—bicycle advocacy, obesity, environmental health, health calculators and quizzes, endurance racing, and even links to Ron Jones's heroes: the late great Norm Hoffman and the endlessly fit Jack LaLanne. Ron is truly a pioneering spirit and force for the everyday fitness warrior as well as for world-class athletes.

Seiza Bench

These meditation benches are for those whose knees, hips, or ankles rebel a bit too much in the cross-legged seated meditation posture. With a Seiza bench, you can easily sit in a supported kneeling position and keep your spine straight during your session. Many New Age bookstores and online catalogs, such as www.huggermugger.com or www.yogaprop.com, offer Seiza benches.

Shakuhachi Flute Music

Although I don't want you to become attached to it, *Shakuhachi Meditation Music* by Stan Richardson is a fantastic background to periodically use during your zazen sessions. It is traditional Japanese flute music that has been used for seven hundred years to help still the mind and awaken attention. The 2-CD set is sold at most New Age bookstores or online bookstores such as www.amazon.com. Or contact Sounds True at 800-333-9185.

Sunrider International

Sunrider has earned its designation as "The Official Nutrition Program of Wholistic Fitness." For the past twenty years, I've depended upon Sunrider as my key source for my core nutrition, weight management, and skin care. Sunrider just makes sense for wise yogic and fitness warriors. The hallmark product of Sunrider is Calli Beverage, a tealike product that cleanses cells and decreases bodyfat. The products are cruelty-free, eco-friendly, internationally available, and are of super-high concentration and integrity. Some people are scared by Sunrider's direct marketing approach. Their fear is unfounded. You can join Sunrider for free as a "customer" instead of a "distributor" and buy all the products at wholesale.

The strength of these herbs has pulled me through hundreds of hard-core multisport WF workouts, whittled my bodyfat to 2.3 percent, and kept it there for years. They've kept my immune system so strong that I've never seen the inside of a doctor's office since getting on them in 1983. Not even the slightest sickness afflicts me more than once a year, if that. These herbs have steadily increased my flexibility while improving my strength. Even after a career in extreme outdoor conditions, Sunrider's regenerative powers have kept my skin looking and feeling years younger than my chronological age. These herbs defeated an early addiction to Diet Coke and were huge in making sure I didn't screw myself up on drugs. Potent as they are, these herbs are food-grade quality, known as "royal" herbs in China. They are meant to be eaten every day, and the longer you eat them, the better and healthier you become.

I personally know Dr. Chen. He has chi. Today, his company has grown into one of the largest direct marketing businesses in the world, but the quality of Dr. Chen's herbs have only grown better as the availability of quality soil and water to produce potent, concentrated whole foods grows ever more precious. Take a tour of the company at www.sunrider.com.

If you want to get into these herbs, I recommend contacting a certified Wholistic Fitness teacher (through www.wholisticfitness.com) before becoming a member of Sunrider. Having one of my teachers guide you through their vast ocean of herbs and herbal products is valuable. There are many products, but only a few are core to our path. Costs range from $40 to $400 monthly. There is no need to add Sunrider products to your diet; just switch poorer quality foods with Sunrider products.

Verve

Excellent clothes for a WF warrior. Rock climb, work out, meditate, or do yoga in these clothes and you'll probably grow to cherish them as much as Kathy and I do. Verve is owned by Christian Griffith, my ol' rock climbing bro from Boulder, Colorado, who is now a living legend in the sport climbing world. 303-443-7010. Tell him Ilg sent you.

Water

Where would you be without a fresh, quality supply of it? Learn and take action:

www.epa.gov
www.preventingharm.org
www.cleanwateraction.org
www.waterforpeople.org

GLOSSARY

Aerobic: in the presence of oxygen, normally refers to metabolism utilizing oxygen.

Ai Imawa: a form of Taoist yoga. A series of twelve ancient, healing postures that also act as a precursor to Tai Chi and other forms of movement meditation. These postures teach you how to relate and move with chi, or life force.

Anaerobic: In the absence of oxygen, normally refers to nonoxidative metabolism.

Aparigraha: Freedom from hoarding, greediness, and collecting.

Asana: Any of the various poses of Hatha Yoga. In Sanskrit, means "seat."

Ashtanga yoga: Classically, the eight limbs of yoga as described by Patanjali. Also refers to the vinyasa style of hatha yoga forwarded by Krishnamacharya from the *Yoga Korunta,* and then popularized by Sri K. Pattabhi Jois.

Asrama: A yogic term distinguishing the four consecutive twenty-five-year phases of a human life.

Atman: The individual soul.

Bodhisattva: An enlightened being who renounces entry into heaven for the sake of continuing to help all sentient beings.

Body composition: The balance of the major structural components of the body: fat, muscle, and bone.

Brahman: The supreme soul.

Cagers: Term used by devoted bicycle commuters to describe people addicted to driving cars.

Chakras: In Sanskrit, means "wheel." In yoga, usually refers to energy centers or concentrations located along the spine in approximate relation to the curves of the spine as well as the neural plexuses.

Chi: Chinese word meaning the vital energy, life force, or cosmic spirit that animates all things.

Chrondomalcia: Aching pain behind the kneecap often caused by muscle imbalance or compression that pulls the kneecap sideways out of alignment.

Cleansing breath: A deep nasal inhale followed by a mouth exhale. Helps to lower heart rate and energize the body during athletic or stressed situations.

Concentric: A muscle contraction that shortens muscle fibers.

Dharma: Usually relates to the central notion of Buddhism that sees dharma as the cosmic law that expresses universal truth.

Dhyana: Sustained concentration, flawless attention. Patanjali describes three basic levels of concentration. The first is if the mind can flow uninterrupted toward the same object for twelve seconds. If that concentration is sustained for twelve times twelve seconds (2:24), that is meditation or dhyana. When dhyana can be continued for twelve times two minutes and twenty seconds (28:48), lower samadhi, or bliss union with Atman, is attained. There are several levels of samadhi.

Dojo: In Zen, "Hall of the Way." A training room for spiritual practice.

Dragon: In Ai Imawa philosophy, any force or matter (including aspects of ourselves) that tends to pull us away from our natural, peaceful serenity and wisdom.

Drala: Tibetan word meaning natural wisdom.

Ego: In this book, describes that aspect of mind that delineates reality into notions of personal separateness such as "I" and "mine." It is the thought form of duality, which sees reality as comprised of self and other.

Engaged-cardio warriorism: A conscious effort to integrate cardio fitness and activity into one's lifestyle for purposes of spiritual growth and universal empathy.

Extreme: In outdoor athletics, a term used to describe a situation or sport where severe injury or death may occur if one screws up.

False grip: In strength training, where thumbs are placed on same side of barbell as the fingers.

Gassho mudra: A prayer hand posture where the palms are held together at the level of the chest. Traditional gesture in Zen for greeting, gratitude, request, veneration, or supplication. In yoga, this gesture is known as namaskar, or anjali mudra.

Green Tara: In Tibetan Buddhism, Green Tara is the female aspect of enlightenment. Green Tara guides novice practitioners along the path of awakening. She encourages victory over inner obstacles and fear.

Garhasthya asrama: The second twenty-five-year span of human aging: years twenty-five to fifty. A phase of life where our focus is life in the home and our aim is the acquisition of goods and security.

Gi: A martial arts uniform.

Hatha yoga: The combination of two limbs of the yoga sciences: pranayama (breath control) and asana (steady poses) to balance the solar (ha) and lunar (tha) energies in the human body/mind system.

Higher self: Opposite of ego: true knowledge. The intuitive wisdom that sees no separation between self and reality.

High Performance Yoga: A subdivision of Wholistic Fitness created by Steve Ilg. A unique form of power yoga blended with Western sport physiology notions.

Ida: One of the three principal nadis (channels of energy) in the body related with the left nostril governing the channel of lunar, or yin, energy.

Kata: A martial arts dance form usually done as a meditation in motion.

Kin hin: In Zen, a walking meditation done between periods of formal sitting practice. Can be done slowly or rapidly or in between.

Kirtan: Ritual or communal chanting in honor of God. Often a main spiritual medium for bhakti yogis.

Kundalini: The primordial cosmic energy that lies dormant within each individual until it is awakened by meditation and yoga techniques. Resides in the sushumna. Also known as shakti in Hinduism.

Lactate threshold: A component of exercise physiology. Generally described as that level of sustained work whereby the blood lactate does not diminish as more of it is produced by the exercising muscles. Supposedly, this threshold is increased with training. Consistent data is almost impossible to find since results of tests fluctuate with variables such as food ingested, time of day, etc.

Macronutrients: Protein, carbohydrates, and fats.

Mantram, or mantra: A sacred syllable, word, phrase, or prayer repeated as a form of meditation.

Meridians: Subtle energy channels in the body.

Metaphysical: That which is beyond the known laws of physics. Refers to the unknown but intelligent forces latent in the human mind.

Micronutrients: Nutritional elements that are not classified as macronutrients, such as vitamins, minerals, enzymes, enzymatic cofactors, and antioxidants.

Nadis: Channels of energy in the body. Yoga chiefly uses the three primary ones: sushumna, ida, and pingala.

Niyamas: The second limb of yoga; five disciplines to purify the inner self: saucha (purity), santosha (contentment), tapas (inner drive), svadhyaya (study of self), and ishvara pranidhana (dedication to God).

Nordic skiing: Skiing where the heel is not fastened to the ski. Often called cross-country skiing. Nordic skiing also includes free-heeled jumping.

Patanjali: An enigmatic figure(s) presumably active in the second century B.C. His insightful but practical guidelines toward body/mind liberation are still considered the epitome of classical yogic methodology.

Periodizational training: A process of cyclic, structured training periods to produce a desired training effect.

Pingala: One of the three principal nadis (channels of energy) in the body related with the right nostril governing the channel of solar, or yang, energy.

Plyometrics: Athletic training system that concentrates on the development of fast-twitch muscles and explosive power.

PowerBar: The original athletic energy food. A longtime sponsor of Steve Ilg. www.powerbar.com or 800*58*POWER. Wholistic Fitness approved.

Prajnaparmita: Buddhism; "the book of Divine Wisdom."

Prana: Sanskrit term meaning breath of life. The cosmic energy that animates all living things.

Pranayama: Sanskrit translation includes "controlling the breath of life." Commonly regarded as "the science of breath." Breathing exercises, often combined with the practice of mantra or asana, to facilitate personal health and spiritual progress.

Pratyahara: Withdrawal of the mind from the domination of the senses and sensual attraction; the fifth stage of yoga.

Rinpoche: A Tibetan Buddhist religious master or guru. Means "none above." Also known as a *lama*.

Sadhana: Spiritual practice, or one's path toward self-mastery.

Samadhi: The culmination of many yogic traditions, which results in a superconscious state. Blissful absorption. The end of the dualistic mind. Patanjali describes several samadhic levels of which nirvikalpa is the highest.

Samsara: In yogic terms, the cycle of birth, death, and rebirth that we are all subject to as long we do not realize our unity with the universe (Atman).

Sangha: A community of like-minded people helping one another in their spiritual aspirations.

Sanskrit: "The language of the gods." Today a "dead" language like Latin, but remains the sacred language of Hindus and yogis. A highly differentiated terminology exists in Sanskrit, which embodies the various stages of meditation, consciousness levels, and various mental and spiritual processes, most of which have no equivalent in European languages. Also, Sanscrit.

Santosha: Contentment; natural delight.

Serial distortion: A state of malalignment resulting from a loss of functional integrity.

Shanti: Sanskrit for peace. Refers to the peaceful nature attained through spiritual/inner work once one realizes that he or she is imperishable consciousness, not the mortal body, which is susceptible to death.

Shakti: Also known as Kali or Durga, she is a Hindi personification of the force of god (Brahman); wife of Shiva.

Shiva: The third divinity in the Hindu trinity (Brahma and Vishnu being the others). Known for being the popular destroyer of ignorance. Married to Shakti.

Sport-specificity: The act of focusing upon one sport to the exclusion of healthy body/mind balance.

Stupa: A focal point in Buddhist temples, usually with a pointed, ornate top. Originally used as a memorial to store relics, the stupa serves as a reminder of the awakened state of mind.

Sunrider: "The Official Nutrition Program of Wholistic Fitness." A company that Steve Ilg depends upon for high-quality, preservative- and cruelty-free herbal whole foods and personal-care products. www.sunrider.com.

Supine: Lying on the back or having the face upward.

Sushumna or susumna: The main nadi (channel of energy), situated inside the spinal column.

Tao: The natural, omnipresent flow of the UniVerse. In China, literally means, "the Way."

Transition phase: One of three Wholistic Fitness strength training phases occurring within every repetition in the gym. The other two are yin (slow, lengthening movement) and yang (explosive, shortening movement).

Uddiyana: A pranayamic technique wherein the diaphragm is lifted toward the chest region while the abdominal organs are drawn toward the spine.

Ujjayi: A pranayamic technique especially suited for asana practice whereby deep nasal breathing is controlled by a conscious narrowing of the throat, producing a "hissing" sound.

Vinyasa: Refers to several asanas linked together in a flow sequence.

Wholistic Fitness: A pioneering body/mind approach to personal fitness training created in 1982 by Steve Ilg. Students of this path practice Five Fitness Disciplines (Strength, Cardio, Yoga, Meditation, Nutrition) and Four Lifestyle Principles (Breath and Posture, Mindfulness, Appropriate Action, and Practice). www.wholisticfitness.com.

Wu-wei: Taoist term meaning unmotivated action or effortless effort.

Yamas: The first limb of yoga; five disciplines to purify the outer or ethical self: ahimsa (nonviolence), satya (truth), asteya (nonstealing), brahmacharya (appropriate use of sensual and sexual energy), and aparigraha (nonhoarding).

Yang: The male aspect of the Tao. Chinese term meaning the sunny side of a mountain. Relates to masculine, active, creative, bright, and hard. In Wholistic Fitness terms, yang also means the explosive, forceful, and shortening qualities of an exercise movement.

Yin: The female aspect of the Tao. Chinese term meaning the shady side of a mountain. Relates to feminine, passive, receptive, dark, and soft. In Wholistic Fitness terms, yin also means the more controlled, poetic, or lengthening qualities of an exercise movement.

Yoga Korunta: An ancient Sanskrit manuscript in which Vamana Rishi describes a lengthy and intricate system of hatha yoga that was then forwarded by Krishnamacharya and his students.

Yoga squat or yogi squat: A natural common body position done squatting close to the ground, heels flat, buttocks near the ground.

Zazen: In Zen, formal sitting practice. Main vehicle used to attain enlightenment.

BIBLIOGRAPHY

Beginning to See, Sujata. Berkeley: Celestial Arts, 1987. A handwritten collection of insights and sketchings delightfully steer the reader toward the value of meditation.

Being Nobody, Going Nowhere, Ayya Khema. Boston: Wisdom, 1987. Using this and her other book, *When the Iron Eagle Flies,* the path of meditative insight is available to anyone.

Beyond Therapy: The Impact of Eastern Religions on Psychological Theory and Practice, Guy Claxton. Dorset: Prism/Unity, 1996.

The Bhagavad Gita. Choose any translation that appeals to you and devour this stunning, historical yogic love poem.

BodyMind, Ken Dychtwald. New York: Tarcher/Putnam, 1977. Established classic in the field, which integrates Eastern wisdom with body/mind connections.

Discovering the Body's Wisdom, Mirka Knaster. New York: Bantam New Age, 1991. A pragmatic and well-researched guide to body-centered therapies.

The Future of the Body: Explorations into the Further Evolution of Human Nature. Michael Murphy. Los Angeles: Tarcher, 1993.

Health at the Crossroads: Exploring the Conflict between Natural Healing and Conventional Medicine, Dean Black. Springville, VT: Tapestry Press, 1988.

Job's Body: A Handbook for Bodywork, Deane Juhan. Barrytown, NY: Station Hill, 1987. The, I mean *the* book for body reference.

Meditation in Action, Chogyam Trungpa. Boston and London: Shambala, 1991. Keep this little jewel near you at all times. It is full of insight to help you stay awake throughout your day.

Plyometrics: Explosive Power Training, James Radcliffe and Robert Farentinos. Champaign, IL: Human Kinetic Publishers, 1999. An ideal guide for understanding plyometrics. Includes routines for many sports and excellent descriptions.

Returning to Silence: Zen Practice in Daily Life, Dainin Katagiri. Boston and London: Shambala, 1988. Katagiri Roshi says, "Don't expect enlightenment—just sit down!" This book is based on this Zen master's dharma talks to his students at the Minnesota Zen Meditation Center.

Shambala, the Sacred Path of the Warrior, Chogyam Trungpa. Boston and London: Shambala, 1988. A beautiful but very practical articulation of principles that guide one toward enlightened conduct in an often troubling and chaotic world.

Sound Health: The Music and Sounds That Make Us Whole, Steven Halpern. New York: Harper & Row, 1985. Pioneering study of the effects of music and sound on the body, mind, and spirit. Halpern ushered in the New Age, cellularly based genre that set the vibratory stage for later house/trance music.

Spontaneous Healing: How to Discover and Enhance Your Body's Natural Ability to Maintain and Heal Itself, Andrew Weil. New York: Ballantine Books, 1995.

The Tibetan Book of Living and Dying, Sogyal Rinpoche. New York: HarperCollins, 1993. Mandatory reading for those genuinely interested in learning how to live and die elegantly and consciously.

The Way of the Shaman, Michael Harner. New York: Bantam New Age, 1980.

Wheels of Life, Anodea Judith. St. Paul, MN: Llewellyn, 1987. A rigorously updated and comprehensive treatment on chakral science.

The Wholeness Principle, Stephano Sabetti. Sherman Oaks, CA: Life Energy Media, 1986. Oxygen charges, orgones, microstreamers, morphic field energies, it's all in there.

Yoga: Mind and Body, Sivananda Yoga Vedanta Center. London: Dorling Kindersley, 1996. A gorgeous, big book that details the Sivananda approach to yoga.

Zen Mind, Beginner's Mind, Shunryu Suzuki. Weatherhill, 1970. The best of the best.

With an incredible five world championship performances in four physiologically diverse outdoor sports, Steve Ilg earned the title "The world's fittest human" from *Ultra Cycling* and was twice featured on the cover of *Outside* magazine. His internationally acclaimed path of Wholistic Fitness has blazed the field of mind/body fitness training since 1982. His work is now regularly featured in all forms of the popular media.

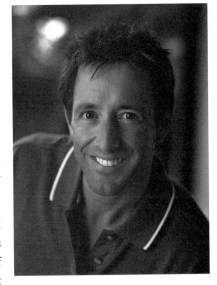

A licensed coach with the United States Cycling Federation (USCF), a Registered Yoga Teacher (RYT) through the international Yoga Alliance, with over five thousand teaching hours, and certified personal trainer through National Health Club Association (NHCA), Coach Ilg's free-thinking, East-meets-West wisdom has consistently produced national, world, and Olympic champions in several sports, while simultaneously providing a spiritual depth and joy to the lives his work touches.

In an era where "image is everything" the authenticity of the centered counsel and grounded teachings from this humble mountain yogi is greatly needed by all who struggle to navigate the spiritual terrain of lifestyle fitness. This top-selling author, poet, and extreme athlete left his beloved Southwest mountains as part of his own spiritual practice to spread his life message of personal balance through lifestyle fitness. Steve currently lives, practices, and teaches Wholistic Fitness and High Performance Yoga from Los Angeles with his wife, Kathy.

For information on becoming a formal online student or teacher of Wholistic Fitness and High Performance Yoga, or to learn more about Coach Ilg's other services, products, and special events visit www.wholisticfitness.com or www.HighPerformanceYoga.com.